Nutrient-Gene Interactions *in* Cancer

Nutrient-Gene Interactions *in* Cancer

Edited by
Sang-Woon Choi
Tufts University
Boston, Massachusetts

Simonetta Friso
University of Verona
Verona, Italy

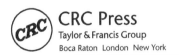

CRC Press
Taylor & Francis Group
Boca Raton London New York

CRC Press is an imprint of the
Taylor & Francis Group, an **informa** business

Published in 2006 by
CRC Press
Taylor & Francis Group
6000 Broken Sound Parkway NW, Suite 300
Boca Raton, FL 33487-2742

ISBN-13: 978-0-367-45385-5 (pbk)
ISBN-13: 978-0-8493-3229-6 (hbk)

Library of Congress Card Number 2005052931

Library of Congress Cataloging-in-Publication Data

Nutrient-gene interactions in cancer / Sang-Woon Choi, and Simonetta Friso.
     p. cm.
  Includes bibliographical references and index.
  ISBN 0-8493-3229-X (alk. paper)
  1. Cancer--Nutritional aspects. 2. Gene expression 3. Genetic regulation. I. Choi, Sang-Woon. II. Friso, Simonetta.

RC268.45.N86 2005
616.99'4042--dc22
                                        2005052931

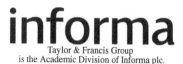
Taylor & Francis Group
is the Academic Division of Informa plc.

Visit the Taylor & Francis Web site at
http://www.taylorandfrancis.com

and the CRC Press Web site at
http://www.crcpress.com

Preface

In the era of ancient Greek medicine, based on the theory of the four equal and universal elements posited by Empedocles, Hippocrates postulated that disease is caused by *isonomia*, an imbalance in the four body humors: blood, phlegm, black bile, and yellow bile. Later on, Galen introduced four human basic temperaments that reflect the humors and influence the susceptibility to disease: the sanguine, buoyant type; the phlegmatic, sluggish type; the melancholic, dejected type; and the choleric, quick-tempered type. Thereafter, both Western and Oriental medicines have tried to categorize humans into different types for the sake of treatment efficacy and have believed that these different types affect physiology, pathology, diagnosis, treatment, and prognosis of diseases. These old classifications were based on physical shapes or tempers (phenotypic expression), whereas modern medicine classifies humans according to their genotypes, which may be predictive for the risk of certain diseases as well as helpful for the design of better strategies for disease prevention and treatment.

Early research regarding the relationship between diet and cancer was based on the idea that cancer is caused by an overexposure to a specific diet. With a more clear understanding gained in recent years that cancer is a genetic disease, as shown by the molecular aberrations occurring in cancer cells, most of the studies have focused more specifically on the effect of particular nutrients on the expression of genes related to carcinogenesis. However, the presence of inherited mutations or defective genes is not sufficient to determine the phenotype, and finding aberrant genes does not guarantee, by itself, the onset of clinically manifested disease. Most recently, the complete mapping of the human genome and sophisticated molecular technologies have accelerated research on the relationship between nutrients and genes. Consequently, compelling evidence from epidemiological and experimental observations has suggested that the risk of certain cancers is different from one genotype of critical genes to another and has supported the idea that the interaction between nutrients and genes is one of the most important mechanisms by which nutrients modulate carcinogenesis.

This book specifically focuses on the interrelationships between nutrients and genes in cancer, which, we believe, highlights that nutrients have not just one simple function in cancer development but, more notably, that nutrition is one of the most important factors, which serves as a modulator for cancer growth through the interaction with specific genes. A deeper understanding of such a relationship also has contributed to the detection of a new strategy for cancer chemoprevention. In this book we have endeavored to provide a comprehensive and systematic review of the latest information regarding the role of nutrients and genes interactions on cancer development, with the aim of also providing specific examples of well-known interactions between nutrients and genes with a defined pathogenetic role in clinical manifestations of different cancer diseases.

The first part of the book includes chapters on the basic elements of biology and pathobiology of gene–nutrient interactions with a focus on mechanisms and biomarkers. The following chapters describe in detail specific gene–nutrient interactions that are considered, in the current knowledge, the most striking examples of the interaction between genetics, epigenetics, and nutrition in many different types of cancer. Each chapter also describes the currently available methodologies to evaluate each nutrient and gene interaction. This section is designed both for basic-science investigators as well as for clinicians who manage cancer patients, with the intent of presenting useful tools to address the clinical implications of the gene–nutrient interaction field in medical nutrition and oncology. In contemporary medicine, oncologists have an increasing appreciation for this promising subject, as do many other specialists and scientists encountering the emerging field of nutrition and genetics interactions. The last chapter of the book emphasizes the directions research is taking and the implications of fostering further investigation. Included will be new perspectives in this rapidly growing area of medical science.

We are deeply grateful to each one of our esteemed authors, who are among the leading authorities in the field. We know that this project required more time and effort than anticipated, and we are truly thankful to them for their dedication and their remarkable contributions. We would also like to thank Taylor & Francis for providing an arena to discuss this topic. Appreciation goes also to our admired readers for their interest, present and future, in this unique and fascinating field. With this book we aim to give them a perspective on what is presently known, as well as the challenge of what is as yet unknown. Indeed, the attempt at improving our knowledge is a precious part of the marvelous adventure of the mind which is seeking the simplicity and beauty of the truth through the little secrets of science.

About the Editors

Sang-Woon Choi graduated from the College of Medicine, Seoul National University and received postgraduate training in internal medicine and gastroenterology at the Seoul National University Hospital in Korea. He obtained a master's degree in 1988 and a Ph.D. degree in 1992 from the same university. His research interest during that time was the relationship between hepatitis B virus and primary liver cancer, both of which were prevalent in Korea.

To pursue a particular interest in the relationship between nutrition and cancer, he joined the Jean Mayer USDA Human Nutrition Research Center at Tufts University in 1993 and is now a research scientist and assistant professor of nutrition. Over the past 12 years, Dr. Choi's research has focused on the question of how one-carbon nutrients, such as folate and vitamin B_{12}, modulate the process of carcinogenesis, especially how these nutrients and genes interact in colorectal carcinogenesis and the potential chemopreventive properties of one-carbon nutrients. His work has involved studies aimed at identifying the molecular mechanisms by which the effect of folate depletion is mediated and by which folate supplementation prevents this effect. He has focused primarily on basic mechanisms such as DNA methylation and nucleotide synthesis, each of which is a major function of one-carbon metabolism.

Simonetta Friso is university scientist and assistant professor of internal medicine at the University of Verona School of Medicine and Surgery in Italy. She graduated in 1991 from the University of Verona School of Medicine and Surgery with a thesis on red blood cell cotransport systems. She subsequently specialized in internal medicine at the Verona University Hospital and wrote her thesis on emergent risk factors for thrombophilia. During this course of study, she dedicated her research to molecular mechanisms of coagulation factors and thromboembolic diseases.

A doctoral thesis on gene–nutrient interactions within one-carbon metabolism and effects on DNA methylation was the topic of her doctoral thesis for her Ph.D. in experimental hematology from the National University of Milan, and was the beginning of her work in the field of gene–nutrient interactions and epigenetics. She developed her interest in the area of nutrition and genetics as a visiting scientist at the Jean Mayer USDA Human Nutrition Research Center at Tufts University between 1998 and 2002. Author of several research articles, she received the 2002 Hamish N. Munro Postdoctoral Fellowship Award in Boston in 2002 for outstanding scientific research on folate metabolism, genetics, and DNA methylation, and the Carlo Procacci Award for excellence in basic research in the emerging field of one-carbon metabolism and epigenetics in Italy in 2005.

Over the past several years, she has focused her research work on identifying the molecular mechanisms of interrelationships between nutrients and genes, and her major interest has been dedicated to the effect of B-vitamins and polymorphic genes within one-carbon metabolism on DNA methylation, a major epigenetic feature of DNA involved in carcinogenesis.

Contributors

Moray J. Campbell
University of Birmingham Medical
  School
Birmingham, United Kingdom

Sang-Woon Choi
Jean Mayer USDA Human Nutrition
  Research Center on Aging at
  Tufts University
Boston, Massachusetts

Kay W. Colston
St. George's University of London
London, United Kingdom

Roberto Corrocher
University of Verona School of
  Medicine
Verona, Italy

Jay H. Fowke
Vanderbilt University Medical Center
Nashville, Tennessee

Simonetta Friso
University of Verona School of
  Medicine
Verona, Italy

Edward Giovannucci
Harvard School of Public Health
Boston, Massachusetts

David W. Hein
University of Louisville School of
  Medicine
Louisville, Kentucky

La Creis Renee Kidd
University of Louisville School of
  Medicine
Louisville, Kentucky

Stacey King
Jean Mayer USDA Human Nutrition
  Research Center on Aging at
  Tufts University
Boston, Massachusetts

Shelly C. Lu
Keck School of Medicine
University of Southern California
Los Angeles, California

Robert C.G. Martin
University of Louisville School of
  Medicine
Louisville, Kentucky

M. Luz Martínez-Chantar
CIC–Biogune
Bizkaia, Spain

John C. Mathers
Human Nutrition Research Centre
University of Newcastle
Newcastle-upon-Tyne, United
  Kingdom

José M. Mato
CIC–Biogune
Bizkaia, Spain

Jason H. Moore
Dartmouth Medical School
Lebanon, New Hampshire

Claire E. Robertson
Imperial College London
London, United Kingdom

Helmut K. Seitz
Salem Medical Centre
University of Heidelberg
Heidelberg, Germany

Felix Stickel
Bern University
Bern, Switzerland

Patrick J. Stover
Cornell University
Ithaca, New York

Cornelia M. Ulrich
Fred Hutchinson Cancer Research Center
University of Washington
Seattle, Washington

Paolo Vineis
Imperial College London
London, United Kingdom

Xiang-Dong Wang
Jean Mayer USDA Human Nutrition
  Research Center on Aging at
  Tufts University
Boston, Massachusetts

Table of Contents

1 Nutrient and Gene Interactions in Cancer

Edward Giovannucci

CONTENTS

1.1　INTRODUCTION

The idea that diet and nutrition play an important role in carcinogenesis is not new. Much has been learned in this area during the past several decades through traditional epidemiological methods, but many questions remain unanswered. The present is a particularly exciting time for researching how genetic and nutritional factors interact to influence the risk of various cancers. With new methods that help us better identify genetic susceptibility, clearer answers are likely to emerge in the field of nutrition and cancer. The first part of this chapter will briefly summarize the role of various epidemiological strategies that are used to understand cancer causation and prevention. In particular, the strengths and weaknesses of various epidemiological approaches will be described. Building upon this, the second part of the chapter will examine how our evolving understanding of genetic susceptibility can be integrated into traditional epidemiological methods to help refine our understanding of diet, nutrition, and cancer.

1.2　TYPES OF EPIDEMIOLOGICAL STUDIES

A summary of the major epidemiological designs, including important strengths and weaknesses, that have been used in the study of nutrition and cancer is given in Table 1.1. The studies can be divided into observational studies, which encompass

TABLE 1.1
Study Designs Addressing the Effect of Diet on Human Cancer

Study Design	Methods	Potential Strengths/Limitations
Ecological	Comparison of cancer rates in populations having different dietary patterns by assessing per capita intake of specific nutrients and relating them to cancer incidence or mortality; migrant studies compare cancer rates in immigrants to a new region or country with different diets	Examines a wide range of exposures and population diets, which may be more stable over time than individual diets; diet is only one of many variables that differ among populations, so the potential for confounding is great; intakes may be biased when based on food disappearance rather than actual intakes
Case–control	Earlier, prediagnostic diets as reported by patients with a particular type of cancer (or their proxies for fatal cancers) are compared with diets during a comparable time period reported by cancer-free controls; controls can be typically hospital-based patients with other medical conditions or individuals chosen randomly from the underlying population at risk	Useful for rare cancers, although difficult to implement for rapidly developing fatal cancers; confounding other factors cannot be excluded in observational (nonrandomized studies); recall bias can result when patients systematically differ from the controls in their dietary recall; selection bias can occur if controls do not accurately represent the population from which the cases arise; in hospital-based studies, selection bias can arise if the conditions for which controls are hospitalized are related to diet; in population-based case–control studies, response rates may be low for controls, leading to selection bias
Cohort (prospective or follow-up)	Diets and other factors are determined in individuals who are then followed for cancer; cancer rates are compared, for example, in high-fat vs. low-fat groups, controlling for potentially confounding factors	As for case–control studies, confounding factors cannot be definitively excluded, but selection bias and recall bias are unlikely to occur; cohort studies for cancer must generally enroll tens or even hundreds of thousands of participants, and then follow them for many years, with high follow-up response rates necessary for valid inference
Intervention	Incidence of cancer or a surrogate endpoint is compared in two groups randomized to specific interventions vs. placebo	The only study design that can definitely exclude confounding; compliance with substantial dietary changes is difficult for many people; subjects cannot be easily blinded to the treatment or placebo; optimal dosages (e.g., of supplemental nutrients) and dose–response relationships can be difficult to ascertain; duration of intervention required is generally unknown, but it may be decades for specific cancers

ecological and analytic case–control and cohort studies, and intervention studies. In principle, the distinction between observational and intervention studies is most critical because, in essence, causality can be "proved" only in the context of a randomized intervention trial. This is generally well appreciated by most researchers, but if results from randomized clinical trials are accepted uncritically and observational studies are relegated as inferior studies, important insights may be missed. Ultimately, when considering a nutrient–disease relationship, it is best to consider the total evidence, ranging from *in vitro* studies, animal studies, human metabolic studies, ecological and analytic epidemiological studies, and intervention studies. When the various lines of evidence are viewed as complementary and the strengths and limitations of each approach are appreciated, the most correct answers are likely to emerge. The strengths and limitations in human study designs are discussed here.

1.3 ECOLOGICAL STUDIES

Ecological studies can be quite useful in enhancing our understanding of nutrition and cancer. These studies have been critical in establishing that most, if not all, human cancer types exhibit marked variation by geographic region and that rates are susceptible to change over time. Interestingly, although overall cancer rates among adults vary only modestly worldwide, the types of cancers are dramatically different across populations [1,2]. In general, in most affluent countries, particularly in North America and Europe, cancers of the lung, colon, breast, and prostate predominate, whereas in less-affluent regions and the Far East, cancers of the stomach, liver, oral cavity, esophagus, and uterine cervix are the most common. In addition, cancer incidence rates have been shown to be highly dynamic; for example, immigrants who move from countries with low rates of specific cancers to countries with high rates typically attain the rates characteristic of the new country, or the reverse [3–5]. The time required to attain the new rate, which can vary, may provide important clues as to how quickly exposure to the new factor may influence cancer rates.

In general, ecological studies can provide invaluable information regarding diet and cancer. The large variations in cancer rates around the world and changes over time illustrate rather conclusively that many cancers are potentially avoidable if we were able to identify and remove the causal factors or increase the exposure to protective factors. Although genetic factors undoubtedly influence the development of various malignancies, the changes in cancer rates that occur within countries demonstrate the importance of noninherited factors. As discussed in the preceding text, ecological studies can also indicate the potential time frame of exposures becoming important and what time period may be required to obtain optimal benefits. For example, this time can range from several decades in the case of colon cancer to about three generations for breast cancer [5–8]. Finally, ecological studies may provide clues to dietary and nutritional factors that may account for many of these variations in cancer rates. For example, early observations that national rates of colon, breast, and prostate cancers are strongly correlated with aspects of diet such as per capita consumption of fat generated the hypothesis that fat consumption or some close correlate accounts for the excess of these cancers in Western or economically developed countries [9].

Given the strong suggestions from ecological studies and animal studies that dietary manipulations can influence tumorigenesis [10], three important questions need to be addressed: Which dietary factors are actually important determinants of human cancer? What is the nature of the dose–response and temporal relationships? What other factors, environmental or genetic, modify the relationship?

Ecological studies may help establish the framework of these questions but are probably unable to provide the most precise answers. The most important drawback in ecological studies is that the populations for which rates of specific cancers vary tend to differ markedly in many characteristics, rendering it difficult, if not impossible, to identify the precise causal factors. For example, rates of colon cancer tend to be low in agrarian populations and high in affluent populations. Not surprisingly, if we compare colon cancer rates across populations, we find that they are highly correlated with consumption of fat, animal protein, and meat. However, correlations with body mass, attained height, and level of physical activity, to name a few, are also likely to exist. These factors may work together to some extent to influence cancer risk: high availability of meat and fat, coupled with little need for physical activity, could lead to higher growth rates in childhood (thus, greater height) and greater body mass in adulthood. Subsequent exposure to growth factors such as insulin and insulin-like growth factors throughout the life span could enhance cancer risk [11]. Although this knowledge may be theoretically useful, it does not answer specific questions such as whether a reduction of the percentage of energy in fat from 45% to 30% in adulthood lowers the risk of colon or breast cancer in U.S. postmenopausal women. Such a specific question is unlikely to be adequately addressed by ecological studies. For example, rapid gains in height during the last several decades [12] have corresponded with increases in breast cancer rates; thus, one conclusion from ecological studies is that energy restriction sufficient to restrict attained height could lower breast cancer rate; population per capita dietary fat intake could simply be a correlate of this phenomenon.

1.4   ANALYTIC EPIDEMIOLOGY: CASE–CONTROL AND PROSPECTIVE COHORT STUDIES

Regarding observational studies, the case–control and prospective cohort studies may be better suited to address such a question as that of the percentage of energy from fat in relation to the aforementioned postmenopausal breast cancer risk. These studies assess dietary intake at the individual level in the population of interest by using dietary assessment methods that are generally more precise than ecological studies, which often rely on food disappearance data. For example, in ecological studies, when we compare a high-fat-consuming to a low-fat-consuming population, the comparison may actually be high fat intake/sedentary/obese vs. low fat intake/active/lean. In analytic epidemiological studies, we may better address the question of whether this reduction in fat composition influences cancer risk independently of body mass and physical activity. Of course, in any observational study, ecological or analytic, fat may be a correlate of another behavior or dietary factor, but in order to determine a potentially independent role of fat, analytic studies generally have three distinctive advantages. First, individuals within a population are likely to be more homogeneous with respect to many factors, including genetic factors, than are populations worldwide. For fat intake in adults, within the U.S., for example, relatively weak correlations are observed for height, body mass index, and physical activity, whereas across populations these are strongly linked. Second, in analytic studies, potentially confounding factors can be assessed and dealt with statistically. Third, as discussed later in this chapter (Section 1.7), genetic approaches could complement the study of nutrition and cancer in analytic studies.

Of course, important requirements of epidemiological studies are that diet and other characteristics such as physical activity be adequately measured. Relationships between diet, nutrition, and cancer incidence can be evaluated by collecting data on dietary intake, by using biochemical indicators of dietary factors, or by measuring body size and composition. In most epidemiological studies, food frequency questionnaires have been used to assess diet because they provide information on the usual diet over an extended period of time, which is of most interest in the study of cancer. In addition, these questionnaires are efficient for use in large populations. Although no method can perfectly assess dietary intake over a range of foods and nutrients, these questionnaires are sufficiently valid based on comparisons with more detailed assessments of diet (such as detailed dietary records) and biochemical indicators [13]. Biochemical indicators of diet can be useful in some situations, such as for the measure of carotenoids, but for many dietary factors of interest, such as total fat, fiber, and carbohydrates, no useful indicators are currently available. Some biomarkers, such as multiple 24-h urinary samples to assess long-term sodium intake, for example, may be available, but they are generally not practical for large-scale studies. DNA specimens have been collected from participants in many studies, and these allow for the examination of gene–diet interactions.

Historically, the bulk of epidemiological knowledge on diet and cancer has been obtained from case–control studies. However, a number of large prospective cohort studies of diet and cancer in various countries are now generating data and are increasing our knowledge of the role of diet and nutrition in cancer. All else being equal, prospective studies have the distinct advantage over case–control studies of avoiding potential recall bias or selection bias (see Table 1.1). If exposure data are collected after the diagnosis of cancer, various systematic biases may occur. For example, cancer patients may think more carefully about their past exposures and may recall their dietary habits differently from controls. Further, in case–control studies valid selection of controls requires they be a random sample of individuals who, if they had developed the cancer of interest, would have been identified as a case in that study. Selection bias may occur if, for example, selected disease-free controls with less healthy lifestyles are less likely to participate in a study. In general, the lower the response rate for controls, the more the concern for bias, even though acceptable ranges of response rates have not been established.

The primary advantage of prospective cohort studies over case–control studies is that they collect dietary and exposure information prior to the diagnosis of cancer. Although some measurement error in dietary recall or biochemical measures in determining long-term intake is inevitable, in a prospective study this error should likely be nondifferential or independent with regard to case–control status. In essence, many individuals are likely to over- or underreport a particular factor (food or nutrient), but because all of the study participants are cancer free at the time of reporting, these errors will be, on average, the same for individuals who eventually get cancer and those who remain cancer free. This over- and underreporting adds nondifferential measurement error and would tend to weaken any true observation, that is, weaken the nutrient–cancer signal, but generally this would not cause an association that did not exist to spuriously emerge. Thus, a significant association observed in a prospective study, in general, is weighted more than that in a case–control study. On the other hand, when an association is not observed in either case–control or cohort studies, it is important to examine critically how precise the dietary assessment measure was, when diet was assessed in relation to disease outcome, the range of intake in the population, the sample size, and other factors that may have obscured a true association. Unlike recall or selection bias, which is more of a concern for case–control studies, these factors are relevant to all study designs.

Approximately 60 prospective cancer cohort studies with over 10,000 participants each are currently ongoing worldwide. Many of these studies have collected extensive data on dietary intake. Relatively few of them are decades old, and many have only recently begun publishing findings. Most of these studies, except for a few such as the Nurses' Health Study and the Health Professionals Follow-Up Study, are based on a single dietary measure at baseline. Over the past decade, several prospective cohort studies have reported weaker or null associations between various dietary factors and cancer risk compared to findings reported previously from case–control studies. For example, findings from prospective studies of gastrointestinal cancers and fruits and vegetables are generally weaker than results suggested by previous case–control studies [14]. Also, unlike case–control studies, which suggest a moderate increase in breast cancer risk associated with higher fat intake in adulthood [15], prospective studies have not confirmed this finding [16,17]. The reasons for these differences are not clear. A potential explanation is that the relationships were overestimated in case–control studies if individuals with cancer systematically recalled their prediagnosis diet erroneously, either because they had a preconception about how diet might influence disease or their current diet changed because of cancer. The possibility of recall and selection bias has not been extensively addressed, but some data suggest that these occur in real-life situations [18].

Other methodological issues, such as limited ranges of dietary intakes in the cohort studies, could be relevant. However, this factor is unlikely to explain the differences between the case–control and cohort studies because this limitation applies to both types of studies. Perhaps of relevance is the fact that more potential confounders have been extensively measured and controlled for in prospective studies, suggesting that some associations in some of the earlier case–control studies were confounded. For example, recent evidence suggests that obesity, physical inactivity, tobacco use, and alcohol increase the risk of colon cancer [19]; generally, these confounders were not controlled for in many earlier studies, which were typically case–control studies.

Two large consortium projects may help resolve many questions regarding nutrition and cancer. The Pooling Project of Prospective Studies of Diet and Cancer Cohorts [20] is a collaborative effort of researchers from more than 16 cohorts in 6 countries. European Prospective Investigation of Cancer (EPIC) [21] is a multicenter cohort study of approximately 500,000 participants from 22 participating European centers. Combined, these studies include over one million study participants. These studies will enable researchers to evaluate a wide range of dietary intakes across populations, to have greater statistical power to examine differences in diet effects among potentially susceptible subgroups of the participants, and to evaluate consistency in results among the various subpopulations.

1.5 CONFOUNDING

The major theoretical limitation for any observational study, whether ecological, case–control, or cohort, is the possibility of confounding. Confounding results when the apparent effect of one exposure on risk is not causal but is brought about by its correlation with another causal factor [22]. For a factor to be a confounder in a particular study, it must be a causal risk factor for the specific disease and it must be correlated with the exposure (e.g., nutrient) of interest. Confounding is not a constant characteristic across all populations, but depends on the correlations within a specific population. For example, if individuals who consume fewer vegetables are more likely to be smokers, then smoking history could confound the relationship between vegetable intake and lung cancer risk. However, if in another population the proportion of smokers does not vary across levels of vegetable intake, it will not be a confounder. The potential importance of a confounder is proportional to its degree of correlation with the factor of interest and to the strength of the association with cancer. For example, tobacco use is always an important confounder to consider in lung cancer studies because of its very strong association with lung cancer. In general, confounding is an important issue to consider in nutritional epidemiology because dietary factors are often highly correlated. For example, saturated fat and monounsaturated fat tend to be positively correlated in many populations, and dietary fiber and total fat intake are generally inversely correlated.

In analytic studies, several strategies are utilized to minimize the influence of confounding. In dietary-based studies, confounding is usually dealt with through statistical analysis. An "adjusted relative risk" is a weighted, pooled average of the relative risk across different categories or levels of the confounder. For example, the association between high vs. low fat intake on cancer risk can be compared across subgroups of specific levels of smoking (e.g., nonsmokers, past smokers, current smokers who smoke 1 to 10 cigarettes/day, 11 to 20 cigarettes/day, and more than 21 cigarettes/day), and the adjusted relative risk will represent some average of the relative risks between diet and cancer among these groups. The epidemiologist must anticipate potential confounders, measure them in detail, and then use the appropriate statistical models in controlling for them. "Residual confounding," or incomplete control for confounding, occurs when information on a confounding factor is measured crudely. For example, only categorizing smoking history as "ever" vs. "never" would fail to distinguish among levels of smoking in current smokers and when past smokers may have quit. Because comprehensive knowledge of disease risk factors is rare, the possibility of uncontrolled confounding persists. The goal of the epidemiologist is to assess the plausibility of uncontrolled confounding, often by doing some types of sensitivity analyses. For example, if calcium is found to be a protective factor for a particular cancer, the plausibility of the findings are enhanced if calcium from both dairy products and supplements are associated with lower risk; if, for example, only dairy and not supplementary calcium is associated with lower risk, one would suspect that some factor other than calcium that is present in dairy products causally lowers risk.

1.6 RANDOMIZED INTERVENTION TRIALS

Confounding is best addressed in randomized intervention studies, in which random assignment of treatment naturally controls for known or unknown confounders. One of the most well-known intervention studies in cancer prevention involved β-carotene. Epidemiological observational studies suggested that diets high in β-carotene were associated with lower risk of lung cancer [23]. This evidence led to several intervention trials to study lung cancer risk. The results from these studies were in sharp contrast to what had been hypothesized: two trials using 20 to 30 mg of β-carotene supplements reported increased risk of lung disease [24], whereas in a third trial, 50 mg every other day did not influence lung cancer risk [25]. This is an example of the potentially powerful capability of randomized interventions to resolve a question — in this case, whether β-carotene could lower the risk of lung cancer.

Despite the major theoretical advantage of randomized intervention studies, which is the ability to control for known and unknown confounders, these studies have theoretical, ethical, and practical limitations. Null findings may simply reflect that the outcome measure or the duration, dose, or form of the nutrient under investigation was not appropriate to test the research question. For example, for β-carotene, most of the epidemiological evidence came from populations consuming approximately 2 to 5 mg/d, and high risk was generally at the lower end of this range. If a threshold exists for a benefit of β-carotene, it is possible that most individuals in the trials had little potential to benefit from additional β-carotene. Furthermore, the doses of 20 to 30 mg of β-carotene supplements used in these studies far exceed dietary doses. In epidemiological studies, which often generate the rationale for an intervention study, the comparison includes individuals with very low intakes of a nutrient (e.g., the bottom quintile of a population); in contrast, an intervention trial typically adds a certain dose of a nutrient to a population not generally selected for low intake. In fact, as relatively health-conscious individuals may be more likely to enroll in intervention studies, perhaps few individuals at the low end of intake, who are most likely to benefit, are enrolled. This problem could be avoided if trials preselected individuals who are most likely to benefit from an intervention given their diet (for example, those with lowest β-carotene intakes), although this is not often feasible or done.

Other limitations exist: First, surrogate endpoints for cancer development, which are often used in trials, may not encompass the whole spectrum of carcinogenesis over which dietary factors may act. For example, for colon cancer chemoprevention, a standard design is to identify patients who have just had an adenoma removed and to randomize them for several years, with the endpoint being whether or not any new adenomas are discovered upon surveillance colonoscopy. [26,27] This design may be excellent at examining factors that influence early aspects of colorectal carcinogenesis but may not be effective in studying factors that promote the progression of small adenomas to large adenomas, and large adenomas to cancers. Second, for intervention studies of dietary factors, blinding participants to an intervention, such as a low-fat diet, is difficult; it is more feasible for the study of micronutrients, which can be formulated into pills. For large-scale interventions, compliance and crossover may be issues, and the differences in intervention and control diets may narrow as the study progresses. Third, isolated nutrients taken in pill form may not have the same biological effect as foods supplying the nutrient, because food sources contain numerous other dietary factors that may act additively or synergistically to influence carcinogenesis. Fourth, for ethical reasons, intervention trials cannot evaluate dietary factors hypothesized to increase cancer risk. Further, many dietary factors that have hypothesized benefits for various cancers also have potential benefits for other chronic diseases, particularly cardiovascular disease. If a benefit is established for cardiovascular disease, it may be unethical to induce a long-term deprivation of a factor among those randomized to the placebo group. Finally, individuals who volunteer to participate in trials may often differ in relevant ways from the general population, restricting generalizability of the results. For all of these reasons, knowledge of cancer risk in humans is usually based on observational studies and the total evidence from several study designs. When feasible, randomized trials can provide powerful evidence to a diet or nutrient–cancer hypothesis.

1.7 THE COMBINED STUDY OF GENETICS AND NUTRITION IN EPIDEMIOLOGICAL STUDIES

The study of diet, nutrition, and cancer is complex, for many of the reasons summarized in the preceding sections. Mostly in the past decade or so, genetic factors have become incorporated into nutritional studies. Undoubtedly, studies combining nutrition and genetics will continue to proliferate in the future, as the costs of genotyping continue to come down. As more and more data are generated, it is increasingly important to have a conceptual framework to study what are often termed *gene and nutrient interactions*. The focus of the rest of this introductory chapter is to consider how the study of genetics can be incorporated into nutritional epidemiology and what insights can be generated by these studies.

What exactly is a nutrient–gene interaction in regard to cancer risk? In simple terms, it is the concept that the actions of a nutrient may differ according to specific genotypes, usually in a physiological or metabolic pathway related to carcinogenesis. There are a number of relevant pathways that dietary and nutritional factors could influence, which could increase or decrease the probability that a cancer will develop. For example, oxidative damage to DNA, which is likely to increase the rate of mutations, could enhance carcinogenesis. Many genes are involved in antioxidant defenses [28]. It is plausible, if not likely, that genetic variation in genes that influence important antioxidant enzymes could make an individual more or less susceptible to a relative deficiency of an antioxidant nutrient. Some dietary factors, such as polyunsaturated fats and iron, may enhance carcinogenesis, and nutrients that are cofactors for antioxidant enzymes, such as selenium or copper, or small-molecule antioxidants such as vitamin C and vitamin E may be beneficial. Conceptually, it would seem that the overall effect of the dietary antioxidants on cancer risk would be at least in part dependent on a specific genotype associated with antioxidation.

Taking into account gene–nutrient interactions can yield important insights and enhance the traditional approaches used in nutritional epidemiology. It is important to remember that the ultimate goal in nutritional epidemiology is to establish a cause–effect relationship between a specific nutrient (or food or dietary pattern) and cancer. The study of a gene–environment interaction may help immensely in establishing a causal relationship. To consider how integrating genetic and nutrient factors can be informative, it is useful to consider three of the important limitations of traditional studies of nutrition and cancer. The first limitation is that relative risks comparing high to low intake of a nutrient have been relatively modest in magnitude (for example, < 1.5 or < 2), and, thus, are not always consistent. Modest-sized associations are more likely to have been produced by bias and confounding. The second limitation is that intercorrelations among foods and nutrients make it difficult to be confident in concluding that a factor has truly an independent causal effect rather than acting as a surrogate of a correlated factor. A third important limitation is that carcinogenesis for many cancers typically requires a long time, perhaps several decades, and for many study designs it is difficult to obtain an estimate of dietary intake in the distant past, such as decades before the cancer diagnosis.

One of the criteria in establishing causality is the strength of the association. In general, the stronger the magnitude of the relative risk, the more likely that an association is causal rather than a result of bias or uncontrolled confounding. Consider, for example, a nutritional factor deficiency that increases the relative risk (RR) of a specific cancer fivefold in a genetically susceptible group but has no effect in the remaining population. In this case, the RR in the total population will be largely dependent on the proportion of susceptible individuals. For example, if half the individuals in the population have the susceptible genotype, the overall RR in the total population would be around 2.5, but if only 10% have the susceptible genotype, the RR would be around 1.4. In essence, the larger the number of nonsusceptible individuals, the more diluted the RR will be. As a general rule, in a reasonably well-designed study with no obvious major flaws, an RR of 5 would be considered strong evidence for causality; an RR of 2.5, moderately strong evidence; and an RR of 1.4, relatively weak evidence. Note that an RR of 1.4 could still be quite important from a public health perspective for a common exposure and a common endpoint; however, if the question of causality remains, it would be difficult to make recommendations confidently for this putative nutritional factor.

In nutrition and cancer epidemiological studies, there are many examples of factors with RRs of around 1.4. One of the main reasons that some risk factors for various cancers (e.g., tobacco, alcohol, and infectious agents) are well established and generally noncontroversial as causal is that the magnitude of the RR tends to be large. These results are based primarily on observational data rather than randomized studies, illustrating that nonrandomized observational studies can, in principle, generate data that lead to scientific consensus regarding causality. However, for nutritional factors, it may possibly be the exception rather than the rule that very high RRs will be observed, particularly for common, multifactorial cancers such as colon, breast, and prostate cancer. However, if a genetic subgroup for which the RR is high is consistently observed in many studies, a stronger case for causality can be made, at least for the susceptible group. A related advantage in addition to yielding stronger RRs is that if a bias, such as recall bias, is responsible for an association, this bias is likely to be the same across genotype because individuals would generally be unaware of their genotype. If a dietary risk factor is only apparent for one genotype, this is unlikely to be the result of bias because it is unlikely that only individuals with a specific genotype (unknown to them) would have recall bias.

The second important and related limitation in studies of nutrition and cancer is that strong intercorrelations among foods and nutrients reduce our confidence about whether an observed association with a nutrient is causal or whether the nutrient is acting as a surrogate of another correlated factor. Genetic studies offer a way to overcome this obstacle by contributing complementary evidence for an association that is unlikely to suffer from the same confounding factors. This point is best illustrated with an example: Some epidemiological evidence suggests that low folate intake or status may increase the risk of colon cancer; in general, the RR is around 1.5 for low vs. high folate, but whether this association is causal is not yet settled [29]. The enzyme methylenetetrahydrofolate reductase (MTHFR) is at a critical branch point that directs the folate pool toward remethylation of homocysteine to methionine at the expense of thymidylate synthesis (see Figure 1.1). A

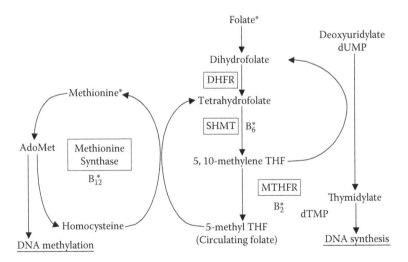

FIGURE 1.1 One-carbon metabolism involves a number of nutrients (indicated by *). MTHFR is at a critical juncture, directing folate into the pathway required for methylation (including DNA methylation) or DNA synthesis.

single-nucleotide polymorphism of the *MTHFR* gene (*677C→ T*) is associated with an alanine-to-valine substitution and with reduced enzyme activity [30], and thus this polymorphism is critical in directing folate pools into different pathways. The mutant *677TT* variant has generally been associated with reduced colon cancer risk, especially when the folate status is adequate and alcohol intake (an antifolate) is low [29]. Because the only known function of this enzyme is related to folate, its association with colon cancer strongly suggests that folate is indeed important in cancer risk because if folate status did not influence cancer risk, this genotype should be unassociated with risk. It is highly unlikely that a potential confounding factor for folate intake (e.g., intake of another correlated vitamin) would also confound a genetic factor such as a *MTHFR* genotype. Thus, the nutritional and genetic evidence are quite complementary in pointing to the importance of folate.

The same example illustrates another potential use of studying gene–environment interactions, that is, it provides insights into mechanisms in which nutrients may be acting. Individuals with the *MTHFR 677TT* genotype, if they have adequate folate intake, tend to accumulate appreciable levels of 5,10-methyleneTHF intracellularly, whereas those with *CC* and *CT* genotypes have their folate largely in the 5-methyl-THF form [31] (Figure 1.1). When levels of 5,10-methyleneTHF are low, misincorporation of uracil for thymidine may occur during DNA synthesis [32], leading to increased frequency of chromosomal breaks [33]. Thus, when folate is adequate, the *TT* genotype may be beneficial in enhancing the pool of 5,10-methyleneTHF. However, the *TT* genotype and poor folate (or high alcohol) intakes disrupt methylation reactions, including DNA methylation, as a result of inadequate levels of 5-methyl-THF [34]. In theory, alterations in DNA synthesis and DNA methylation could be important for carcinogenesis. The finding that individuals who are adequate in folate and who have the *MTHFR 677TT* genotype seem to be overall at the lowest risk suggests some benefit in having higher levels of 5,10-methyleneTHF, whereas the potentially increased risk associated with folate-poor states associated with the *MTHFR 677TT* genotype suggests a deleterious effect of reduced methylation.

The third way that the study of genetic factors in relation to cancer risk is helpful in establishing relationships between diet and cancer is that a genetic factor would represent a constant "exposure" and thus provide insights into a longer-term effect, including any influence during childhood, adolescence, and early adulthood. By their nature, most epidemiological studies are skewed toward studying factors that tend to act late in carcinogenesis. Epidemiologists do not discount early-acting effects and, in fact, for breast cancer, most acknowledge that many important events in carcinogenesis are likely to act during the early years, decades before the clinical diagnosis of cancer. Diets and exposures later in life are emphasized for practical reasons; it is unclear how well older adults can report on early diet, and if a cohort is started in children, one would have to await many decades to study cancer endpoints. Because a genetic factor would be operative throughout the life span, it may provide insight into early events. As an example, insulin-like growth factor-1 (IGF-1) levels during the growth phase may increase the risk of certain cancers, possibly explaining the positive correlation between height and these cancers [35]. However, IGF-1 levels in epidemiological studies have been typically measured in middle-aged and older individuals, and these are unlikely to correlate well with the high levels of IGF-1 that peak in adolescence. If, for example, a genetic factor that is a strong determinant of the magnitude of the IGF-1 peak during adolescence is identified, testing this genotype in relation to cancer risk may prove more feasible than actually measuring IGF-1 levels in adolescence and correlating these with cancer risk in adulthood.

1.8 PUBLIC HEALTH IMPLICATIONS OF NUTRIENT–ENVIRONMENT INTERACTIONS

Gene–environment interactions may provide important insights into whether a nutrient is causally associated with cancer risk. This knowledge obviously may have important chemical or public health implications, but the appropriate actions may not always be straightforward. An obvious question is: If a gene–nutrient interaction is established, should individuals be genotyped and their diets targeted based on the results? Several important factors must be taken into account, including the strength of the specific interaction, how common the outcome is, and the likely effect of the nutrients on overall health. For example, a recent study suggested a strong interaction between genetic polymorphism in manganese superoxide dismutase (MnSOD) and various potential antioxidants (selenium, vitamin E, and lycopene) in regard to prostate cancer risk (Figure 1.2) [36]. In essence, men with the variant genotype are much more sensitive to the effects of these antioxidants; in going from low to high intakes of all three compounds combined, there was an almost tenfold differential

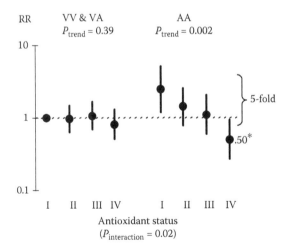

FIGURE 1.2 Risk of prostate cancer associated with manganese superoxide dismutase (MnSOD) genotype modified by prediagnostic levels of plasma antioxidant combinations. Dots represent relative risks (RR) and bars represent 95% confidence intervals (CI). Total prostate cancer: 496 cases and 402 controls; *95% CI (for group I) = 1.21 to 5.20; 95% CI (for group IV) = 0.27 to 0.94; among AA men, group IV vs. I RR = 0.20, 95% CI = 0.09 to 0.49. (From Li, H. et al., Manganese superoxide dismutase polymorphism, prediagnostic antioxidant status, and risk of clinical significant prostate cancer, *Cancer Res.*, 65, 2498, 2005. With permission.)

in the risk of advanced prostate cancer. Assuming these results are confirmed, should men be genotyped for this factor and then dietary recommendations be made based on the results? This is difficult to answer at this point. For very-high-risk genotypes, such as *BRCA* mutations and breast cancer risk, specific recommendations based on genotype are likely to be appropriate. For more moderate associations, the answer remains unclear. Although the results for the *MnSOD* genotype suggest that a group of men may exist that would particularly benefit from specific recommendations for increased intakes of these antioxidants, even men without the genotype experienced a more modest benefit. Moreover, these antioxidants may be beneficial for many other conditions, so perhaps ensuring high intakes could benefit individuals regardless of genotype. Also, any potential adverse effects of these nutrients cannot be ignored.

If a specific nutritional factor is deemed to be beneficial and there are no likely adverse effects on other conditions, the most appropriate action may possibly be to increase population levels. This action may be achieved by fortification (increasing folic acid in the food supply to prevent neural tube defects is one example). Alternatively, food and supplement manufacturers could be encouraged voluntarily or by mandate to adjust levels in their products (for example, remove trans fatty acids, add vitamin D in milk, and reduce sodium levels in processed foods). These passive approaches could possibly reach more people and would influence individuals' intakes positively. On the other hand, if genotyping indicates important adverse effects of obtaining too much of a nutrient, then knowledge of a specific genotype may be helpful for an individual's decision making. For example, higher iron intakes may be beneficial for menstruating women but not for individuals who have the genetic tendency to accumulate iron in excess [37].

An additional point concerns a methodological issue as to how interaction is usually tested in epidemiological settings. Because statistical models often used in cancer epidemiology (for example, proportional hazards regression or logistic regression) are based on multiplicative effects, multiplicative interaction is typically what is tested for statistically. To illustrate, assume a genetic factor triples a woman's risk of breast cancer and a specific nutrient deficiency doubles risk, but this doubling is statistically independent of the genetic factor. This situation would not constitute multiplicative interaction, as the magnitude of the effect on the RR scale of the nutrient is the same across genotypes. However, as the person with the high-risk genotype has a threefold increase in overall risk, a deficiency of the nutrient would be relatively more important (quantitatively, three times more important) than for the individual with the low-risk genotype. Thus, from a practical perspective it may behoove the high-risk individual to be even more diligent, even though no statistical interaction was determined in this case.

1.9 SUMMARY AND CONCLUSION

The study of nutrition and cancer is difficult for a variety of reasons. Epidemiological studies have contributed much to our knowledge, but various study designs have limitations. Although a randomized controlled intervention is the gold standard and can be powerful when a clear association is demonstrated, many factors could contribute to a null result for a nutrient–cancer association even if a true relationship exists. Furthermore, interventions cannot always be conducted for practical, financial, and ethical reasons, so most information for a nutrient–cancer association in humans will come from observational epidemiological studies. Each design — ecological, case–control, and cohort study — can offer important insights, although cohort studies are generally considered to be the most reliable because collecting dietary data before the development of cancer avoids many potential biases. Worldwide there are about 60 ongoing prospective studies that have a dietary component. A small fraction of these also have biological samples, which can be used to study biomarkers of specific nutritional factors (e.g., carotenoids and fatty acids) or nutritionally mediated biomarkers (e.g., insulin and insulin-like growth factors). These studies are yielding important data and will continue to do so.

The incorporation of studying genetics to complement nutritional factors in studies that have biological samples will provide an important adjunct to the nutritional component. By considering genetic susceptibility, stronger associations in certain genetically defined subgroups are likely to arise. Studies incorporating nutrition and genetics are likely to generate more conclusive findings regarding whether an association is causal, because the magnitude of an association is a critical criterion in considering whether the association is causal. Such studies may also help identify potential mechanisms or pathways through which certain risk or protective factors may be acting. Ultimately, the more important role of studying gene–environment interactions is to help establish causality of a nutrient–disease relationship. Public health and clinical implications such as whether to assess individual genotypes remain to be established.

The excitement of studying gene–nutrition interactions should be tempered with four final suggestions that are important to follow for optimally informative studies. First, studies must be quite large and include many cancer cases to have the adequate data required to examine nutrient–gene interactions. Often, this might involve the pooling of data from a number of large studies. Second, as the numbers of potential comparisons proliferate as nutrients are crossed with genetic factors, many false-positive results will arise, so replication of results is imperative. Third, methods to consider the simultaneous effects of many potentially relevant genes in a pathway (e.g., one-carbon pathway genes beyond *MTHFR*), not to mention nutrient–nutrient interactions, are poorly developed, so innovations in this area of data analysis are required. Finally, the ability to sequence many genes efficiently is important, but it remains equally imperative to acquire sound nutritional and other exposure information to adequately consider gene–nutrient interactions. In the past, genetic data may have been rate limiting but, over time, having complementary nutritional data may become the limiting factor, given the difficulties and cost of acquiring them.

REFERENCES

1. Parkin, D.M. et al., *Cancer Incidence in Five Continents,* Vol. VI, International Agency for Research on Cancer Scientific Publications, No. 120, Lyon, 1992.
2. Parkin, D.M., Cancer in developing countries, *Cancer Surv.,* 19–20, 519, 1994.

3. Haenszel, W. and Kurihara, M., Studies of Japanese migrants. I. Mortality from cancer and other diseases among Japanese in the United States, *J. Natl. Cancer Inst.,* 40, 43, 1968.

4. Buell, P., Changing incidence of breast cancer in Japanese-American women, *J. Natl. Cancer Inst.,* 51, 1479, 1973.

5. Shimizu, H. et al., Cancers of the prostate and breast among Japanese and white immigrants in Los Angeles County, *Br. J. Cancer,* 63, 963, 1991.

6. Thomas, D.B. and Karagas, M.R., Cancer in first and second generation Americans, *Cancer Res.,* 47, 5771, 1987.

7. Kolonel, L.N. et al., Nutrient intakes in relation to cancer incidence in Hawaii, *Br. J. Cancer,* 44, 332, 1981.

8. Ziegler, R.G. et al., Migration patterns and breast cancer risk in Asian-American women, *J. Natl. Cancer Inst.,* 85, 1819, 1993.

9. Armstrong, B. and Doll, R., Environmental factors and cancer incidence and mortality in different countries, with special reference to dietary practices, *Int. J. Cancer,* 15, 617, 1975.

10. Boissonneault, G.A., Elson, C.E., and Pariza, M.W., Net energy effects of dietary fat on chemically induced mammary carcinogenesis in F344 rats, *J. Natl. Cancer Inst.,* 76, 335, 1986.

11. Giovannucci, E. et al., Height, predictors of C-peptide and cancer risk in men, *Int. J. Epidemiol.,* 33, 217, 2004.

12. Micozzi, M.S., Functional consequences from varying patterns of growth and maturation during adolescence, *Horm. Res.,* 39 (Suppl. 3), 49, 1993.

13. Willett, W.C., *Nutritional Epidemiology,* 2nd ed., Oxford University Press, New York, 1998.

14. International Agency for Research on Cancer, Fruits and Vegetables, in *IARC Handbook of Cancer Prevention,* IARC Press, Lyon, France, 2003.

15. Howe, G.R. et al., Dietary factors and risk of breast cancer: combined analysis of 12 case-control studies, *J. Natl. Cancer Inst.,* 82, 561, 1990.

16. Hunter, D.J. et al., Cohort studies of fat intake and the risk of breast cancer: a pooled analysis, *N. Engl. J. Med.,* 334, 356, 1996.

17. Smith-Warner, S.A. et al., Types of dietary fat and breast cancer: a pooled analysis of cohort studies, *Int. J. Cancer,* 92, 767, 2001.

18. Giovannucci, E. et al., A comparison of prospective and retrospective assessments of diet in the study of breast cancer, *Am. J. Epidemiol.,* 137, 502, 1993.

19. Giovannucci, E., Modifiable risk factors for colon cancer, *Gastroenterol. Clin. N. Am.,* 31, 925, 2002.

20. Smith-Warner, S.A. et al., Methods for Retrospective Pooling of Results of Studies: The Pooling Project of Prospective Studies of Diet and Cancer, Submitted.

21. Riboli, E. and Kaaks, R., The EPIC project: rationale and study design, *Int. J. Epidemiol.,* 26, S6, 1997.

22. Last, J.M., *A Dictionary of Epidemiology,* Oxford University Press, Oxford, 1983.

23. Panel on Dietary Antioxidants and Related Compounds, Food and Nutrition Board, Institute of Medicine, *Dietary Reference Intakes for Vitamin C, Vitamin E, Selenium, and Carotenoids,* National Academy Press, Washington, D.C., 2000.

24. Food and Nutrition Board, Institute of Medicine., *Dietary Reference Intakes for Calcium, Phosphorus, Magnesium, Vitamin D, and Fluoride,* National Academy Press, Washington, D.C., 1997.

25. Hennekens, C.H. et al., Lack of effect of long-term supplementation with beta carotene on the incidence of malignant neoplasms and cardiovascular disease, *N. Engl. J. Med.,* 334, 1145, 1996.

26. Bostick, R.M., Human studies of calcium supplementation and colorectal epithelial cell proliferation, *Cancer Epidemiol. Biomarkers Prev.,* 6, 971, 1997.

27. Schatzkin, A. and Gail, M., The promise and peril of surrogate end points in cancer research, *Nat. Rev. Cancer,* 2, 19, 2002.

28. Ames, B.N., Gold, L.S., and Willett, W.C., The causes and prevention of cancer, *Proc. Natl. Acad. Sci. U.S.A.,* 92, 5258, 1995.

29. Giovannucci, E., Epidemiologic studies of folate and colorectal neoplasia: a review, *J. Nutr.,* 132, 2350S, 2002.

30. Frosst, P. et al., A candidate genetic risk factor for vascular disease: a common mutation in methylenetetrahydrofolate reductase (letter), *Nat. Genet.,* 10, 111, 1995.

31. Bagley, P.J. and Selhub, J., A common mutation in the methylenetetrahydrofolate reductase gene is associated with an accumulation of formylated tetrahydrofolates in red blood cells, *Proc. Natl. Acad. Sci. U.S.A.,* 95, 13217, 1998.

32. Wickramasinghe, S.N. and Fida, S., Bone marrow cells from vitamin B_{12}- and folate-deficient patients misincorporate uracil into DNA, *Blood,* 83, 1656, 1994.

33. Blount, B.C. et al., Folate deficiency causes uracil misincorporation into human DNA and chromosome breakage: implications for cancer and neuronal damage, *Proc. Natl. Acad. Sci. U.S.A.,* 94, 3290, 1997.

34. Friso, S. et al., A common mutation in the 5, 10-methylenetetrahydrofolate reductase gene affects genomic DNA methylation through an interaction with folate status, *Proc. Natl. Acad. Sci. U.S.A.,* 99, 5606, 2002.

35. Giovannucci, E., Nutrition, insulin, insulin-like growth factors and cancer, *Horm. Metab. Res.,* 35, 694, 2003.

36. Li, H. et al., Manganese superoxide dismutase polymorphism, prediagnostic antioxidant status, and risk of clinical significant prostate cancer, *Cancer Res.,* 65, 2498, 2005.

37. Heath, A.L. and Fairweather-Tait, S.J., Health implications of iron overload: the role of diet and genotype, *Nutr. Rev.,* 61, 45, 2003.

2 Candidate Mechanisms for Interactions between Nutrients and Genes

John C. Mathers

CONTENTS

2.1 INTRODUCTION

Although every nucleated cell in a particular human body contains the same genetic information that encodes around 20,000 to 25,000 genes, different cell types express a different complement of genes at particular stages of the life course and in response to variations in the environment to which the cell or the person is exposed. On average, each open reading frame in the human genome produces two to three different proteins, for example, by alternative splicing of the primary transcript, so that the potential number of proteins in the human proteome is considerably greater than the number of genes in the genome. Therefore, the key to normal function and maintenance of homeostasis is the ability to express the appropriate consortium of genes and to synthesize the appropriate proteome and metabolome in each cell type at the correct time. Aberrant gene expression is fundamental to the aging process and to the development of most, if not all, diseases, including cancer. Gene expression can be regulated at any of at least seven potential control steps: (1) chromatin structure, (2) initiation of transcription, (3) processing of the transcript, (4) transport to the cytoplasm, (5) translation of mRNA, (6) mRNA stability, and (7) protein activity stability [1].

2.2 NUTRITIONAL MODULATION OF GENE EXPRESSION

2.2.1 Effects on Transcription

Although posttranscriptional regulation of gene expression is known (see Section 2.2.2), it is believed that most temporal and tissue-specific regulation of gene expression occurs at the level of transcription initiation through both *cis*-acting control elements and *trans*-acting factors [2].

2.2.1.1 *Cis*-Acting Elements

Cis-acting elements are DNA sequences normally in the vicinity of structural portions of genes that are required for gene expression, but some *cis*-acting elements can be hundreds or thousands of base pairs (bp) up- or downstream of initiation sites. Nutrient-sensitive response elements are examples of *cis*-acting control elements that can influence gene expression by direct interaction with nutrients including retinoic acid, vitamin D, and zinc [2]. For example, when zinc concentrations in the cell are high, the metalloregulatory protein metal-response element-binding transcription factor-1 (MTF-1) binds zinc via its zinc-finger domain, translocates to the nucleus where it binds to metal-response elements in the promoter regions of target genes including those that encode metallothionein (MT), the zinc-transporter-1 (ZnT-1), and the gamma-glutamylcysteine synthetase heavy chain (gammaGCShc) [3]. These proteins then modulate "free" zinc in the cell because MT functions as an intracellular metal chelator (which binds zinc with high affinity via its cysteine-rich domains), ZnT-1 transports zinc out of the cell, and gammaGCShc controls the rate-limiting step in glutathione biosynthesis, another zinc chelator [3].

2.2.1.2 Transcription Factors Are *Trans*-Acting Factors

Transcription factors (TFs) are proteins that bind to DNA at specific promoter or enhancer sites, where they regulate transcription. TFs display particular motifs including helix-turn-helix (which binds the major groove in DNA), zinc fingers (structural platforms for DNA binding), and leucine zippers (facilitate TF binding with other TFs). These *trans*-acting factors include the peroxisome proliferators-activated receptors (PPARs), the CCAAT/ enhancer-binding proteins (C/EBPs), the signal transducers and activators of transcription (STATs), and the sterol regulatory element binding proteins (SREBPs). Because they may act as ligands for these receptors, nutrients can regulate the expression of transcription factors and so alter gene expression. For example, the PPARs (which are members of the nuclear hormone receptor superfamily) regulate gene expression by binding specific ligands and heterodimerization with other members of the superfamily prior to DNA binding and activation of transcription of a wide range of target genes involved in many key cell functions including proliferation, differentiation, and apoptosis [4]. There are at least three PPARs (designated α, β [also known as δ] and γ) with characteristically different expression in different tissues. For example, PPARα is expressed in muscle, liver, and blood vessel walls and PPARγ in adipose tissue and colon, whereas PPARβ is expressed ubiquitously. The gene encoding PPARγ can produce three different isoforms via use of different promoters and alternative splicing, with the PPARγ_2 isoform being particularly responsive to nutritional status [2]. Fatty acids and their derivatives, the eicosanoids, are natural ligands for PPARs that dimerize with their obligate heterodimeric partner retinoic X receptor alpha (RXRα) before binding with the promoter of a target gene and switching on transcription [4].

2.2.1.3 Epigenetic Modifications

Epigenetics describes noncoding changes to the genome that are transmitted through mitosis and alter gene expression. These epigenetic markings include posttranslational modifications of histones (methylation, acetylation, phosphorylation — described as "decoration"), and DNA methylation. Nucleosomes consist of 146 bp of DNA wrapped around an octet of histones, two copies each of histones H2A, H2B, H3, and H4. One nucleosome is joined to the next by a 60-bp DNA linker associated with a single molecule of histone H1. In addition to its role in packaging DNA tendrils into the nucleus, chromatin provides an information store (additional to the information encoded in the primary DNA sequence) and offers an important means of regulating gene expression. Approximately 1% of the DNA bases in the human genome is accounted for by 5-methylcytosine (m^5C), which occurs predominantly in CpG dinucleotides. The promoter regions of about half of human genes contain CpG islands, which are contiguous windows of 500 or more base pairs in which the G:C content is at least 55% and the observed-over-expected CpG frequency is at least 0.65 [5]. During cell division, methylation patterns in the parental strand of DNA are maintained in the daughter strand by the action of DNA methyltransferase 1 (DNMT1), which catalyzes the transfer of a methyl group from S-adenosylmethionine (AdoMet; the universal methyl donor) to the 5' position on cytosine residues [6]. Unlike cytosines elsewhere in the genome, those in CpG islands are normally unmethylated and are associated with euchromatin and gene expression. To a first approximation, chromatin, which is in a relatively open form allowing access by the transcriptional factors (TF) and associated proteins, is transcriptionally active, whereas genes are silent in the relatively condensed heterochromatin (see Gilbert et al. [7] for update). Such regulation of gene expression is essential for normal cell function, and both aging and the development of a wide range of diseases, including cancers, are associated with (some undoubtedly caused by) abnormal gene expression due to altered epigenetic marking of the genome.

Several nutrients, including methionine, choline, vitamins B_6 and B_{12}, riboflavin, folate, and zinc, are essential components of the pathways for synthesis of AdoMet for methylation of DNA and other cell macromolecules [6]. In theory, a deficiency of any of these nutrients could affect DNA methylation and, hence, modulate gene expression. Although it has been demonstrated that folate depletion and supplementation can affect genomic DNA methylation of lymphocytes [8–11] and the colonic mucosa [12] in human volunteers, as yet there is no evidence that such global modification of epigenetic marking is accompanied by changes in methylation of CpG islands in regulatory regions of genes or is responsible for changes in gene expression in humans [13]. However, supplementation of viable yellow agouti (A^{vy}) mouse dams with a combination of folic acid, vitamin B_{12}, choline, and betaine increased CpG methylation at the A^{vy} locus in DNA from all tissues studied (tail, brain, liver, and kidney) and altered the coat color of the offspring, presumably by switching off expression of the *agouti* gene [14].

The short-chain fatty acid butyrate, which is present in the large bowel in low millimolar concentrations as an end-product of carbohydrate fermentation by the resident bacteria, is a potent inhibitor of histone deacetylase [15] and induces widespread changes in gene expression [16]. Regulation of gene expression by epigenetic mechanisms is likely to involve cooperation between changes in DNA methylation and histone decoration [17]. A recent study has demonstrated that ligation of both arteries of the pregnant rat, which induces uteroplacental insufficiency and fetal malnutrition characteristic of intrauterine growth retardation, resulted in increased acetylation of histone H3, DNA hypomethylation, and reduced expression of cystathionine-β-synthase and methionine adenosyltransferase in the liver of offspring at birth [18]. The epigenetic changes persisted to at least 21 d after birth, and the authors speculated that their surgical insult affected hepatic one-carbon metabolism and, thus, DNA methylation, thereby altering chromatin dynamics and leading to sustained changes in hepatic gene expression [18]. Novel opportunities for investigating the influence of nutrients on epigenetic events are outlined by Oommen et al. [19].

2.2.2 Posttranscriptional Control of Gene Expression

The observation that changes in gene expression at the level of mRNA do not always correlate with changes in abundance (or activity) of the corresponding protein is evidence of posttranscriptional controls on gene expression that may be influenced by the nutritional status of the cell [2]. These controls are exercised via noncoding regions of the gene present in the 3′ and 5′ untranslated regions (UTRs) of the mRNA. For example, intracellular concentrations of iron regulate the synthesis of both ferritin (a multifunctional protein involved in the detoxification, storage, and transport of iron) and of transferrin (required for uptake of iron by cells) via a conserved sequence of 28 nucleotides known as the iron-responsive element (IRE) [20]. The mRNA for the transferrin receptor contains five IREs in its 3′-UTR, which, in the absence of iron, bind *trans*-acting transcription repressor proteins known as iron regulatory proteins (IRPs), prevent the mRNA from being degraded and therefore ensure continued synthesis of the transferrin receptor protein. When iron supply is adequate, the IRPs are released from the IREs, further transcription is prevented, the mRNA is destabilized, and production of the protein is curtailed to prevent further uptake of potentially damaging iron by the cell [2].

2.2.3 POSTTRANSLATIONAL MODIFICATION

The classical example of a nutrient necessary for the posttranslational modification of proteins, and hence for their function, is the role of vitamin K in the carboxylation of proteins involved in blood clotting (Factors II [prothrombin], VII, IX, and X) and of osteocalcin and matrix gamma-carboxyglutamyl (Gla) protein — the latter is an inhibitor of extracellular matrix calcification in arteries and in the epiphyseal growth plate. Vitamin K is an essential cofactor for the carboxylase, which, in the presence of O_2 and CO_2, catalyzes the conversion of glutamate residues to Gla residues [21]. More recently, evidence has emerged that fatty acids may regulate the expression of genes at a posttranslational locus. Incubation of macrophages in oleic-acid-containing media stimulated the secretion of APOE and altered the glycosylation pattern of the protein. This effect appeared to be protein specific because oleic acid did not alter glycosylation of interleukin 6 secreted from these cells [22]. Glycosylation plays a key role in a diverse range of cellular process including protein folding in the endoplasmic reticulum, targeting of newly synthesized lysozymes to the lysosome, recruitment and activation of cells during inflammation, cell-recognition processes, and the adhesion of microbes to host cells [23]. The resurgence of interest in these posttranslational decorations of glycoproteins and proteoglycans is stimulating interest in the development of array-based methods for surveying the glycome and proteome [23] and could be important tools in investigations of the potential regulatory role of oleic acid, or other nutrients, in other posttranslational glycosylation events.

2.3 IMPACT OF GENOTYPE ON RESPONSES TO NUTRIENTS

In addition to the key role that dietary factors play in regulating gene expression, an individual genotype impacts the way in which cells and tissues respond to nutrients (the science of nutrigenetics) and therefore are fundamental to understanding interindividual differences in nutritional needs [24]. There appear to be about 2 million single nucleotide polymorphisms (SNPs) in the human genome with around 100,000 SNPs distinguishing one individual from another. Although many of these SNPs are in "junk" regions of DNA with no known implications for gene expression, others occur within coding regions or in regulatory regions of genes and may result in altered gene expression or in the translation of proteins with altered characteristics. Although there is a potentially huge number of interactions between SNPs in individual genes and environmental agents including dietary factors, several examples have been studied that establish the importance of such interactions in explaining interindividual differences in responses to nutritional exposure or to nutritional interventions (Table 2.1). Most studies in this area have taken a "candidate gene" approach and examined responses of individuals carrying specific versions of genes (known, or suspected, to be modifiers of disease risk) to altered nutritional exposure. For example, it is now clear that responses in blood lipids concentrations to changes in the amount or type of fat in the diet are influenced by SNPs in the

TABLE 2.1

Examples of Nutrient Interactions with Genotype That Have Implications for Human Health

Gene	SNP/Isoform	Nutrient
MTHFR	C677T	Folate, alcohol
APOE	E_2, E_3, E_4	*n*-3 PUFA
APOA1	–75(G/A)	PUFA
GPX4	3′-UTR	Selenium
HFE	C282Y, H63D, S65C	Iron

genes encoding lipoproteins [25]. Similarly, SNPs in proinflammatory cytokine genes modulate the lipid-lowering effects of fish oil in healthy men [26].

Carriage of the *TT* version of the common polymorphism (*677 C→T*) in the *MTHFR* gene that encodes methylenetetrahydrofolate reductase, a key enzyme in folate metabolism, is associated with raised plasma homocysteine concentrations and increased risk of ischemic heart disease. In contrast, *TT* carriers appear to have a lower risk of colorectal cancer (CRC), especially if their intake of folate is adequate and they consume little or no alcohol [27]. There is marked geographic and ethnic variation in genotype frequencies for *MTHFR 677 C→T* [27], which may help explain the diversity in findings on the relationship between folate intake and CRC risk.

Cellular defenses against reactive oxygen species (ROS) include glutathione peroxidases (GPXs), catalase, and superoxide dismutase (SOD). The mitochondrial form of SOD (MnSOD) is synthesized in the cytosol and posttranslationally modified for transport into the mitochondrion. Within the mitochondrial targeting sequence, a *T→C* transition leads to a Val→Ala amino acid change at position 9, which is predicted to result in a change to the secondary structure of the protein and to cause inefficient targeting of MnSOD to the mitochondrion [28]. Both pre- and postmenopausal women who are homozygous for the unusual variant (MnSOD^Ala/Ala) have a higher risk of breast cancer in some [29–31], but not all, studies [32]. However, higher intakes of vegetables and fruits, or greater dietary antioxidant intake, may reduce the risk of breast cancer in women carrying the Ala/Ala form of the gene (Table 2.2), possibly because the greater availability of other antioxidants may compensate for the putatively less efficient mitochondrial MnSOD.

Intervention studies provide stronger evidence of causality than do observational studies but, until recently, most intervention studies investigating SNP–diet interactions have used retrospective genotyping, which limits the extent to which it is possible to infer causality. Prospective genotyping, together with the use of randomized, placebo-controlled trials, have the potential to provide powerful evidence of diet–gene interactions, but the design, logistic, and practical issues associated with such studies, especially if SNPs in more than one gene are being investigated, are formidable [33].

TABLE 2.2
Reduction in Odds Ratio for Breast Cancer in Premenopausal Women Homozygous for a Single-Nucleotide Polymorphism in Manganese Superoxide Dismutase with Higher Intakes of Fruits and Vegetables

Food	Low Intake[a]	High Intake[a]	Reference
Fruits and vegetables	6.0	3.2	29
Total vegetables	2.6	1.5	31
Total fruits	2.4	1.5	31

Note: Reference population for calculation of odds ratios were women carrying the Val/Val and Val/Ala forms [29] or Val/Val form [31] of MnSOD.

[a] Intakes were dichotomized at the median into low and high intakes.

2.4 MECHANISMS BY WHICH FOOD CONSTITUENTS MAY INFLUENCE CARCINOGENESIS

Genomic damage resulting in aberrant gene expression is the fundamental cause of all cancers. Such damage includes mutations, aberrant epigenetic marking (global DNA hypomethylation, hypermethylation of CpG islands in the promoter regions of genes, and changes to the pattern of posttranslational modifications of histones), chromosomal damage (e.g., loss, rearrangements, and aneuploidy), and telomere shortening (Figure 2.1). Because both external agents and normal cell functions, such as mitosis, subject the genome to frequent and diverse insults, the human cell has evolved a battery of defense mechanisms that (1) attempt to minimize such damage (including inhibition of oxidative reactions by free radical scavenging and the detoxification of potential mutagens), (2) repair the damage, or (3) remove severely damaged cells by shunting them into apoptosis [33]. When such defenses fail and a tumor becomes established, further genomic damage and further alterations in gene expression enable the tumor to grow, to cope with anoxia, to develop a novel blood supply (angiogenesis), to escape from the confines of its initiation site, and to establish colonies elsewhere in the body (metastasis). All of these processes are potentially modifiable by components in foods and by nutritional status (Table 2.3 and Table 2.4) [34]. In addition, interactions between dietary (and other environmental or lifestyle) factors and genetic makeup (seen principally in the assembly of single-nucleotide polymorphisms [SNPs], which is unique to each individual and which confers greater or less susceptibility) contributes to interperson differences in cancer risk. The simple model in Figure 2.2 illustrates how these factors combine to modify risk. Note that for most cancers, time is among the strongest etiological factors, which provides support for the hypothesis that the accumulation of genomic damage is fundamental to carcinogenesis, i.e., during aging there is deterioration in genomic maintenance [35].

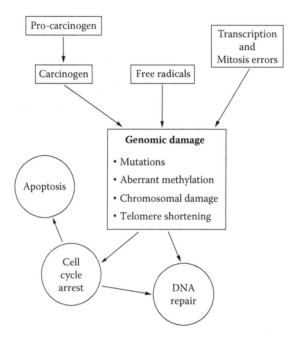

FIGURE 2.1 Tumors may arise if damage to the genome is unrepaired. All of these processes may be influenced by nutrition. (From Mathers, J.C., The biological revolution — towards a mechanistic understanding of the impact of diet on cancer risk, *Mutat. Res.*, 551, 43, 2004. With permission.)

TABLE 2.3
Dietary Factors That May Reduce Cancer Risk by Preventing DNA Damage

Mechanism	Molecular Targets	Dietary Factors
Inhibit activation of carcinogens	Cytochrome P450	Tea
	Cyclooxygenases	Salicylates, *n*-3 PUFA, flavonoids
Detoxify activated carcinogens	Glutathione-*S*-transferase	Glucosinolates
Inhibit carcinogen uptake	Bile acids	Calcium
Enhance DNA repair	Multiple DNA repair systems	Selenium
Inhibit free radical DNA damage	Free radicals	Tea, soy isoflavones, antioxidant nutrients
Reduce inflammation	NFκB	Salicylates, *n*-3 PUFA, reduced energy intake

Source: Adapted from Steele, V.E., Current mechanistic approaches to chemoprevention of cancer, *J. Biochem. Mol. Biol.*, 36, 78, 2002.

2.4.1   NUTRITION, INFLAMMATION, AND CANCER RISK

One of the clearest examples of the link between inflammation and cancer is the approximately tenfold greater risk of CRC in those with ulcerative colitis (UC) [36].

TABLE 2.4
Dietary Factors That May Help Prevent Cancer by Modulating Cell Proliferation

Mechanism	Molecular Targets	Dietary Factors
Induce apoptosis	Caspase activity	Retinoids
	Histone deacetylase	Butyrate, diallyl sulfide
Cell cycle arrest	Topoisomerase II?	Selenium, diallyl sulfide, genistein
Induce terminal differentiation	TGFβ	Vitamin D, retinoids
Alter DNA methylation	DNA methyltransferase 1	Epigallocatechin-3-gallate, folate, selenium
Enhance immunosurveillance	—	Butyrate, probiotics (?)
Inhibit angiogenesis	VEGF expression	Retinoids, salicylates, n-3 PUFA, butyrate

Source: Adapted from Steele, V.E., Current mechanistic approaches to chemoprevention of cancer, *J. Biochem. Mol. Biol.*, 36, 78, 2002.

CRC risk in those with UC increases exponentially with the duration of the disease and also increases with the extent and severity of the inflammation [37,38]. Cancers at other sites including the bladder, lung, skin, esophagus, and pancreas are also associated with chronic inflammatory diseases [39]. Evidence from both naturally occurring (e.g., the cotton-top tamarin) and chemically induced animal models of colitis [40] supports the concept that inflammation may be causal for CRC. Inflammation-associated genes including cyclooxygenase-2 (*COX-2*) and nitric oxide synthase-2 (*NOS-2*), which are elevated in inflamed mucosa, are also elevated in colonic tumors [36]. When the $Apc^{\Delta716}$ mouse (which develops multiple intestinal adenomas spontaneously) was crossed with a mouse in which the *COX-2* gene was knocked out, there was a huge reduction in numbers of intestinal neoplasms. A similar, albeit less dramatic, response was seen when the activity of the COX-2 enzyme was inhibited using a COX-2 selective drug [41]. Both observational [42] and intervention studies [43,44] in humans demonstrate that frequent and prolonged consumption of nonsteroidal antiinflammatory drugs (NSAIDS) such as aspirin may prevent adenoma formation and/or progression to CRC in some individuals.

The oxidative stress that accompanies chronic inflammation may play a mechanistic role in the greater cancer risk through genomic damage by the reactive oxygen and nitrogen species (RONS) generated by inflammatory cells [36]. In the gut epithelium, the inflammatory response may be mediated by activation of the transcription factor NF-κB, which switches on expression of proinflammatory cytokines, adhesion molecules, growth factors, and COX-2 [45]. In unstimulated cells, NF-κB is confined to the cytoplasm, where it dimerizes with the IκB family of inhibitory proteins. Phosphorylation of IκB results in the release of NF-κB and its translocation to the nucleus, while IκB is ubiquitinated and degraded in the proteasome. Nutrients with key roles in protection of the genome against oxidative stress, e.g., selenium (via the role of selenocysteine in selenoproteins including the glutathione peroxidases

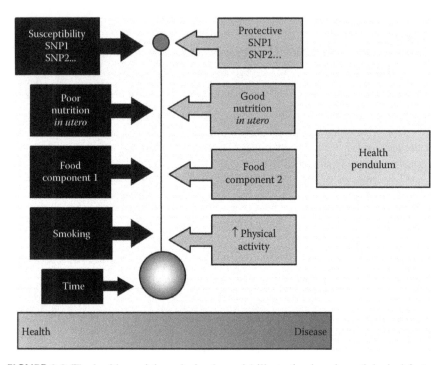

FIGURE 2.2 The health pendulum. A simple model illustrating how key etiological factors influence cancer risk. For a given individual, the position over the health–disease continuum from which the pendulum is suspended depends on the genetic makeup (indicated as the inherited collection of "susceptibility" and "protective" genes). Nutrition *in utero* and postnatal lifestyle interact with genetic makeup to further modify risk. For most common cancers, risk increases with age. (Adapted from Mathers, J.C., Pulses and carcinogenesis: potential for the prevention of colon, breast and other cancers, *Br. J. Nutr.,* 88, Suppl. 3, S273, 2002.)

[46]) and vitamins C and E and food components that have antiinflammatory activity, e.g., *n*-3 long-chain polyunsaturated fatty acids [45] would be expected to help prevent cancer development. Recent work has shown that a variety of food-derived compounds including resveratrol (from grapes) and curcumin (from cumin seeds) that have potent antiinflammatory properties suppressed tumor cell growth and suppressed NF-κB-regulated reporter gene expression and expression of COX-2 [47].

2.4.1.1 Intestinal Bacteria

Recent studies have shown that the intestinal microflora may have an important role to play not only in inflammation but also in the increased risk of CRC in individuals with UC or other inflammatory bowel diseases. [37] Colonic bacteria may contribute to loss of mucosal integrity and may trigger the NF-κB pathway in macrophages, resulting in increased expression of a battery of proinflammatory agents. In addition, through the binding of yet-to-be-identified factors, derived from intestinal bacteria, to the Toll-like receptors (TLRs) on the apical membrane of colonocytes, the NF-κB pathway is activated and expression of survival signals (such as the antiapoptotic protein BCL-$_{XL}$) is switched on [37]. This may provide damaged (initiated) cells with a defense against apoptosis and so facilitate tumor development. The short-chain fatty acid (SCFA) butyrate (which is present in the colonic lumen in low millimolar concentrations as an endproduct of bacterial fermentation of carbohydrates) has been shown to exert antiinflammatory actions when used in rectal enemas for the treatment of UC [48]. It is now known that butyrate inhibits NF-κB activation in colonic adenocarcinoma cells and suppresses expression of NF-κB-responsive proinflammatory cytokines *in vitro* [49,50]. Administration of butyrate by rectal enema to UC patients for up to 8 weeks resulted in a decrease in NF-κB translocation to the nucleus in lamina propria macrophages and less mucosal inflammation [51]. These results suggest that there may be a robust mechanistic basis for attempts to modulate the colonic luminal environment through the use of pro- and prebiotics for the treatment of inflammatory conditions and for the prevention of CRC. Probiotic bacteria may displace pathogenic species from the colon, thus helping to maintain mucosal immunity and barrier function [45]. Prebiotics (which are usually carbohydrates) may alter the production of SCFA, in addition to affecting the balance of bacterial species. There is evidence that bacterial fermentation of some carbohydrates, in particular starches, results in increased production of butyrate but understanding of the factors that determine the amounts and pattern of SCFA produced in the human colon remains limited [52]. Mechanistic studies on intestinal bacterial metabolism aimed at production of additional butyrate offer the promise of novel means of manipulating the intestinal lumen to prevent adverse inflammatory responses and, hence, the risk of CRC.

2.4.1.2 Obesity

The association between obesity and increased risk of cancer at a number of sites including colon, female breast, endometrium, and esophagus has long been recognized [53]. Central adiposity has been shown, recently, to be a risk factor for bowel cancer in both men and women [54], suggesting that the distribution of body fat, in addition to its quantity, may influence tumorigenesis. The mechanisms responsible for this increased risk have not been elucidated, but putative mechanisms include altered carcinogen metabolism, increased DNA damage, poorer DNA repair capacity, and higher concentrations of growth factors such as insulin-like growth factor-1 (IGF-1) [53]. Obesity and other conditions resulting in chronically elevated blood insulin concentrations result in higher concentrations of free (bioavailable) IGF-1 in blood, which, together, inhibit synthesis of sex-hormone-binding globulin in the liver, leading to higher circulating concentrations of androgens and estrogens. Higher circulating concentrations of estrogens may also occur via aromatization of androstenedione to estrone in the adipose tissue of postmenopausal women [53], with adverse consequences for risk-hormone-sensitive tumors, e.g., breast and endometrial cancer.

However, the recent observation that circulating mononuclear cells in obese individuals are in a proinflammatory state with greater intranuclear NF-κB binding and increased transcription of proinflammatory genes regulated by NF-κB [55] provides an alternative explanation for the positive relationship between body fatness and cancer risk. In addition to its role as a significant risk factor for many chronic diseases including rheumatoid arthritis, Alzheimer's disease, osteoporosis, periodontitis, and cardiovascular disease [56], the recognition that an aberrant inflammatory response in the obese may predispose to cancer should help focus research on dietary and other agents that may prevent excessive inflammation as well as on the development of effective strategies for the prevention and treatment of obesity.

2.5 NUTRITIONAL MODULATION OF DNA DAMAGE AND REPAIR

DNA damage resulting in aberrant gene expression is fundamental to tumor initiation and development. Because oxidative damage to DNA is known to be mutagenic, micronutrients such as the vitamins A, C, and E and trace minerals including zinc, selenium, and manganese, which prevent oxidative damage (antioxidants), are potentially anticarcinogenic [57]. This is supportive of the epidemiological evidence, which is "persuasive" that diets rich in fruits and vegetables are protective against cancers at a number of sites including the colorectum [58]. However, as yet, there is no unequivocal evidence that antioxidant supplements will reduce cancer risk. Indeed, major intervention studies giving high doses of β-carotene to middle-aged male smokers or to those previously exposed to asbestos had no protective effect against cancer. Worse, there was a significantly greater incidence of lung cancer among those supplemented with β-carotene [59]. The reason for this unexpected adverse effect is not known, but it could be that at the very high dose given in this trial, β-carotene acted as a pro- rather than an antioxidant. Certainly, β-carotene has antineoplastic effects *in vitro*, where it has been shown to suppress the growth of CRC cells in a dose-dependent manner by inducing cell cycle arrest at G_2-M and by promoting apoptosis [60].

Both observational and intervention studies support the hypothesis that low selenium intake increases cancer risk [46]. There are several possible mechanisms through which optimal selenium status may help reduce cancer risk, including (1) its key role as a structural component of the selenoproteins, the GPXs, which protect cell macromolecules against damage by peroxides, (2) altered carcinogen metabolism, (3) enhanced immunosurveillance, (4) induction of apoptosis, (5) suppression of angiogenesis, and (6) enhanced DNA repair (see the following paragraph) [46]. Selenium is present in the human diet in both inorganic (principally selenite) and organic (selenocysteine and selenomethionine) forms, and it remains uncertain whether specific forms, or food sources, of selenium have superior antineoplastic properties [46,61].

The genome in every cell is exposed continually to damage by both exogenous and endogenous factors, and humans have evolved a range of DNA repair mechanisms that sense and repair different kinds of DNA damage. Cells with DNA damage may arrest at the G_1-S cell cycle checkpoint when damage is sensed by the protein product of the *ATM* gene. This information is signaled to *TP53* and results in increased concentrations of the tumor suppressor protein p53, which, in its tetrameric form, is a transcription factor. Signals from both oxidative stress and DNA strand breaks are integrated by p53 [62] and hence lead to cell cycle arrest to allow time for DNA repair or to divert the cell into apoptosis [63]. The major types of DNA repair in mammalian cells include one-step repair, base excision repair, nucleotide excision repair, DNA mismatch repair, and recombinational repair. Clearly enhancing the effectiveness of these repair mechanisms would be an advantage in helping the cell defend the genome against potentially mutagenic damage. Recent research suggests that in addition to their role in cancer prevention through radical scavenging, antioxidants may be antineoplastic through upregulating DNA repair [64]. The best evidence in this area is for the role of selenium (in the form of selenomethionine), which appears to induce base excision repair via p53 activation in normal human fibroblasts *in vitro* [65]. p53 and several of the proteins involved in base excision and nucleotide excision repair are zinc finger or zinc-associated proteins, and adequate zinc status is essential to ensure optimal function of these proteins [66]. There is now evidence from a human intervention trial that improved nutrition may enhance DNA repair in humans *in vivo*. Collins et al. [67] supplemented the diet of healthy human volunteers with kiwifruit for 3 weeks and observed reduced endogenous oxidation of purines and pyrimidines and enhanced base excision repair by lymphocytes. In a study of this kind, it is not possible to ascertain the molecular mechanism for the enhanced base excision repair in those consuming supplemental kiwifruit, but these exciting observations should encourage others to investigate the underlying mechanisms and the potential for enhancement for each DNA repair mechanism by other dietary factors. Tentative evidence that low folate status may limit the cell's capacity for nucleotide excision repair has emerged recently from a human epidemiological study [68].

2.6 DEVELOPMENTAL ORIGINS OF CANCER

There is now substantial epidemiological evidence that poor growth *in utero*, especially when followed by rapid growth in infancy or childhood, is associated with above average risk of a range of diseases including coronary heart disease, type 2 diabetes, stroke, and hypertension [69]. Experimental studies in animal models in which intrauterine growth is limited by maternal undernutrition provide evidence that this association may be causal [70]. These and other observations underpin the concept of developmental plasticity whereby a given genotype can give rise to a range of phenotypes depending on the environmental conditions to which the fetus and growing child are exposed [71]. This has stimulated extensive research to uncover the mechanisms of cellular (or tissue) "memory" through which early life environmental experiences are "recorded" and which result in altered gene expression and aberrant function decades later. Numerous possible mechanisms for this "memory" have been proposed including epigenetic changes, alterations in organ structure, clonal selection of particular cell populations, apoptotic remodeling, and metabolic differentiation (reviewed by Mcmillen and Robinson in Reference 70). Recent studies using a model in which intrauterine growth retardation was induced by ligating both uterine arteries of the pregnant rat have shown that this nutritional insult resulted in major changes to one-carbon metabolism characterized by increased hepatic concentrations of homocysteine, S-adenosylhomocysteine, and methionine [18]. These metabolite disturbances were accompanied by genomewide DNA hypomethylation, altered CpG methylation of a number of genes, and altered gene expression including downregulation of DNMT1, Bcl-2, methionine adenosyl transferase, and cystathionine-β-synthase and increased expression of p53 [72,18]. The involvement of epigenetic mechanisms in these differential patterns of gene expression is reinforced by the finding of increased histone H3 acetylation, and the authors speculate that the aberrant chromatin structure induced by fetal malnutrition may be the basis for altering the functional responses of the genome to subsequent environments [18]. The impact of alterations in genome-wide DNA methylation and in the pattern of CpG methylation of regulatory regions of genes during *in utero* or early postnatal life on risk of cancer has yet to be investigated.

Although there is a wealth of evidence from many animal models that energy restriction can increase longevity [73] and reduce cancer risk [74], there appears to be little information about the impact of fetal and neonatal growth on cancer development in humans. Frankel et al. [75] reported a positive association between childhood energy intake and adult mortality from cancer, and investigation of the same cohort suggested that men (but not women) who had long legs in childhood (a surrogate for better diet and socioeconomic circumstances) had significantly increased cancer mortality [76]. Given the key role of nutrition in influencing fetal and neonatal growth resulting in potentially lifelong alterations in epigenetic marking of the genome, further work on the developmental origins of cancer seems attractive.

2.7 CONCLUDING REMARKS

From the public health perspective, the epidemiological evidence linking diet with cancer risk has been very encouraging, but it has proved difficult, using conventional epidemiological methodology, to identify which dietary factors, in what amounts and over which time periods, are most important in modulating risk [33]. The rapid expansion of understanding of the molecular events in cancer development, the recognition that aberrant gene expression is fundamental at all stages from tumor initiation to metastasis, and the realization that dietary factors interact with the genome to determine gene expression are the basis for today's rapid advances in understanding of the mechanistic links between food choices and cancer risk. Although much useful information is emerging from *in vitro* and animal model studies, there are still rather few data from appropriately designed human studies. For most cancer sites, such studies are limited by the lack of reliable surrogate endpoints but the application of "omics" technologies offers a novel approach to identifying patterns of gene expression that will distinguish cells predisposed to tumor development and may offer targets for dietary interventions to arrest or reverse aberrant gene expression.

REFERENCES

1. Villard, J., Transcription regulation and human diseases, *Swiss Med. Wkly.* 134, 571, 2004.
2. Roche, H.M. and Mensink, R.P., Molecular aspects of nutrition, in *Nutrition and Metabolism*, Gibney, M.J., Macdonald, I.A., and Roche, H.M., Eds., Blackwell Science, Oxford, 2003, chap. 2.
3. Andrews, G.K., Cellular zinc sensors: MTF-1 regulation of gene expression, *Biometals*, 14, 223, 2001.
4. Morrison, R.F. and Farmer S.R., Nutrition and adipocyte gene expression, in *Nutrient-Gene Interactions in Health and Disease*, Moustad-Moussa, N. and Berdanier, C.D., Eds., CRC Press, Boca Raton, FL, 2001, chap. 2.
5. Laird, P.W., The power and the promise of DNA methylation markers, *Nat. Rev. Cancer,* 3, 253, 2003.
6. Christman, J.K., Diet, DNA methylation and Cancer, in *Molecular Nutrition,* Zempleni, J. and Daniel, H., Eds., CABI Publishing, Wallingford, 2003, chap. 16.
7. Gilbert, N. et al., Chromatin architecture of the human genome: gene-rich domains are enriched in open chromatin fibers, *Cell*, 118, 555, 2004.
8. Jacob, R.A. et al., Moderate folate depletion increases plasma homocysteine and decreases lymphocyte DNA methylation in postmenopausal women, *J. Nutr.*, 128, 1204, 1998.
9. Rampersaud, G.C. et al. Genomic DNA methylation decreases in response to moderate folate depletion in elderly women. *Am. J. Clin. Nutr.,* 72, 998, 2000.
10. Shelnutt, K.P. et al., Methylenetetrahydrofolate reductase 677CT polymorphism affects DNA methylation response to controlled folate intake in young women, *J. Nutr. Biochem.*, 15, 554, 2004.
11. Pufulete, M. et al., Folic acid supplementation increases genomic DNA methylation in patients with colorectal adenoma, *Gut,* 54, 648, 2005.
12. Kim, Y.-I. et al., Effects of folate supplementation on two provisional molecular markers of colon cancer: a prospective, randomized trial, *Am. J. Gastroenterol.*, 96, 184, 2001.
13. Mathers, J.C., Reversal of DNA hypomethylation by folic acid supplements: possible role in colorectal cancer prevention, *Gut,* 54, 579, 2005.
14. Waterland, R.A. and Jirtle, R.L., Transposable elements: targets for early nutritional effects on epigenetic gene regulation, *Mol. Cell. Biol.*, 23, 5293, 2003.
15. Boffa, L.C. et al., Suppression of histone deacetylation in vivo and in vitro by sodium butyrate, *J. Biol. Chem.,* 253, 3364, 1978.
16. Williams, E.A., Coxhead, J.M., and Mathers, J.C., Anti-cancer effects of butyrate: use of microarray technology to investigate mechanisms, *Proc. Nutr. Soc.,* 62, 107, 2003.
17. Robertson, K.D., DNA methylation and chromatin — unraveling the tangled web, *Oncogene*, 21, 5361, 2002.
18. MacLennan, N.K. et al., Uteroplacental insufficiency alters DNA methylation, one-carbon metabolism, and histone acetylation in IUGR rats, *Physiol. Genomics,* 18, 43, 2004.
19. Oommen, A.M. et al., Roles for nutrients in epigenetic events, *J. Nutr. Biochem.,* 16, 74, 2005.
20. Dhar, M.S., Ferritin: a novel human ferritin heavy-chain mRNA is predominately expressed in the adult brain, in *Nutrient-Gene Interactions in Health and Disease*, Moustad-Moussa, N. and Berdanier, C.D., Eds., CRC Press, Boca Raton, FL, 2001, chap. 18.

21. Suttie, J.W., Synthesis of vitamin K-dependent proteins, *FASEB J.*, 7, 445, 1993.
22. Huang, Z.H., Gu, D., and Mazzone, T., Oleic acid modulates the post-translational glycosylation of macrophage ApoE to increase its secretion, *J. Biol. Chem.*, 279, 29195, 2004.
23. Feizi, T. and Chai, W., Oligosaccharide microarrays to decipher the glyco code, *Nat. Rev. Mol. Cell. Biol.*, 5, 582, 2004.
24. Mathers, J.C., Chairman's introduction: what can we expect to learn from genomics? *Proc. Nutr. Soc.*, 63, 1, 2004.
25. Ordovas, J.M., The quest for cardiovascular health in the genomic era: nutrigenetics and plasma lipoproteins, *Proc. Nutr. Soc.*, 63, 145, 2004.
26. Markovic, O. et al., Role of single nucleotide polymorphisms of pro-inflammatory cytokine genes in the relationship between serum lipids and inflammatory parameters, and the lipid-lowering effect of fish oil in healthy males, *Clin. Nutr.*, 23, 1084, 2004.
27. Sharp, L. and Little, J., Polymorphisms in genes involved in folate metabolism and colorectal neoplasia: a HuGE review, *Am. J. Epidemiol.*, 159, 423, 2004.
28. Sutton, A. et al., The Ala16Val genetic dimorphism modulates the import of human manganese superoxide dismutase into rate liver, *Pharmacogenetics*, 13, 145, 2003.
29. Ambrosone, C.B. et al., Manganese superoxide dismutase (*MnSOD*) genetic polymorphisms, dietary antioxidants, and risk of breast cancer, *Cancer Res.*, 59, 602, 1999.
30. Mitrunen, K. et al., Association between manganese superoxide dismutase (*MnSOD*) gene polymorphism and breast cancer risk, *Carcinogenesis*, 22, 827, 2001.
31. Cai, Q. et al., Genetic polymorphism in the manganese superoxide dismutase gene, antioxidant intake, and breast cancer risk: results from the Shanghai Breast Cancer Study, *Breast Cancer Res.*, 6, R647, 2004.
32. Tamimi, R.M. et al., Manganese superoxide dismutase polymorphism, plasma antioxidants, cigarette smoking, and risk of breast cancer, *Cancer Epidemiol. Biomark. Prev.*, 13, 989, 2004.
33. Mathers, J.C., The biological revolution — towards a mechanistic understanding of the impact of diet on cancer risk, *Mutat. Res.*, 551, 43, 2004.
34. Steele, V.E., Current mechanistic approaches to chemoprevention of cancer, *J. Biochem. Mol. Biol.*, 36, 78, 2002.
35. DePinho, R.A., The age of cancer, *Nature*, 408, 248, 2000.
36. Itzkowitz S.H. and Yio, X., Inflammation and cancer IV. Colorectal cancer in inflammatory bowel disease: the role of inflammation, *Am. J. Physiol. Gastrointest. Liver Physiol.*, 287, G7, 2004.
37. Clevers, H., At the crossroads of inflammation and cancer, *Cell*, 118, 671, 2004.
38. Rutter, M. et al., Severity of inflammation is a risk factor for colorectal neoplasia in ulcerative colitis, *Gastroenterology*, 126, 451, 2004.
39. Coussens, L.M. and Werb, Z., Inflammation and cancer, *Nature*, 420, 860, 2002.
40. Seril, D.N. et al., Oxidative stress and ulcerative colitis-associated carcinogenesis: studies in humans and animal models, *Carcinogenesis*, 24, 353, 2003.
41. Oshima, M. et al., Suppression of intestinal polyposis in Apc delta 716 knockout mice by inhibition of cyclooxygenase 2 (Cox-2), *Cell*, 87, 803, 1996.
42. Baron, J.A. and Sandler, R.S., Nonsteroidal anti-inflammatory drugs and cancer prevention, *Annu. Rev. Med.* 51, 511, 2000.
43. Sandler, R.S. et al., A randomized trial of aspirin to prevent colorectal adenomas in patients with previous colorectal cancer, *New Engl. J. Med.*, 348, 883, 2003.
44. Baron, J.A. et al., A randomised trial of aspirin to prevent colorectal adenomas, *New Engl. J. Med.*, 348, 891, 2003.
45. Philpott, M. and Ferguson, L.R., Immunonutrition and cancer, *Mutat. Res.* 551, 29, 2004.

46. Whanger, P.D., Selenium and its relationship to cancer: an update, *Br. J. Nutr.*, 91, 11, 2004.
47. Takada, Y. et al., Non-steroidal anti-inflammatory agents differ in their ability to suppress NF-κB activation, inhibition of expression of cyclooxygenase-2 and cyclin D1, and abrogation of tumor cell proliferation, *Oncogene*, 23, 9247, 2004.
48. Scheppach, W. et al., Effect of butyrate enemas on the colonic mucosa in distal ulcerative colitis, *Gastroenterology*, 103, 51, 1992.
49. Inan, M.S. et al., The luminal short-chain fatty acid butyrate modulates NF-κB activity in a human colonic epithelial cell line, *Gastroenterology*, 118, 724, 2000.
50. Segain, J.P. et al., Butyrate inhibits inflammatory responses through NFκB inhibition: implications for Crohn's Disease, *Gut*, 47, 397, 2000.
51. Lührs, H. et al., Butyrate inhibits NF-κB activation in lamina propria macrophages of patients with ulcerative colitis, *Scand. J. Gastroenterol.*, 37, 458, 2002.
52. Mathers, J.C., Smith, H., and Carter, S., Dose-response effects of raw potato starch on small-intestinal escape, large bowel fermentation and gut transit time in the rat, *Br. J. Nutr.*, 78, 1015, 1997.
53. Calle, E.E. and Thun, M.J., Obesity and cancer, *Oncogene*, 23, 6365, 2004.
54. Moore, L.L. et al., BMI and waist circumference as predictors of lifetime colon cancer risk in Framingham study adults, *Int. J. Obesity*, 28, 559, 2004.
55. Ghanim, H. et al., Circulating mononuclear cells in the obese are in a proinflammatory state, *Circulation*, 110, 1564, 2004.
56. Kornman, K.S., Martha, P.M., and Duff, G.W., Genetic variations and inflammation: a practical nutrigenomics opportunity, *Nutrition*, 20, 44, 2004.
57. Ames, B.N. and Wakimoto, P., Are vitamin and mineral deficiencies a major cancer risk? *Nat. Rev. Cancer*, 2, 694, 2002.
58. Department of Health, Nutritional Aspects of the Development of Cancer, Report on Health and Social Subjects 48, The Stationery Office, London, 1998.
59. Alpha-Tocopherol, Beta Carotene Cancer Prevention Study Group, The effect of vitamin E and beta-carotene on lung cancer incidence and other cancers in male smokers, *N. Engl. J. Med.*, 330, 1029, 1994.
60. Palozza, P. et al., Induction of cell cycle arrest and apoptosis in human colon adeno-carcinoma cells by β-carotene through down regulation of cyclin A and Bcl-2 family proteins, *Carcinogenesis*, 23, 11, 2002.
61. Rayman, M.P., The use of high-selenium yeast to raise selenium status: how does it measure up? *Br. J. Nutr.*, 92, 557, 2004.
62. Liu, Y. and Kulesz-Martin, M., p53 protein at the hub of cellular DNA damage response pathways through sequence-specific and non-sequence-specific DNA binding, *Carcinogenesis*, 22, 851, 2001.
63. Mathers, J.C., Nutrients and apoptosis, in *Molecular Nutrition*, Zempleni, J. and Daniel, H., Eds., CABI publishing, Wallingford, 2003, chap. 6.
64. Brash, D.E. and Havre, P.A., New careers for antioxidants, *Proc. Natl. Acad. Sci. U.S.A.*, 99, 13969, 2002.
65. Seo, Y.R., Sweeney, C., and Smith, M.L., Selenomethionine induction of DNA repair response in human fibroblasts, *Oncogene*, 21, 3663, 2002.
66. Ho, E., Zinc deficiency, DNA damage and cancer risk, *J. Nutr. Biochem.*, 15, 572, 2004.
67. Collins, A.R. et al., Nutritional modulation of DNA repair in a human intervention study, *Carcinogenesis*, 24, 511, 2003.
68. Wei, Q. et al., Association between low dietary folate intake and suboptimal cellular DNA repair capacity, *Cancer Epidemiol. Biomark. Prev.*, 12, 963, 2003.

69. Barker, D.J., The developmental origins of well-being, *Philos. Trans. R. Soc. Lond. B,* 359, 1359, 2004.
70. Mcmillen, I.C. and Robinson, J.S., Developmental origins of the metabolic syndrome: prediction, plasticity and programming, *Physiol. Rev.,* 85, 571, 2005.
71. Bateson, P. et al., Developmental plasticity and human health, *Nature,* 430, 419, 2004.
72. Pham, T.D. et al., Uteroplacental insufficiency increases apoptosis and alters p53 gene methylation in the full-term IUGR rat kidney, *Am. J. Physiol. Regul. Integr. Comp. Physiol.,* 285, R962, 2003.
73. Weindruch, R. and Walford, R.L., *The Retardation of Aging and Disease by Dietary Restriction,* C.C. Thomas, Springfield, IL, 1998.
74. Ross, M.H. and Bras, G., Lasting influence of early caloric restriction on prevalence of neoplasms in the rat, *J. Natl. Cancer Inst.,* 47, 1095, 1971.
75. Frankel, S. et al., Childhood energy intake and adult mortality from cancer: the Boyd Orr cohort study, *Br. Med. J.,* 316, 499, 1998.
76. Gunnell D.J. et al., Childhood leg length and adult mortality: follow up of the Carnegie (Boyd Orr) survey of diet and health in pre-war Britain, *J. Epidemiol. Community Health,* 52, 142, 1998.
77. Mathers, J.C., Pulses and carcinogenesis: potential for the prevention of colon, breast and other cancers, *Br. J. Nutr.,* 88 (Suppl. 3), S273, 2002.

3 Biomarkers for Nutrient–Gene Interactions

Claire E. Robertson and Paolo Vineis

CONTENTS

3.1 DIETETIC MODIFICATION OF CANCER RISK
AND RELEVANT BIOMARKERS

Relationships between diet and cancer are complex and still only partially understood
[1]. Interactions among various potential mechanisms involved in carcinogenesis
and foods and nutrients have been proposed; these include the formation of DNA
adducts, DNA repair, promoter methylation, and gene–environment interactions. The
roles that specific foods and nutrients play in these mechanisms are discussed in
this chapter.

3.1.1 FRUIT, VEGETABLES, AND DECREASED CANCER RISK:
PUTATIVE MECHANISMS

3.1.1.1 Oxidative DNA Damage (8-OHdG)

Free radicals, which are produced naturally in the body, can cause oxidative damage
of DNA, lipids, proteins, and other cell constituents, contributing to the onset of
cancers and other chronic diseases [2]. Oxidative damage to DNA plays a major
role in carcinogenesis, and all living cells have defense mechanisms in place to
counter this. The simplest involves foods and nutrients with antioxidant properties,
which work by intercepting free radicals to become less reactive radicals, preventing
cellular damage [2,3]. Such effects have stimulated considerable research efforts
aiming to establish the potential chemopreventive properties of antioxidants. Epidemiological studies have utilized controlled supplementation intervention study
designs to investigate what effects antioxidant compounds such as vitamin C, vitamin
E, carotenoids, and various natural foods (e.g., tomatoes and carrot juice) have on
oxidative stress biomarkers [3]. Oxidative damage to DNA, commonly evaluated
using markers such as 8-hydroxy-2'-deoxyguanosine (8-OHdG) and the comet assay,
has been assessed as a pathway to carcinogenesis [2]. Results from short-term
intervention studies are mixed; however, some interesting and potentially important
findings have been identified.

Changes in DNA 8-hydroxy-2'-deoxyguanosine (8-OHdG) in relation to diet
have been assessed in several experimental investigations. In one randomized crossover design study, 32 nonsmoking healthy subjects consumed two liquid formula
diets as their sole source of nutrition for 10 d with energy requirements and weight
monitored to maintain constancy. Prior to randomization, the subjects consumed a
carotenoid-rich solid diet containing 5 servings of fruits and vegetables per day for
5 d. This was followed by randomization to two different liquid-formula diets that
were significantly different in contents of polyunsaturated fats (PUFA) and vitamin
A and vitamin E. Contrary to the hypothesis that the leukocyte 8-OHdG/deoxy-
guanoside (dG) ratio would be lower following consumption of the low PUFA, high
vitamin A and vitamin E compared to the high PUFA, low vitamin A and vitamin
E liquid-formula, no changes were evident. However, a 22% decrease in 8-OHdG/dG
ratio was observed when baseline values were compared to those at the end of the

study, irrespective of the order of randomization, with a significant downward trend of leukocyte 8-OHdG (test for trend: $p = 0.04$) [4].

Huang et al. [5] investigated the effects of antioxidant vitamins on oxidative DNA damage in a double-blinded, placebo-controlled, 2×2 factorial trial. They recruited 184 healthy, nonsmoking adults to determine what effects supplementary vitamins C and E — taken alone or combined — have on urinary excretion of 8-OHdG. Participants were randomized to four groups: placebo, vitamin C only, vitamin E only, and combined vitamin C and vitamin E supplementation, for a mean duration of 2 months. Following supplementation, no significant differences in 8-OHdG (ng/mg creatinine) between groups were found. Fruit and vegetable intake and serum ascorbic acid concentrations, however, were inversely associated with urinary 8-OHdG (p trend = 0.02 and 0.016, respectively), with the beneficial effects associated with the fruit and vegetable intake becoming evident after consumption of at least three medium servings per day [5].

Following publication of clinical and epidemiological study results outlining an inverse relationship between fruit and vegetable consumption and cancer occurrence [6], Thompson et al. [7] completed an intervention study to determine whether increased consumption would reduce biomarkers of oxidative cellular damage. The full study protocol was completed by 28 women. A 3-d food record kept by all participants at baseline found the women to consume an average of 5.8 (80 g) servings of fruit and vegetables each day. Protocols aimed to increase average daily consumption to 12 servings/d using a recipe-based diet, while examining the concurrent effects on biomarkers 8-OHdG, 8-isoprostane F-2alpha, and malondialdehyde, in blood and urine. Significant elevations in all plasma carotenoids were identified following the intervention, ranging from 12.3% for β-cryptoxanthin ($p = 0.032$) to 77.5% for α-carotene ($p = 0.001$). The intervention most notably reduced lymphocyte 8-OHdG (21.5%) and urinary 8-EPG (35%) concentrations. This was more pronounced when preintervention plasma concentrations of α-carotene were low, with no significant changes in lymphocyte 8-OHdG evident in those with high preintervention α-carotene concentrations. This work illustrated that high intakes of whole fruit and vegetables decrease markers of DNA oxidation and lipid peroxidation and, therefore, could potentially reduce cancer risk. The ability of individual antioxidants to cause these effects, however, was not addressed [7].

The capacity of lymphocytes supplemented with antioxidant micronutrients β-carotene, lutein, or lycopene to recover from DNA damage, induced *in vitro* by treatment with H_2O_2, was tested by Torbergsen and Collins [8]. Eight healthy volunteers aged 24 to 34 yr were given supplements of lutein (15 mg/d), lycopene (15 mg/d), and β-carotene (15 mg/d), each for 1 week and each separated by a 3-week wash out. DNA damage was measured using the comet assay (single-cell gel electrophoresis) after 0, 2, 4, 6, 8, and 24 h. Following β-carotene supplementation, a significantly enhanced recovery from DNA damage was evident; however, no such effects were evident following lutein or lycopene supplementation. Whereas β-carotene was shown to enhance recovery from oxidative damage, this was attributed by the authors to the demonstration of an antioxidant protective effect against additional damage induced by atmospheric oxygen, rather than a stimulation of DNA repair [8].

As shown in these and other studies, there is some evidence linking diet to DNA damage (in particular, DNA oxidation and lipid peroxidation), which could be relevant to the mechanisms of cancer onset. Limitations surrounding this kind of work are generally associated with measurement errors obscuring associations between the measured risk and protective factors and the outcome [1]. Dietary information, for example, is notoriously difficult to obtain with accuracy [9,10], and the reliability of biomarkers is sometimes uncertain [2,4,11].

3.1.1.2 Bulky DNA Adducts and Mutagen Sensitivity

When chemicals from cigarette smoke or ingestion of burnt meat, for example, attach to DNA, DNA adducts are formed. These can alter structure and biological processes, including replication, transcription, and repair functions. If they are not repaired, or are repaired incorrectly, DNA adducts can eventually lead to mutations, and ultimately, cancer. Adducts are particularly relevant if they are formed in an oncogene or tumor suppressor gene. Bulky adducts are a broad class of adducts formed by aromatic compounds.

The relationship of fruit and vegetable consumption to DNA-adduct formation was examined in a case–control study on bladder cancer [12]. The level of WBC-DNA adducts was shown to decrease with increasing levels of vegetable consumption ($p = 0.027$) in the controls. In addition, the association between case–control status and the level of adducts (below or above the median value) was stronger in subjects who consumed less than one portion of vegetables/d (odds ratio [OR] = 7.80, 95% confidence interval [CI] = 3.0–20.3) than in heavy consumers (OR = 4.98 for consumers of two portions/d; OR = 1.97 for consumers of three or more portions/d). The results from this study suggest that increasing the intake of fruit and vegetables may protect against bladder cancer by preventing DNA adduct formation in WBCs [12]. However, detailed assessments are required to prove this association and to clarify the mode of action.

In another Italian study among healthy subjects, strong inverse associations emerged between levels of DNA adducts and plasma retinol ($p = 0.02$), α-tocopherol ($p = 0.04$), and gamma-tocopherol ($p = 0.03$), but not carotenoids (except a borderline inverse association with β-carotene, $p = 0.08$) [13].

A series of studies, reported by Mooney and Perera [14], investigated the relationships between plasma levels of micronutrients (including antioxidants), genetic polymorphisms, and carcinogen-DNA adducts in WBCs. A cross-sectional analysis of 159 heavy smokers enrolled in a smoking cessation program, for example, found polycyclic aromatic hydrocarbon (PAH-DNA) adducts to be inversely associated with plasma levels of retinol ($\beta = -0.93$, $p = 0.01$), β-carotene ($\beta = -0.18$, $p = 0.09$) and α-tocopherol ($\beta = -0.28$, $p = 0.21$). The association between smoking-adjusted plasma β-carotene levels and DNA damage was significant only in subjects lacking the glutathione S-transferaseM1 (GSTM1) detoxification gene ($\beta = -0.30$, $p = 0.05$, n = 75). There was a statistical interaction between β-carotene and α-tocopherol:

when β-carotene was low, α-tocopherol had a significant protective effect (β = –0.78, p = 0.04) on adducts. A subset of 40 subjects who had quit smoking displayed a strong inverse relationship between adducts and vitamins (retinol, α-tocopherol, and zeaxanthin), but only in subjects with the GSTM1 null genotype [14]. Because there was no effect of GSTM1 genotype alone, these results suggest that some individuals may be at increased risk of DNA damage due to a combination of low plasma antioxidant and micronutrient levels and susceptible genotypes (see also Section 3.4.1).

Evidence demonstrating how DNA repair can be modified by dietary components is suggestive. Several functional tests have been developed to explore individual DNA repair capacity (see [15] for a detailed description). Classically, lymphocytes from cancer patients and controls are treated with a clastogen (a substance that causes breaks in chromosomes, resulting in the gain, loss, or rearrangement of chromosomal segments) and the number of chromosome breaks is counted (mutagen sensitivity test). A greater proportion of breaks is usually found in such cases, and is consequently interpreted as an expression of a limited repair capacity. The repair capacity thus explored appears to be modified by several exposures or personal habits, including, for example, alcohol intake and smoking status. In cultured lymphocytes, antioxidants such as α-tocopherol exhibited a dose-dependent protective effect, preventing bleomycin-induced chromosomal damage [16]. A study of 25 healthy individuals, Kucuk et al. [17] also found strong inverse correlations between plasma nutrients and the mutagen sensitivity assay. Mean monthly inverse correlations were evident for β-carotene (r = –0.76) and total carotenoids (r = –0.72), with a positive association found for triglyceride levels (r = 0.60). This relationship was not evident in a randomized double-blind trial conducted by Hu et al. [18], where the effects of α-tocopherol supplementation on DNA repair activity were measured using ADPRT (a repair enzyme) or UDS (unscheduled DNA synthesis) tests (which assess DNA repair capacity).

As shown here, intakes of whole fruit and vegetables and supplementary antioxidant micronutrients suggest links with DNA adducts and, possibly, with DNA repair, indirectly measured by the mutagen sensitivity tests. They are, consequently, potentially linked to cancer risk; however, the evidence for this is not yet conclusive.

3.1.2 HIGH MEAT CONSUMPTION AND INCREASED RISK OF COLORECTAL CANCER

3.1.2.1 Heterocyclic Aromatic Amines (HAA) and HAA Adducts

Several epidemiological studies have suggested that eating red meat may be associated with an increased risk of colon cancer [19]. The pyrolysis (decomposition of a chemical by extreme heat) of amino acids resulting from cooking at high temperatures and direct contact between meat and cooking surfaces, leads to the formation of a group of compounds known as HAA [20]. These HAA are highly mutagenic and have been found to induce tumors in several sites in different animal species. Feeding experiments in mice, for example, have induced tumors of the liver, lung, fore-stomach, and colon, as well as leukemias and lymphomas. In rats, the colon is the most frequently targeted, with the small intestine and liver also affected. 2-amino-1-methyl-6-phenylimidazo-(4,5-b)-pyridine (PhIP) is particularly interesting because it explains 85% of the mutagenic activity associated with fried beef, and has been classified as a probable carcinogen for humans (with sufficient evidence in experimental animals) by an International Agency for Research on Cancer (IARC) Working Group [21].

Adducts formed by HAA can be measured using several different methods. The major adduct of PhIP is N-(deoxyguanosin-8-yl)-PhIP. One study evaluated the formation of PhIP–DNA adducts in lymphocytes obtained from 76 incident colorectal cancer patients identified as likely to be exposed to dietary PhIP (i.e., meat consumers). Adduct levels were not significantly higher in smokers, young subjects, or high meat consumers; however, high vegetable intake significantly reduced PhIP–DNA adducts (Mann–Whitney U, $p = 0.044$) [22].

In contrast to bulky DNA adducts as summarized above, which indicate exposure to a whole group of aromatic compounds, the PhIP adducts are specific for a single exposure, and, therefore, more relevant to the study of the relationships between dietary habits and cancer. Further research on the role of HAA, through molecular epidemiology, could contribute considerably to the understanding of diet-related human cancer.

3.1.2.2 N-Nitroso Compounds

One explanation for the association between red meat and colorectal cancer found in some epidemiological studies is the presence of N-nitroso compounds (NOC) formed within the colon [23]. NOC are formed from the reaction between amides and nitrosating agents. In the anaerobic large bowel, nitrate is reduced by the colonic flora to nitrite, from which nitrosating agents may be formed. Meat intake increases the level of nitrogenous residues reaching the colon so that meat might be expected to increase levels of NOC in the colon. Fecal NOC excretion consistently increased when high red meat diets were consumed [23–25], and a dose–response curve was evident [24,25]. The intake of an equivalent amount of white meat had no effect on fecal excretion of NOC in volunteers [25]. Heme is probably responsible for the endogenous formation of NOC, because administration of heme iron led to a significant increase in fecal NOC, whereas, inorganic iron had no detectable effect [26]. NOC are potent carcinogens in experimental animals.

3.1.3 SINGLE NUTRIENTS: FOLATE

3.1.3.1 Evidence and Strength of Association from Cohort Studies

Folate is a water-soluble B vitamin, which is involved in red blood cell maturation and participates in nucleic acid synthesis. It is also probably the single most important nutrient shown to be associated with cancer risk in epidemiological studies. A key enzyme involved in folate metabolic pathways is 5,10 methylenetetrahydrofolate reductase (MTHFR) (see Figure 3.1). The involvement of folate in metabolic pathways is complex, and perturbations to these have been identified as likely to

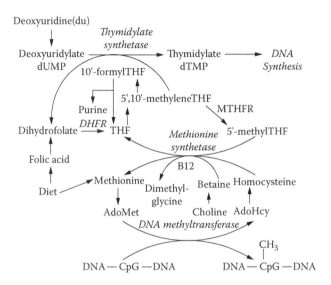

FIGURE 3.1 Simplified scheme of folate metabolism involving DNA synthesis and methylation. B12 — vitamin B_{12}; DHFR — dihydrofolate reductase; CH3 — methyl group; CpG — cytosine-guanine dinucleotide sequence; MTHFR — methylenetetrahydrofolate reductase; AdoHcy — S-adenosylhomocysteine; AdoMet — S-adenosylmethionine; THF — tetrahydrofolate. (From Kim, Y.I., Folate, colorectal carcinogenesis, and DNA methylation: lessons from animal studies. *Environmental and Molecular Mutagenesis* 44: 10–25, 2004. With permission.)

lead to aberrant cell growth and, consequently, to increased cancer risk. Folate has been most commonly associated with cervical, colon, and breast cancers; however, increasing research interest in this nutrient has extended to additional sites including the lung, pancreas, stomach, esophagus, blood tissue, skin, and endometrium [27]. Two mechanisms are proposed to be involved in the relationship between folate deficiencies and cancer. Deficiency causes a reduced concentration of intracellular S-adenosylmethionine (AdoMet), a compound utilized in DNA methylation and, therefore, associated with DNA stability and mutagenesis. In addition, via their central role in DNA synthesis and repair, folate deficiencies have been thought to cause an imbalance in DNA precursors, uracil misincorporation into DNA, and chromosome breakage [27].

As shown in Table 3.1, cohort studies suggest that a low dietary intake or plasma concentrations of folate increases the risks from several cancers, particularly for breast and colorectal cancer.

Also, vitamin B_6 and vitamin B_{12} have biological roles potentially associating them with cancer. Both vitamin B_6 and vitamin B_{12}, act as coenzymes synthesizing purines and thymidylate for DNA synthesis. Deficiencies lead to chromosome breakages and disrupted DNA repair via misincorporation of uracil. If vitamin B_{12} and folate are deficient, availability of AdoMet for DNA methylation is reduced, thereby influencing gene expression. Because of probable effects such as (and not limited to) these, Zhang et al. [28] examined the effects of folate, vitamin B_6, and vitamin

TABLE 3.1
Folate Intake or Plasma Levels and Risk of Breast or Colorectal Cancer:
Evidence from Cohort Studies

Cancer Site	Results	Interactions	Authors, Year
Ovary	Highest vs. lowest quartile of intake; RR = 0.67, 95% CI = 0.43 – 1.04, p(trend) = 0.08	Ethanol	Larsson et al. [31]
Breast	Highest quintile of plasma folate vs. lowest intake; RR = 0.73, 95% CI = 0.50–1.07, p(trend) = 0.06	Alcohol > 15 g/d; RR = 0.11, 95% CI = 0.02–0.59	Zhang et al. [28]
Breast	Women		Feigelson et al. [29]

Dietary folate (µg/d)	RR	95% CI
<178.8	1.00	
178.8 to <230.9	1.11	0.95–1.30
230.9 to <294.3	1.10	0.93–1.29
294.3+	1.07	0.91–1.27

Cancer Site	Results	Interactions	Authors, Year
Breast	Low folate intake and high alcohol; RR = 1.43 95% CI = 1.02–2.02	Estrogen receptor status	Sellers et al. [30]
Proximal colon	High folate and high vitamin B_{12} intake; RR = 0.59, 95% CI = 0.39 – 0.89; high folate and high vitamin B_6 intake; RR = 0.65, 95% CI = 0.50–0.84	High folate and low alcohol intake; RR = 0.44, 95% CI = 0.22–0.89	Harnack et al. [50]
Colon	Total dietary folate intake highest vs. lowest quintile; men RR = 0.73, 95% CI = 0.46–1.17, p(trend) = 0.03; women RR = 0.68, 95% CI = 0.39–1.20, p(trend) = 0.18		Konings et al. [32]
Rectum	Highest vs. lowest quintile intake, (men); RR = 0.66, 95% CI = 0.35 – 1.21, p(trend) = 0.03		Konings et al. [32]
Colorectal	High vs. low quintile of intake; RR = 0.86, 95% CI = 0.65–1.13, p(trend) = 0.14		Flood et al. [51]
Colorectal	Highest compared with the lowest quintile intake, (women); RR = 0.6, 95% CI = 0.4–1.1, p(trend) = 0.25		Terry et al. [49]

B_{12} on the risks of breast cancer. From the Nurses Health Study, 712 incident cases and matched controls were recruited and relative risks from breast cancer calculated with adjustment for known risk factors including age at menarche, family history of breast cancer, body mass index (BMI), and alcohol intake. Higher plasma folate and vitamin B_6 levels were significantly associated with lower breast cancer risk, with adjusted relative risk (RR) of 0.73 (95% CI = 0.50–1.07) for plasma folate, and RR of 0.70 (95% = CI 0.48–1.02) for vitamin B_6. No appreciable changes were evident after exclusions for cases diagnosed within 2 yr of blood collection, or after controlling for menopausal status; however, the inverse association between plasma folate and breast cancer risk was stronger in women consuming alcohol in excess of one drink (15 g/d: RR = 0.11 (95% CI = 0.02–0.59), compared to RR = 0.72 (95% CI = 0.49–1.05) for those consuming less than 15 g/d.

3.1.3.2 Alcohol and Folate

The association between folate, alcohol, and breast cancer risk has also been studied by Feigelson et al. [29] to determine whether there is any interaction between alcohol and folate on incident breast cancer. Incident cases (N = 1303) were recruited from the American Cancer Society Prevention Study II Nutrition Cohort, and the effects of dietary folate, total folate (i.e., diet plus supplement intakes), methionine, and alcohol on breast cancer incidence were investigated. Ethanol intake was positively associated with breast cancer risk at intakes greater than or equal to 10 g/d (p for trend = 0.01), and in the highest category of consumption (greater than or equal to 15 g/d), RR = 1.26 (95% CI = 1.04–1.53). No associations were evident between alcohol intake and folate use, and no association was evident between folate and breast cancer risk. These results are consistent with work completed by other researchers [28,30].

The relative risk of epithelial ovarian cancer in the highest vs. lowest quartiles of folate intake was 0.67 (95% CI = 0.43–1.04; p for trend = 0.08) among 266 incident cases occurring in the Swedish Mammography Cohort. In those who consumed in excess of 20 g alcohol per week, relative risk increased (RR = 1.00, 95% CI = 0.59–1.70) in comparison with the lowest alcohol consumers, indicating that folate may play a role in reducing risk from ovarian cancer, particularly among alcohol consumers [31]. In addition, an average 35% reduction in risk from developing colorectal cancer was evident in subjects with high, compared to low, folate intakes [32].

Additional research is necessary to completely understand the mechanisms of folate in reducing cancer risk, in particular its interaction with alcohol intake and other nutrients. However, current evidence suggests that achieving adequate circulating levels of folate is beneficial for cancer risk reduction in numerous sites.

3.2 GENETIC SUSCEPTIBILITY

Highly penetrant mutations in genes that are directly involved in carcinogenesis and confer a high risk of cancer in carriers represent the tail of a distribution of individual susceptibility to carcinogenesis [33]. Less penetrant susceptibility may be conferred by common variants in the same cancer genes (single-nucleotide polymorphisms [SNPs]) that have a less disruptive effect on the protein function than the highly penetrant mutations, or by SNPs in genes that mediate the metabolism of carcinogens. DNA-repair genes involved in rare and cancer-inducing conditions such as xeroderma pigmentosum (a genetic condition where even short exposure to ultraviolet light can lead to early death from cancer) also show common polymorphisms whose effects on DNA repair enzymes are mild, and a number of studies suggest that such mild defects in DNA repair predispose to cancer [15,34]. Polymorphisms in metabolic genes such as *CYP1A1, GSTM1, GSTT1, NAT2*, and others are common, low-penetrant conditions in which the function of the protein (an enzyme involved in the metabolism of toxic chemicals or carcinogens) is impaired, with an ensuing greater susceptibility to the effect of environmental toxicants.

The penetrance of a mutation is not entirely an intrinsic characteristic. Rare and highly penetrant mutations in cancer genes may act without interacting with external exposures (usually by direct interference with basic mechanisms of cell replication and differentiation), but gene–environment interactions are intrinsic to the mode of action of many candidate low-penetrance genes. The penetrance of a mutation is determined at least partly by other endogenous factors, including (1) the importance of the function of the protein encoded by the gene (e.g., in crucial metabolic pathways, as in phenylketonuria, or in key regulatory aspects of the cell cycle, as in the case of the *BRCA1* gene); (2) the functional importance of the mutation (e.g., a truncating deletion vs. a mild loss of function due to a point mutation); (3) the existence of alternative pathways that can substitute for the loss of function; and (4) interactions with other genes, including modifying genes. Penetrance will also depend on the somatic mutation rate and interactions with the environment.

3.3 COMBINATION OF GENES AND PATHWAYS

Most genes act in a sequence or in cascades. This is typical, for example, not only of DNA repair genes but also of metabolic genes (phase I enzymes activate carcinogens and phase II enzymes deactivate carcinogens). Genotyping according to pathways is likely to be much more rewarding then genotyping for single SNP, for both biological plausibility and for statistical power. For example, Matullo et al. [35] have investigated the role of SNPs in three DNA repair genes (*XRCC1*-Arg399Gln, exon 10; *XRCC3*-Thr241Met, exon 7; and *XPD*-Lys751Gln, exon 23), and their combinations, in modulating the levels of bulky DNA adducts in a population sample of healthy individuals. DNA-adduct levels were measured as relative adduct level (RAL) per 10^9 nucleotides by ^{32}P-post DNA labeling assay in WBCs from peripheral blood. Such DNA adducts express a particular kind of damage to DNA that is associated with exposure to aromatic chemicals. They found a dose–response relationship between the number of "at-risk" alleles and the levels of adducts ($p = 0.0046$). Individuals with at least 3 variant alleles had a statistically significant odds ratio for being in the highest tertile of adducts compared to those with undetectable adducts (3 alleles, adjusted OR = 5.07, 95% CI = 1.29–19.9; 4 alleles, adjusted OR = 5.03, 95% CI = 1.18–21.45; 5 alleles, adjusted OR = 7.65, 95% CI = 0.94–62.20).

The combined effect of multiple variant alleles may be more important than the investigation of single SNP in modulating DNA repair capacity; hence, the importance of focusing on gene pathways in the study of gene–environment interactions.

3.4 FRUIT, VEGETABLES, AND DECREASED CANCER RISK

3.4.1 HYPOTHESIS I: ROLE OF GSTs

A decreased incidence of carcinomas associated with fruit and vegetable intake may act through chemopreventive compounds, which may be more available to persons homozygous for the deletion genotypes of the glutathione *S*-transferase (*GST*). Frequent consumption of fresh fruit and vegetables, and polymorphisms in the detoxifying enzyme GSTM1, and other metabolic genes have been shown to modulate cancer risk at some sites. In a study in healthy volunteers (subcohort of EPIC), stratification by *GSTM1* genotype showed strong inverse associations of DNA adduct levels with increasing consumption of all vegetables combined ($p = 0.04$), leafy vegetables ($p = 0.004$), raw leafy vegetables ($p = 0.002$), and fish ($p = 0.03$) among 307 GSTM1-null subjects. Strong inverse associations also emerged with estimated dietary intakes of beta-carotene ($p = 0.004$), vitamin E ($p = 0.004$), niacin ($p = 0.02$), and potassium ($p = 0.01$). In contrast, no association emerged among 295 subjects with a *GSTM1*-wild genotype [36].

London et al. [39] examined the relation between total isothiocyanate (ITC) concentrations in urine, collected before diagnosis, and the subsequent risk of lung cancer in a cohort of 18,244 men in Shanghai, China, followed-up from 1986 to 1997. Individuals with detectable ITCs in the urine were at decreased risk of lung cancer (smoking-adjusted RR for lung cancer = 0.65 [95% CI = 0.43–0.97]). This protective effect of ITCs was seen primarily among individuals with homozygous deletion of *GSTM1* (0.36 [0.20–0.63]) and particularly with deletion of both *GSTM1* and *GSTT1* (0.28 [0.13–0.57]). A similar result was replicated in Singapore by Zhao et al. [38]. Their results, in a Chinese female population, were consistent with the hypothesis that ITC is inversely related to the risk of lung cancer and showed that among nonsmokers this effect may be primarily confined to GST-null individuals. Conjugation and elimination of ITCs was enhanced in GST-non-null individuals, relative to GST-null individuals, such that the GST metabolic genotype modified the protective effect of ITCs on lung cancer development.

However, in one study on head and neck cancers, relatively high intake of cooked vegetables (14 or more weekly servings) and legumes (2 or more weekly servings) were associated with increased incidence of the disease (OR = 2.5, 95% CI = 1.1–6.0; OR = 2.5, 95% CI = 1.2–5.2, respectively). This study did not suggest a clear or consistent pattern of modification by GST genotypes of the association between foods and head and neck cancers [39].

3.4.2 HYPOTHESIS II: REPAIR OF OXIDATIVE DNA DAMAGE

The literature on the possible effect of fruit and vegetable intake on DNA repair is still scanty and seems to suggest that the observed changes in DNA repair are not a direct consequence of such intake but rather an indirect effect via antioxidant capacity (see Section 3.1.1). However, the role of DNA repair polymorphisms in relation to 8-OHdG lesions has been postulated, in particular, for the genes *APEX* and *OGG1* (involved in repair of oxidative damage). In a study on the phenotype (not genotype) of OGG, OGG activity was lower in peripheral blood mononuclear cells from case patients than in those from control subjects. After adjustment for age and smoking status, individuals in the lowest tertile of OGG activity had an increased risk of non-small-cell lung cancer compared to individuals in the highest tertile (OR = 4.8, 95% CI = 1.5–15.9). The adjusted OR associated with a unit decrease in OGG activity was statistically significantly increased (OR = 1.9, 95% CI = 1.3–2.8) [40,41].

3.5   HIGH MEAT CONSUMPTION AND INCREASED RISK OF COLORECTAL CANCERS

Metabolic activation of HAA is associated with meat-eating, because urinary metabolites of activated carcinogenic HAA were found in healthy volunteers eating a meat-containing diet but not in patients receiving parenteral alimentation [20]. HAA are metabolized via pathways similar to those for other arylamines (e.g., 4-aminobiphenyl or 2-naphthylamine, i.e., N-acetylation and N-oxidation). N-acetylation is performed by the polymorphic noninducible enzyme *N*-acetyltransferase, under control of the genes *NAT1* and *NAT2*; N-oxidation is performed by CYP1A2, which is an inducible enzyme of the mixed-function oxidase group. A positive association between the rapid acetylator phenotype and the risk of colon cancer has been shown in some studies but not in others (for reviews, see [20,42]). The slow acetylator phenotype appears to exert a strong protective effect, relative to the rapid acetylator phenotype in early studies based on the phenotype. However, in other studies measuring phenotypes, and in studies based on genotype (i.e., on the identification of mutations in the NAT2 gene), no clear association was found [20,42]. For example, in a multicenter case–control study, 490 colorectal cancer patients and 593 controls were genotyped for common polymorphisms and no effect of NATs was found [43].

A particularly accurate study has recently estimated the intake of HAA [44]. Using a population-based case–control study design, 727 (Japanese, Caucasian, or Native Hawaiian) cases and 727 (age, sex, and ethnicity) matched controls were recruited in Hawaii to test the association of preference for well-done red meat and HAA intake with colon and rectal cancers. The modifying effects of NAT2 and CYP1A2 were also investigated. HAA intake was estimated based on consumption of meat and fish for several cooking methods. They found that preference for well-done red meat was associated with an 8.8-fold increased risk of colorectal cancer (95% CI = 1.7–44.9) among ever smokers with the *NAT2* and *CYP1A2* rapid phenotypes, compared to ever smokers with low NAT2 and CYP1A2 activities and who preferred their red meat rare or medium.

3.6   FOLATE

3.6.1   FOLATE AND *MTHFR* POLYMORPHISMS

More than 30 genetic loci have been identified as being involved in folate metabolism. In addition, due to its close links with cobalamine and pyridoxine metabolism, another 15 and 8 genetic loci, respectively, may also be involved in this process [45]. The role of genetic polymorphisms in the folate metabolism pathway has principally considered the effects of MTHFR. This enzyme provides the methyl group required for *de novo* methionine synthesis and, indirectly, for DNA methylation; therefore, it controls DNA stability and mutagenesis [27,46,47]. *MTHFR* has some frequent polymorphisms (*677C→T* and *1298A→C*), which have been studied to establish whether any modifications to cancer risk are associated with the genotype. For both SNPs, the variant allele is associated with reduced enzyme activity *in vitro*, which in the case of *677C→T*, for example, affects the metabolism of folate, consequently increasing homocysteine levels and the risk of colon cancer [45]. The majority of studies display a moderately reduced colon cancer risk associated with high dietary folate intakes or plasma concentrations, with those individuals with the highest folate intakes and the *677TT* homozygous genotype having the lowest cancer risk. An interaction of *MTHFR* SNPs with alcohol intake has also been reported, with high alcohol consumption levels decreasing DNA methylation probably by hindering folate absorption, metabolism, and excretion [28].

Alcohol is interpreted as a cause of increased risk of cancer through its antagonist effects on folate. Giovannucci et al. [48] attempted to gain a better understanding of the interrelationships between alcohol and folate intakes and genetic polymorphisms in folate and alcohol metabolic genes by examining folate, alcohol, and *MTHFR*, and *ADH3* polymorphisms in relation to risk of colorectal adenomas in 379 cases and 726 controls recruited from the Health Professionals Follow-Up Study participants. *MTHFR* genotypes were not found to be appreciably related to risk of adenoma, but a suggestive interaction ($p = 0.09$) was observed between *MTHFR* *677C→>T* and alcohol intake. Men with *677TT* homozygote mutant genotype who consumed 30 + g/d of alcohol had an OR of 3.52 [95% CI = 1.41–8.78] relative to drinkers of less than or equal to 5 g/d with either the *677CC* or *677CT* genotypes [48].

Studies investigating the folate-*MTHFR*-cancer risk relationships have largely shown inverse associations of breast cancer risk with folate intake in all genotype groups, particularly among subjects with the *677TT* genotype [49–51]. A study utilizing data collected from 1236 controls and 1144 cases in the Shanghai Breast Cancer Study investigated whether the inverse associations reported between folate intakes and breast cancer risk was modified by *MTHFR* genotype. The frequencies of the *677T* and *1298C* alleles were 0.41 and 0.18, respectively, in the controls, and similarly in the cases. Compared to those with the *677CC* genotype and high folate, the adjusted OR (95% CI) associated with low folate intake were 1.94 (1.15–3.26), 2.17 (1.34–3.51), and 2.51 (1.37–4.60) for subjects who had *CC, CT,* and *TT* genotypes (p for interaction, 0.05), indicating that *MTHFR 677C→>T* genotype was a statistically significant effect modifier for the association between folate intakes and breast cancer risk [52].

3.6.2 FOLATE AND PROMOTER METHYLATION

DNA methylation is an important epigenetic determinant in gene expression and, therefore, determines the process by which the instructions in genes are converted to messenger RNA, directing protein synthesis [47]. DNA methylation — that is, the covalent addition of methyl groups ($-CH_3$) to cytosine that precedes a guanosine in the DNA sequence (the CpG dinucleotide) — occurs naturally and is thought to have a role in suppressing gene expression. This is called an *epigenetic modification*, because it does not change the structure of DNA, but is heritable and passes from one generation of cells to the next. In mammalian cells, DNA methylation occurs at the 5′-position of cytosine within the CpG dinucleotide. CpG dinucleotides are richer in the promoting regions of genes (CpG islands) and, for this reason, methylation is thought to be involved in gene expression. Hypermethylation of promoter regions is associated with gene transcriptional silencing and is a common mechanism for the inactivation of tumor suppressor genes in human cancer [53]. Hypermethylation is associated with the inactivation of several pathways involved in the cancer process, such as DNA repair (hMLH1, BRCA1, MGMT), cell cycle regulation, apoptosis, and carcinogen metabolism. Key enzymes involved in methylation patterns are DNA methyltransferases (DNMTs).

The effects of folate deficiency on methylation patterns are still another mechanism to explain the relationships between folate intake and cancer. The evidence, however, remains sparse [54]. In particular, the pattern of gene-specific methylation may not be in concert with the overall direction of changes in genomic DNA methylation. In one study, for example, the number of colorectal cancers with at least one gene methylated was higher (84%) in the low folate intake and high alcohol intake group than within the high folate intake and low alcohol intake group (70%; $p = 0.085$). Despite the size limitations of this study (n = 122), it suggests that folate and alcohol intake may be associated with changes in promoter hypermethylation in colorectal cancer [55]. Other nutrients involved in DNA methylation through the one-carbon metabolism cycle are zinc, retinoic acid, selenium, polyphenols, and phytoestrogens. For example, polyphenols from green tea were found to inhibit DNMTs activity, resulting in the reactivation of silenced genes in cancer cells [56].

Nutritional changes during pregnancy could also interfere with the subsequent cancer risk through methylation patterns. Interesting experiments have been completed in mice. The agouti vs. yellow color of the mice hair is determined by methylation patterns. If the agouti gene terminal repeat region is hypermethylated, the mouse is agouti; if it is hypomethylated, the mouse is yellow. When pregnant mice were fed a diet rich in folate and methionine (i.e., in methyl groups), none of the pups born were yellow. Interestingly, the expression of the yellow coat was linked to an increased risk of obesity, adult diabetes, cancer, and mortality [57,58]. In other words, intrauterine exposure to nutrients associated with epigenetic modifications of the genome in the offspring can lead to increased cancer risk.

3.7 CONCLUSION

The integration between epidemiological studies on foods and nutrients, studies of molecular epidemiology on the putative pathways involved in carcinogenesis (in particular oxidative DNA damage), studies on gene–environment interactions, and animal studies (such as those on nutrient deprivation in pregnancy) suggest that both genetic and epigenetic mechanisms are likely to be involved in the effects of diet on cancer risk. The hypotheses that have been formulated so far need further verification in large, well-designed intervention studies and longitudinal investigations.

ACKNOWLEDGMENTS

This paper has been made possible by a grant of the Compagnia di San Paolo (Torino, Italy) to P.V. (ISI Foundation, Progetto Oncologia).

ABBREVIATIONS

8-OHdG	8-hydroxy-2′-deoxyguanosine
AdoMet	S-adenosylmethionine
ADPRT	Repair enzyme
dG	Deoxyguanoside
DNMT	DNA methyltransferase
EPIC	European Prospective Investigation into Cancer
GST	Glutathione S-transferase
GSTM1	Glutathione S-transferase M1
HAA	Heterocyclic aromatic amines
IARC	International Agency for Research on Cancer
ITC	Isothiocyanate
MTHFR	5, 10 methylenetertrahydrofolate reductase
NOC	N-nitrosocompounds
PAH	Polycyclic aromatic hydrocarbon
PhIP	2-amino-1-methyl-6-phenylimidazo-(4,5-b)-pyridine
PUFA	Polyunsaturated fats
RAL	Relative Adduct Level
SNP	Single-nucleotide polymorphisms
UDS	Unscheduled DNA synthesis
WBC	White blood cells

REFERENCES

1. Bingham, S., Riboli, E. Diet and cancer — the European Prospective Investigation into Cancer and Nutrition. *Nature Reviews* 4, 206–215, 2004.
2. Evans, M., Dizdaroglu, M., Cooke, M. Oxidative DNA damage and disease: induction, repair and significance. *Mutation Research* 567, 1–61, 2004.
3. Møller, P., Loft. S. Oxidative DNA damage in human white blood cells in dietary antioxidant intervention studies. *American Journal of Clinical Nutrition* 76, 303–310, 2002.
4. Chen, L., Bowen, P., Berzy, D., Aryee, F., Stacewicz-Sapuntzakis, M., Riley, R. Diet modification affects DNA oxidative damage in healthy humans. *Free Radical Biology and Medicine* 26, 695–703, 1999.
5. Huang, H., Helzlouser, K., Appel, L. The effects of vitamin C and vitamin E on oxidative DNA damage: results from a randomized controlled trial. *Cancer Epidemiology, Biomarkers and Prevention* 9, 647–652, 2000.

6. Steinmetz, K., Potter, J. Vegetables, fruit, and cancer prevention: a review. *Journal of the American Dietetic Association* 96, 1027–1039, 1996.

7. Thompson, H., Heimendinger, J., Haegele, A., Sedlacek, S., Gillette, C., O'Neill, C., Wolfe, P., Conry, C. Effect of increased vegetable and fruit consumption on markers of oxidative cellular damage. *Carcinogenesis* 20, 2261–2266, 1999.

8. Torbergsen, A., Collins, A. Recovery of human lymphocytes from oxidative DNA damage: the apparent enhancement of DNA repair by carotenoids is probably simply an antioxidant effect. *European Journal of Nutrition* 39, 80–85, 2000.

9. Bingham, S. Limitations of the various methods for collecting dietary intake data. *Annals of Nutrition and Metabolism* 35, 117–127, 1991.

10. Goldberg, G., Black, A., Jebb, S.A., Cole, T., Murgatroyd, P.R., Coward, W., Prentice, A.M. Critical evaluation of energy intake data using fundamental principles of energy physiology: 1. Derivation of cut-off limits to identify under-recording. *European Journal of Clinical Nutrition* 45, 569–581, 1991.

11. Loft, S., Poulsen, H. Cancer risk and oxidative DNA damage in man. *Journal of Molecular Medicine* 74, 297–312, 1996.

12. Peluso, M., Airoldi, L., Magagnotti, C., Fiorini, L., Munnia, A., Hautefueille, A., Malaveille, C., Vineis, P. White blood cell DNA adducts and fruit and vegetable consumption in bladder cancer. *Carcinogenesis* 21, 183–187, 2000.

13. Palli, D., Masala, G., Vineis, P., Garte, S., Saieva, C., Krogh, V., Panico, S., Tumino, R., Munnia, A., Riboli, E., Peluso, M. Biomarkers of dietary intake of micronutrients modulate DNA adduct levels in healthy adults. *Carcinogenesis* 24, 739–746, 2003.

14. Mooney, L., Perara, F. Application of molecular epidemiology to lung cancer chemoprevention. *Journal of Cellular Biochemistry* 25, 63–68, 1996.

15. Berwick, M., Vineis, P. Markers of DNA repair and susceptibility to cancer in humans: an epidemiologic review. *Journal of the National Cancer Institute* 92, 874–897, 2000.

16. Trizna, Z., Hsu, T., Schantz, S. Protective effects of vitamin E against bleomycin-induced genotoxicity in head and neck cancer patients in vitro. *Anticancer Research. International Journal of Cancer Research and Treatment* 12, 325–327, 1992.

17. Kucuk, O., Pung, A., Franke, A., Custer, L., Wilkens, L., Le Marchand, L., Higuchi, C., Cooney, R., Hsu, T. Correlations between mutagen sensitivity and plasma nutrient levels of healthy individuals. *Cancer Epidemiology, Biomarkers and Prevention* 4, 217–221, 1995.

18. Hu, J., Roush, G., Berwick, M., Dubin, N., Mahabir, S., Chandiramani, M., Boorstein, R. Effects of dietary supplementation of alpha-tocopherol on plasma glutathione and DNA repair activities. *Cancer Epidemiology, Biomarkers and Prevention* 5, 263–270, 1996.

19. Riboli, E., Lambert, R., Kleihues, P. Nutrition and cancer: a complex relationship. *IARC Scientific Publications* 156, 3–4, 2002.

20. Vineis, P., McMichael, A. Interplay between heterocyclic amines in cooked meat and metabolic phenotype in the etiology of colon cancer. *Cancer Causes Control* 7, 479–486, 1996.

21. International Agency for Research on Cancer IARC Monographs on the Evaluation of Carcinogenic Risks to Humans. Vol. 56. Lyon, 1993.

22. Magagnotti, C., Pastorelli, R., Pozzi, S., Andreoni, B., Fanelli, R., Airoldi, L. Genetic polymorphisms and modulation of 2-amino-1-methyl-6-phenylimidazo [4,5-b] pyridine (PhIP)-DNA adducts in human lymphocytes. *International Journal of Cancer* 107, 878–884, 2003.

23. Bingham, S., Pignatelli, B., Pollock, J., Ellul, A., Mallaveille, C., Gross, G., Runswick, S., Cummings, J., O'Neill, I. Does increased formation of endogenous N-nitroso compounds in the human colon explain the association between red meat and colon cancer? *Carcinogenesis* 17, 515–523, 1996.
24. Bingham, S., Hughes, R., Cross, A. Effect of white versus red meat on endogenous N-nitrosation in the human colon and further evidence of a dose response. *Journal of Nutrition* 132, 3522S–3525S, 2002.
25. Hughes, R., Cross, A., Pollock, J., Bingham, S. Dose dependent effect of dietary meat on colonic endogenous N-nitrosation. *Carcinogenesis* 22, 199–202, 2001.
26. Cross, A., Pollock, J., Bingham, S. Haem, not protein or inorganic iron, is responsible for endogenous intestinal N-nitrosation arising from red meat. *Cancer Research. International Journal of Cancer Research and Treatment* 63, 2358–2360, 2003.
27. Eichholzer, M., Lüthy, J., Moser, U., Fowler, B. Folate and the risk of colorectal, breast and cervix cancer: the epidemiological evidence. *Swiss Medical Weekly* 131, 539–549, 2001.
28. Zhang, S., Willett, W., Selhub, J., Hunter, D., Giovannucci, E., Holmes, M., Colditz, G., Hankinson, S. Plasma folate, vitamin B_6, vitamin B_{12}, homocysteine, and risk of breast cancer. *Journal of the National Cancer Institute* 95, 373–380, 2003.
29. Feigelson, H., Jonas, C., Robertson, A., McCullough, M., Thun, M., Calle, E. Alcohol, folate, methionine, and risk of incident breast cancer in the American Cancer Society Prevention Study II Nutrition Cohort. *Cancer Epidemiology, Biomarkers and Prevention* 12, 161–164, 2003.
30. Sellers, T., Vierkant, R., Cerhan, J., Gapstur, S., Vachon, C., Olson, J., Pankratz, V., Kushi, L., Folshom, A. Interaction of dietary folate intake, alcohol, and risk of hormone receptor-defined breast cancer in a prospective study of postmenopausal women. *Cancer Epidemiology, Biomarkers and Prevention* 11, 1104–1107, 2002.
31. Larsson, S., Giovannucci, E., Wolk, A. Dietary folate intake and incidence of ovarian cancer: the Swedish Mammography Cohort. *Journal of the National Cancer Institute* 96, 396–402, 2004.
32. Konings, E., Goldbohm, R., Brants, H., Saris, W., van den Brandt, P. Intake of dietary folate vitamers and risk of colorectal carcinoma: results from the Netherlands Cohort study. *Cancer* 95, 1421–1433, 2002.
33. Vogelstein, B., Kinzler, K. *The Genetic Basis of Human Cancer.* McGraw-Hill: New York, 1998.
34. Dybdahl, M., Vogel, U., Frentz, G., Wallin, H., Nexo, B. Polymorphisms in the DNA repair gene XPD: correlations with risk and age at onset of basal cell carcinoma. *Cancer Epidemiology, Biomarkers and Prevention* 8, 77–81, 1999.
35. Matullo, G., Peluso, M., Polidoro, S., Guarrera, S., Munnia, A., Krogh, V., Masala, G., Berrino, F., Panico, S., Tumino, R., Vineis, P., Palli, D. Combination of DNA repair gene single nucleotide polymorphisms and increased levels of DNA adducts in a population-based study. *Cancer Epidemiology, Biomarkers and Prevention* 12, 674–677, 2003.
36. Palli, D., Masala, G., Peluso, M., Gaspari, L., Krogh, V., Munnia, A., Panico, S., Saieva, C., Tumino, R., Vineis, P., Garte, S. The effects of diet on DNA bulky adduct levels are strongly modified by GSTM1 genotype: a study on 634 subjects. *Carcinogenesis* 25, 577–584, 2004.
37. London, S., Yuan, J., Chung, F., Gao, Y., Coetzee, G., Ross, R., Yu, M. Isothiocyanates, glutathione S-transferase M1 and T1 polymorphisms, and lung-cancer risk: a prospective study of men in Shanghai, China. *The Lancet* 356, 724–729, 2000.

38. Zhao, B., Seow, A., Lee, E., Poh, W., Teh, M., Eng, P., Wang, Y., Tan, W., Yu, M., Lee, H. Dietary isothiocyanates, glutathione S-transferase M1, -T1 polymorphisms and lung cancer risk among Chinese women in Singapore. *Cancer Epidemiology, Biomarkers and Prevention* 10, 1063–1067, 2001.

39. Gaudet, M., Olshan, A., Poole, C., Weissler, M., Watson, M., Bell, D. Diet, GSTM1 and GSTT1 and head and neck cancer. *Carcinogenesis* 25, 735–740, 2004.

40. Paz-Elizur, T., Krupsky, M., Blumenstein, S., Elinger, D., Schechtman, E., Vivneh, Z. DNA repair activity for oxidative damage and risk of lung cancer. *Journal of the National Cancer Institute* 95, 1312–1319, 2003.

41. Caporaso, N. The molecular epidemiology of oxidative damage to DNA and cancer. *Journal of the National Cancer Institute* 95, 1263–1265, 2003.

42. Ye, Z., Parry, J. Meta-analysis of 20 case-control studies on the *N*-acetyltransferase 2 acetylation status and colorectal cancer risk. *Medical Science Monitoring* 8, 558–565, 2002.

43. Sachse, C., Smith, G., Wilkie, M., Barrett, J., Waxman, R., Sullivan, F., Forman, D., Bishop, D., Wolf, C. A pharmacogenetic study to investigate the role of dietary carcinogens in the etiology of colorectal cancer. *Carcinogenesis* 23, 1839–1849, 2002.

44. Le Marchand, L., Hankin, J., Pierce, L., Sinha, R., Nerurkar, P., Franke, A., Wilkens, L., Kolonel, L., Donlon, T., Seifried, A., Custer, L., Lum-Jones, A., Chang, W. Well-done red meat, metabolic phenotypes and colorectal cancer in Hawaii. *Mutation Research* 506, 205–215, 2002.

45. Little, J., Sharp, L., Duthie, S., Narayanan, S. Colon cancer and genetic variation in folate metabolism: the clinical bottom line. *Journal of Nutrition* 133, 3758S–3766S, 2003.

46. Sharp, L., Little, J. Polymorphisms in genes involved in folate metabolism and colorectal neoplasia: a HuGE review. *American Journal of Epidemiology* 159, 423–443, 2004.

47. Kim, Y. Folate and DNA methylation: a mechanistic link between folate deficiency and colorectal cancer? *Cancer Epidemiology, Biomarkers and Prevention* 13, 511–519, 2004.

48. Giovannucci, E., Chen, J., Smith-Warner, S., Rimm, E., Fuchs, C., Palomeque, C., Willett, W., Hunter, D. Methylenetetrahydrofolate reductase, alcohol dehydrogenase, diet, and risk of colorectal cancer. *Cancer Epidemiology, Biomarkers and Prevention* 12, 970–979, 2003.

49. Terry, P., Jain, M., Miller, A., Howe, G., Rohan, T. Dietary intake of folic acid and colorectal cancer risk in a cohort of women. *International Journal of Cancer* 97, 864–867, 2002.

50. Harnack, L., Jacobs, D.J., Nicodermus, K., Lazovich, D., Anderson, K., Folsom, A. Relationship of folate, vitamin B-6, vitamin B-12, and methionine intake to incidence of colorectal cancers. *Nutrition and Cancer* 43, 152–158, 2002.

51. Flood, A., Velie, E., Chaterjee, N., Subar, A., Thompson, F., Lacey, J.J., Schairer, C., Troisi, R., Schatzkin, A. Fruit and vegetable intakes and the risk of colorectal cancer in the Breast Cancer Detection Demonstration Project follow-up cohort. *American Journal of Clinical Nutrition* 75, 936–943, 2002.

52. Shrubsole, M., Gao, Y., Cai, Q., Shu, X., Dai, Q., Hebert, J., Jin, F., Zheng, W. MTHFR polymorphisms, dietary folate intake, and breast cancer risk: results from the Shanghai breast cancer study. *Cancer Epidemiology, Biomarkers and Prevention* 13, 190–196, 2004.

53. Robertson, K., Wolffe, A. DNA methylation in health and disease. *Natures Reviews in Genetics* 1, 11–19, 2000.

54. Davis, C., Uthus, E. DNA methylation, cancer susceptibility, and nutrient interactions. *Free Radical Biology and Medicine* 229, 988–995, 2004.

55. van Engeland, M., Weijenberg, M., Roemen, G., Brink, M., de Bruine, A., Goldbohm, R., van den Bracht, P., Baylin, S., de Goeij, A., Herman, J. Effects of dietary folate and alcohol intake on promoter methylation in sporadic colorectal cancer: the Netherlands cohort study on diet and cancer. *Cancer Research* 63, 3133–3137, 2003.

56. Fang, M., Wang, Y., Ai, N., Hou, Z., Sun, Y., Lu, H., Welsh, W., Yang, C. Tea polyphenol(-)-epigallacatechin-3-gallate inhibits DNA methyltransferase and reactivates methylation-silenced genes in cancer cell lines. *Cancer Research. International Journal of Cancer Research and Treatment* 63, 7563–7570, 2003.

57. Cooney, C., Dave, A., Wolff, G. Maternal methyl supplements in mice affect epigenetic variation and DNA methylation of offspring. *Journal of Nutrition* 138, 2393S–2400S, 2002.

58. Waterland, R., Jirtle, R. Early nutrition, epigenetic changes at transposons and imprinted genes, and enhanced susceptibility to adult chronic diseases. *Nutrition* 20, 63–68, 2004.

4 Interaction between Folate and Methylene-tetrahydrofolate Reductase Gene in Cancer

Sang-Woon Choi and Simonetta Friso

CONTENTS

4.1 INTRODUCTION

Folate, a water-soluble B vitamin, has attracted increasing interest over the past decade in regard to the relationship between the habitual dietary intake of this nutrient and the risk of cancer. According to epidemiological studies, diminished folate status is associated with cancer of the cervix, colorectum, lung, esophagus, brain, pancreas, liver, prostate, breast, and blood [1–4]. Such a relationship is clearly most compelling for colorectal cancer [1,5], but evidence is beginning to emerge regarding some of the other preceding tissues. Animal models, as well as cell culture studies, have lent considerable support to a true causative relationship between diminished folate status and carcinogenesis [6–8]. Studies in carcinogen-induced models of colorectal carcinogenesis [7] and those in mice genetically predisposed to intestinal tumorigenesis [8] support a dose-dependent effect of dietary folate.

It was 1997, when Ma et al. [9] reported that men carrying, in homozygosity, the *677C→T* polymorphism in the methylenetetrahydrofolate reductase (*MTHFR*) gene have half the risk of developing colorectal cancer compared to homozygous wild-type or heterozygous genotypes. The common polymorphism at position 677 of the *MTHFR* gene causes thermolability and reduced activity of MTHFR, which catalyzes the irreversible conversion of 5,10 methylenetetrahydrofolate to 5-methyltetrahydrofolate. Although a threefold decrease in risk was observed among men with adequate folate levels, protection associated with the polymorphism was largely absent in men with low systemic folate status. This observation suggests that the modulation of cancer risk associated with the polymorphism may be conveyed through folate status.

This chapter will address the evidences of folate and *MTHFR* gene interaction on the risk of colorectal cancer and discuss the mechanisms that appear to constitute the means by which the interaction between folate and *MTHFR* affects colorectal carcinogenesis. The emerging effects of such nutrient–gene interaction on other neoplastic diseases will be also addressed.

4.2 FOLATE AND THE RISK OF COLORECTAL CANCER

Folate is among the most strongly implicated dietary components that convey protection against colorectal cancer. More than 20 epidemiological studies have examined the relationship between folate and colorectal neoplasia, and the overwhelming consensus of these studies indicates that diminished folate status, measured either by dietary folate intake or by blood folate level, is associated with an enhanced risk of colorectal adenomas and cancer [10–17]. In the Nurses' Health Study and the Health Professionals Follow-up Study, Giovannucci et al. reported the most convincing evidence that dietary folate intake was inversely associated with the risk of colorectal cancer [16] as well as colorectal adenoma [17] in a dose-dependent manner in both men and women. This appears to be true when the issue is examined in individuals affected with chronic ulcerative colitis, a condition that carries with it an enhanced risk of folate deficiency and 10-fold to 40-fold increased risk of colorectal cancer compared with the general population [10]. Lashner [11] described that the risk of dysplasia or cancer was found to be significantly decreased by 18% for each 10 ng/mL increase in RBC folate (OR = 0.82; 95% CI, 0.68 to 0.99). In the chemical carcinogen rodent model of colorectal cancer [6,7] and in rodents genetically predisposed to intestinal neoplasia [8], the same effect has been reported. Most plausible mechanisms by which folate depletion enhances the colorectal carcinogenesis are altered biological methylation and decreased thymidylate synthesis, two pathways that are thought to be the common routes through which neoplastic transformation occurs (Figure 4.1) [18].

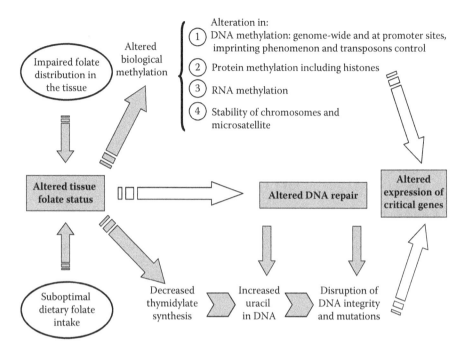

FIGURE 4.1 Molecular effects of folate depletion in carcinogenesis. Quantitative and qualitative alterations in tissue folate status by suboptimal dietary folate and redirecting factors for folate-form distribution such as *MTHFR* genotype, aging, alcohol consumption, and vitamin B_{12} deficiency can affect both biological methylation and neucleotide synthesis, and subsequent epigenetic and genetic changes thereby induce aberrant expression of critical genes for carcinogenesis.

The protective effect of dietary folate has also been reported, thereby providing strong evidence for a true cause-and-effect relationship between folate and colorectal carcinogenesis. In a chemical carcinogen rat model of colorectal cancer, increasing dietary folate up to four times the basal requirement leads to a progressive reduction in the evolution of both microscopic foci of neoplasia [6] as well as macroscopic tumors [7], suggesting a role for folate supplementation in the chemoprevention of colorectal cancer. A recent meta-analysis of 11 prospective epidemiological studies reported a 20% reduction in the risk of colorectal cancer in subjects with the highest folate intake compared to those with the lowest intake [19]. A prospective study conducted in the Nurses' Health Study also showed a marked reduction (RR = 0.25; 95% CI, 0.13 to 0.51) in the risk of colorectal cancer in women using multivitamin supplements exceeding 400 µg folate per day for more than 15 yr compared to those not taking supplementation [20].

Small, placebo-controlled, intervention trials of folate supplementation in humans have been promising, although less than definitive, given the small number of subjects and the inconclusive nature of the primary endpoints [21]. A study involving 60 subjects with colorectal adenoma demonstrated that folate supplementation

(1 mg/d for 2 yr) after polypectomy decreased adenoma recurrence by 46% compared to placebo, although this difference was not statistically significant [15]. A recent folate trial demonstrated that folate supplementation at 2 mg/d for 3 months in 11 subjects with previously resected colorectal adenoma significantly decreased rectal mucosal cell proliferation, a biomarker of colorectal cancer [22]. Several mechanisms have been proposed to explain the protective effects of folate, most of which focus on folate's central role in deoxyribonucleotide synthesis, epigenetic modification, and DNA repair [18].

4.3 IMPORTANCE OF FOLATE AND *MTHFR* GENE IN ONE-CARBON METABOLISM

One-carbon metabolism is a network of interrelated biochemical reactions in which a one-carbon unit from a donor compound is transferred to tetrahydrofolate (THF) for subsequent reduction or oxidation and transfer to other compounds (Figure 4.2). Folate coenzymes in mammalian tissues thereby act as acceptors or donors of one-carbon units in a variety of reactions involving amino acid and nucleotide metabolism [23]. Three of the one-carbon substituted derivatives of THF are each associated with metabolic pathways that are specific to that particular form of the vitamin: 5-methylTHF is needed for methionine synthesis (which is needed for DNA methylation); 5,10-methyleneTHF for thymidylate synthesis; and 10-formylTHF for purine synthesis [24].

Serine hydroxymethyltransferase, a pyridoxal-5'-phosphate (the active form of vitamin B_6)-containing enzyme, catalyzes the reversible transfer of formaldehyde from serine to tetrahydrofolate (THF) to generate glycine and 5,10-methyleneTHF

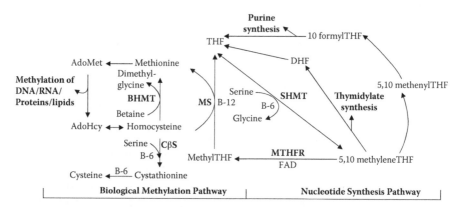

FIGURE 4.2 Folate and methylene-tetrahydrofolate reductase (*MTHFR*) gene in one-carbon metabolism. MTHFR, which irreversibly catalyzes 5,10-methyleneTHF, the primary methyl donor for nucleotide synthesis, to 5-methylTHF, the ultimate methyl donor for biological methylation, sits as a fulcrum between two major pathways, maintaining normal homeostasis of methyl groups in one-carbon metabolism.

[24]. Then, MTHFR irreversibly catalyzes 5,10-methyleneTHF to 5-methylTHF, the primary methyl donor for the remethylation of homocysteine to methionine by methionine synthase.

The methionine synthase reaction plays a major role in methyl group metabolism, as it allows for the reutilization of the homocysteine backbone to be used as a carrier of methyl groups derived primarily from serine (transmethylation pathway). The enzyme contains a cobalamin (vitamin B_{12}) cofactor, and the reaction proceeds via a methylcobalamin intermediate [25]. Methionine, which is regenerated from homocysteine, is then converted to *S*-adenosylmethionine (AdoMet). AdoMet then donates the labile methyl group it obtained from 5-methylTHF to over 80 biological methylation reactions, including the methylation of DNA, RNA, proteins, lipids, and lipoproteins. Homocysteine also condenses with serine to form cystathionine in an irreversible reaction catalyzed by the vitamin-B_6-containing enzyme, cystathionine-β-synthase, which takes part in the transsulfuration pathway. Although the alternative betaine pathway for methionine synthesis may partially compensate, it is nevertheless well known that dietary folate depletion alone is a sufficiently perturbing force to diminish AdoMet pools [26]. Experimental folate depletion in both animals and humans produces demonstrable impairments in biological methylation [27,28].

Folate-derived one-carbon metabolism is also essential for the synthesis of deoxynucleotides (Figure 4.2). Thymidylate synthase catalyzes the transfer of formaldehyde from 5,10-methyleneTHF to the 5′-position of deoxyuridylate, producing deoxythymidylate. In addition, one-carbon moieties at the oxidation level of formate are utilized in *de novo* purine biosynthesis. Because deoxynucleotides are the immediate substrates for the polymerases involved in DNA replication and repair, the fidelity of DNA synthesis is critically dependent on the correct balance and availability of deoxynucleotides [18]. In mammalian cells the *de novo* synthesis of deoxythymidylate from deoxyuridylate is a rate-limiting step for DNA synthesis. In cells, inhibition of folate metabolism results in uracil misincorporation in DNA [29]. This abnormal base substitution in colonic DNA is thought to predispose to mutations [30,31] and DNA strand breaks [32,33]. Repair of uracil residues that are closely spaced on the opposite strands of DNA results in double-strand breaks, deletions [34], chromosomal breaks [35], micronuclei formation [36], and loss of heterozygosity [37]. It has been shown that folate deficiency results in excess uracil incorporation into DNA in the human [32] and animal [38].

Because folate has a critical role in both DNA methylation and DNA synthesis, most studies have focused on these effects. Both alterations in DNA methylation and increased uracil incorporation into DNA have been observed in folate depletion studies in both humans and animals, and both phenomena can be reversed by folate supplementation.

These two pathways, DNA methylation and DNA synthesis, are highlighted by the common polymorphism of the *MTHFR* gene, and the remarkable decrease in the incidence of colorectal cancer associated with it is presumably because the MTHFR reaction sits as a fulcrum between DNA methylation and DNA synthesis, balancing the two pathways and maintaining normal homeostasis (Figure 4.2).

4.4 INTERACTION BETWEEN FOLATE AND *MTHFR* GENE

4.4.1 CHARACTERISTICS OF *MTHFR* GENE POLYMORPHISMS

MTHFR is considered a key enzyme in one-carbon metabolism, because it catalyzes the irreversible conversion of 5,10-methyleneTHF to 5-methylTHF [39]. In 1988, Kang et al. identified a variant of MTHFR that causes enzyme thermolability and reduced activity *in vivo* and *in vitro* [40,41]. The mutant enzyme was associated with elevated total plasma homocysteine concentrations (tHcy), which is to be expected because the conversion of homocysteine to methionine is impaired [39]. The mild hyperhomocysteinemia appears as an indicator of altered one-carbon metabolism. The thermolabile variant of MTHFR is due to a common missense mutation, a cytosine-to-thymine conversion at base pair *677* [41] that results in an alanine-to-valine substitution in the MTHFR amino acid sequence. The prevalence of the valine–valine substitution is rather common, with a frequency of homozygous individuals in about 10 to 20% of North Americans and Europeans [41–43]. Individuals who are homozygous for this variant (*677TT*) have been reported as having 30% of normal enzyme activity, and heterozygotes (*677CT*) have been reported as having 65% of normal enzyme activity [41].

A second common mutation in the *MTHFR* gene at base pair 1298 that results in an adenine-to-cytosine substitution has been described [44,45]. The *MTHFR 1298A→C* variant, which changes a glutamate into an alanine residue and does not confer thermolability [45], has been shown to have biochemical properties that are not markedly distinguishable from those of the *1298AA* wild-type genotype [46]. Further reports on the biochemical relevance of the *1298A→C* mutation showed also that lymphocytes from individuals carrying the mutant *1298CC* genotype have approximately 60% specific wild-type MTHFR activity *in vitro* compared to *1298AA* wild types [45], although this decrease appeared insufficient to affect levels of tHcy [45,47,48]. However, there appears to be an interaction between these two common mutations. When compared with heterozygosity for either the *677C→T* or *1298A→C* mutations, the combined heterozygosity for the *1298A→C* and *677C→T* mutations was associated with reduced *MTHFR* specific activity, higher tHcy concentration, and decreased plasma folate levels. Thus, the combined heterozygosity for both *MTHFR* mutations results in similar features as those observed in homozygotes for the *677C→T* mutation [45].

Yet, the question of whether and to what extent the *1298A→C* polymorphism affects tHcy concentrations is still incompletely answered because the results of several studies are rather controversial [45,47–50] and in most studies the *1298A→C* polymorphism showed no effect on fasting or post-methionine load tHcy concentrations [48]. Besides, it is noteworthy that some authors described even lower tHcy concentrations associated with the *1298CC* genotype [50]. Only one study thus far has shown a trend vs. higher tHcy in *1298CC* mutants taken alone [49]. The most plausible explanation for the different effect of two variants on homocysteine levels is their mode of enzyme regulation. *1298A→C* affects enzyme regulation through AdoMet, an allosteric inhibitor of MTHFR that is known to bind in the C-terminal regulatory domain, whereas *677C→T* is more likely to influence enzyme thermostability more dramatically because of its localization in the N-terminal catalytic domain [51].

These two polymorphisms are usually not present in the same allele (i.e., in "*cis*"), but studies have shown that very rare *MTHFR* alleles have both polymorphisms [47,52]. In a meta-analysis study for the genotype and haplotype distribution of *MTHFR 677C→T* and *1298A→C* polymorphisms, the estimated haplotype frequencies and the fractional contribution of each were *677C/1298A*, 0.37; *677C/1298C*, 0.31; *677T/1298A*, 0.32; and *677T/1298C*, 0.0023 to 0.0034 [53].

4.4.2 MECHANISM OF FOLATE AND *MTHFR* GENE INTERACTION

The *MTHFR 677C→T* polymorphism provides a paradigm for nutrient and gene interaction in carcinogenesis [18,54]. The biological significance of the interaction between folate and this gene is predominantly related to the reduced availability of 5-methylTHF. Consistent with this concept is also the recent observation that the distribution of different coenzymatic forms of folate is altered in *MTHFR 677TT* homozygotes [55,56]. The red blood cells of *677TT* homozygotes showed variable amounts of formylated tetrahydrofolate polyglutamates at the expense of methylated tetrahydrofolates. In contrast, cells from the *677CC* wild-type individuals contained exclusively methylated tetrahydrofolate derivatives [55].

By determination of tHcy concentrations, a strong nutrient–gene interaction was demonstrated in the phenotypic expression of this polymorphism in *MTHFR* [43,57]. Jacques et al. first showed that individuals with the thermolabile MTHFR variant may have a higher folate requirement for the regulation of plasma homocysteine concentrations, highlighting the presence of an interaction between this common polymorphism and folate in homocysteine metabolism [57]. Girelli et al. also reported that subjects with *677TT* with inadequate folate status, as indicated by their blood folate levels being lower than the median (11.5 nmol/l), had 59% increased plasma homocysteine concentrations [43]. An intermediate effect (21%) was also observed in heterozygous (*677CT*) individuals. On the other hand, at adequate folate status there were no differences in plasma homocysteine concentration among the three genotypes. These findings contributed to the opening of a new field of interest for both nutrition and genetics, especially because this relationship between *MTHFR* polymorphism and plasma folate concentrations was implicated as the likely link between the *MTHFR* polymorphism and many diseases including cardiovascular disease, neural tube defects, and cancers. In coronary artery disease, the interaction between *MTHFR* and folate, which defines a higher risk for the disease, is determined by folate levels below certain specific thresholds, which are different for each of the *MTHFR 677C→T* genotypes [58]. The limited availability of methylated folate in carriers of the *677TT* genotype, particularly in conditions of low folate status, significantly impairs the ability of the cell to remethylate homocysteine to methionine, resulting in homocysteine accumulation. Hustad et al. recently showed that vitamin B_2 (riboflavin) concentrations affect this relationship as well, leading to higher homocysteine concentrations only in *677TT* genotypes but not in *677CC* wild types [59].

The presence of such a nutrient–gene interaction between the mutant MTHFR enzyme and folate status is consistent with the recent study of Guenther et al. [51], who evaluated the biochemical structure of mutant MTHFR and explained its tendency to lose its essential flavin cofactor. They used a thermolabile variant MTHFR model expressed in *Escherichia coli* to show that the *MTHFR* mutation results in the exposure of binding sites for the flavin adenine dinucleotide (FAD) cofactor, which otherwise would be embedded in a barrel-like structure. Such exposure results in a weakened enzyme–FAD complex and subsequent loss of activity. The reduced activity of the modified *E. coli* enzyme is attributable to diminished FAD binding, which affects the equilibrium between the more stable tetramer and the less stable dimeric form of the protein. The presence of 5-methylTHF substrates is associated with conformational changes that strengthen the complex, thereby protecting the MTHFR against the loss of its flavin cofactor.

The human enzyme is a dimer rather than a tetramer and contains a domain that allosterically binds the inhibitor *S*-adenosylmethionine. A recent human study demonstrated that once FAD is dissociated from the enzyme, there is a rapid conversion of the dimer to monomers, which is associated with the genotype-related loss of activity. Because both methylTHF and AdoMet can protect the complex against FAD dissociation, folate depletion can further reduce MTHFR activity by decreasing the levels of methylTHF and AdoMet in the *MTHFR 677TT* genotype. These observations also suggest an interaction among FAD, folate, and the *MTHFR* gene [60].

4.4.3 EFFECT OF FOLATE AND *MTHFR* GENE INTERACTION ON DNA METHYLATION

DNA methylation, an essential epigenetic feature of DNA, plays a critical role for gene expression and genomic integrity. In many cancers, aberrant DNA methylation is a universal phenomenon, which can be found from the initial phase of carcinogenesis. Thus, DNA methylation has been regarded as one of the most important mechanisms for carcinogenesis as well as an essential biomarker for cancer research, especially for the folate-related carcinogenesis.

It has been suggested that the cancer protective effect of the common *MTHFR 677C→T* polymorphism in folate-replete conditions is related to the increased availability of 5,10-methyleneTHF, and therefore increased ease of nucleotide synthesis. On the other hand, the increased risk of colorectal cancer apparent in *677TT* individuals with low folate status may be due to the fact that below a certain threshold, the availability of 5-methylTHF for biological methylation becomes severely enough compromised to become the critical determinant of whether the cell is pushed down the pathway towards neoplasia [18]. *MTHFR 677TT* genotypes had a diminished level of DNA methylation compared to those with the 677CC wild-type as shown in a small population [56], as well as in a larger set of subjects [61]. When analyzed according to total folate status, however, only the *677TT* subjects with low levels of folate accounted for the diminished DNA methylation [61,62].

When analyzed according to the folate coenzymatic form distribution, in 677TT subjects DNA methylation status correlated with the methylated proportion of RBC folate [61] and was inversely related to the formylated proportion of RBC folates that are solely represented in 677*TT* individuals. This observation indicates that the *MTHFR* 677*C*→*T* polymorphism influences DNA methylation status through an interaction with different folate form distribution. Thus, the modulation of cancer risk associated with the polymorphism may be conveyed by a shift in proportions of the different coenzymatic forms of folate contained within the cell, thereby changing the balance of biological methylation and DNA synthesis. Qualitative alterations in cellular folate pools related to genotype may also explain how the protective effect associated with the mutant genotype is operable even in the face of plentiful quantities of cellular folate in folate-replete individuals.

On the other hand, carriers of the *1298AA* wild-type genotype showed lower genomic DNA methylation compared to *1298AC* or *1298CC* genotypes. When DNA methylation was evaluated according to plasma folate status, only *1298AA* with low folate levels revealed diminished DNA methylation. Moreover, when the two *MTHFR* polymorphisms were concomitantly evaluated at the low folate status, DNA methylation was reduced only in *1298AA/677TT* compared to *1298AA/677CC* and to *1298CC/677CC* genotypes. However, the high prevalence of *677TT* mutants within the *1298AA* group (79%) and the similar biochemical features of *1298AA/677CC* and *1298CC/677CC* combined genotypes, suggest that the nutrient–gene interaction affecting DNA methylation in *1298AA* is due mainly to the coexistence of the *677TT* genotype, and that the *1298A*→*C* polymorphism may convey its protective effect not through this interaction, but through another pathway in one-carbon metabolism [63]. This finding also suggests that the *MTHFR* 677*C*→*T* polymorphism has a prevalent effect on MTHFR function, and both of them should be evaluated to better define enzyme activity.

Alteration in methylation status within promoter regions is also a very important epigenetic mechanism in gene control [64]. Because methylation of the promoter region generally suppresses transcription, it has been thought that promoter hypomethylation can activate protooncogenes, and promoter hypermethylation can inactivate tumor suppressor genes. In a rodent model of hepatocellular carcinoma, a choline-deficient diet induced hypomethylation of 5′ upstream CpG sites of the *c-myc* gene as well as overexpression of this gene [65]. Interestingly, experimental deficiency of one-carbon nutrients in animals, which showed decreased genomic DNA methylation status, caused a paradoxical (and presumably compensatory) hypermethylation of certain loci [66]. It is of particular interest because the promoter regions of several tumor suppressor genes such as *p16*, *p53*, and *APC* are frequently found to be hypermethylated in cancers [67–69]. Jhaveri et al. also reported that the *H-cadherin* gene, which showed hypermethylation of 5′ sequences in response to folate depletion, was downregulated in human nasopharyngeal carcinoma KB cells [70]. This hypermethylation suppresses expression of the gene, and is, therefore hypothesized to contribute to the evolution of the cancer.

These observations suggest that an altered genomic DNA methylation status due to the interaction between folate and *MTHFR* might modulate the status of promoter specific DNA methylation in cancer-related genes, which contributes to carcinogenesis by changing the expression of those critical genes.

In contrast to the effect of folate and *MTHFR* interaction on DNA methylation, the effect of this interaction on DNA synthesis remains an unsolved problems; there is a hypothesis that the shift toward the formylated form of folate enhances thymidy-late and purine synthesis to protect carcinogenesis, even though two null results under limited experiment condition have been reported in this regard [71,72].

4.5 INTERACTION BETWEEN FOLATE AND *MTHFR* GENE IN COLORECTAL CARCINOGENESIS

In a case–control study conducted in the Health Professionals Follow-up Study, Chen et al. [73] demonstrated that dietary methyl supply is critical among *MTHFR 677TT* individuals. When dietary methyl supply is high, the *MTHFR 677TT* genotype may be at reduced risk of colorectal cancer. In contrast, alcohol consumption, which can deplete 5-methylTHF, abolished the reduced risk. Thereafter, in a nested case–control study in the Physicians' Health Study, Ma et al. [9] demonstrated that the status of folate, one of dietary methyl sources, is also critical to the *MTHFR*-related risk of colorectal cancer. Men with the *MTHFR 677TT* genotype had half the risk of colorectal cancer (OR = 0.49; 95% CI, 0.27 to 0.87) compared to wild or heterozy-gous genotypes. At the adequate folate level, men with *MTHFR 677TT* had a threefold decrease in risk (OR = 0.32; 95% CI, 0.15 to 0.68) compared to wild-type or heterozy-gous genotypes. However, at the low folate level this protective effect disappeared, and the *MTHFR 677TT* genotype even increased colorectal cancer risk [9].

In an incident case–control study Slattery et al. [74] reported the additive effect of vitamin B_6 and vitamin B_{12}, both of which are coenzymes for folate metabolism, to this interaction. High levels of intake of folate, vitamin B_6, and vitamin B_{12} were associated with a 30 to 40% reduction in risk of colon cancer among those with *677TT* compared to those with low levels of intake carrying wild-type genotype.

Marugame et al. [75] also investigated the possible influence of folate status on the risk of colorectal adenoma, a pathological lesion that precedes the onset of colorectal cancer, in individuals with the *MTHFR 677TT* genotype. As compared to subjects with the *677CC* or *677CT* genotype having low plasma folate levels, those with the *677TT* genotype showed a decreased risk of colorectal adenomas when they had high levels of plasma folate (OR = 0.58, 95% CI, 0.21 to 1.61) and an increased risk when they had low folate levels (OR = 2.13, 95% CI, 0.82 to 5.54). On the other hand, there was no clear relationship between plasma folate and colorectal adenoma among those with the *677CC* or *677CT* genotype. These observations suggest a possible interaction between folate and the *MTHFR* genotype on colorectal adenomas. Ulrich et al. [76] also reported that low dietary intake of folate, B_{12}, and B_6 might increase the risk of colorectal adenoma among those with *MTHFR 677TT* as observed in subjects with colorectal cancer.

The second *MTHFR* variant, codon 1298 A to C, is also associated with decreased enzyme activity [45,47] and would be expected to have a similar protective effect on colon cancer risk when folate intake is high. Chen et al. [77] recently reported a weak but statistically not significant inverse relationship between the *1298CC* genotype and colon cancer in the Physician's Health Study, as well as a lack of evidence of modification by folate intake. However, in a population-based case–control study in North Carolina, Keku et al. [78] reported that the *1298CC* genotype was inversely associated with colon cancer in white subjects (OR = 0.5, 95% CI, 0.3 to 0.9), not among African-Americans.

4.6 INTERACTION BETWEEN FOLATE AND *MTHFR* GENE IN OTHER NEOPLASTIC DISEASES

Skibola et al. [79] reported that the *MTHFR 677TT* genotype has a 4.3-fold decreased risk of adult acute lymphoblastic leukemia (ALL) (OR = 0.23; 95% CI, 0.06 to 0.81). An individual with the *MTHFR 1298AC* heterozygous genotype has a three-fold reduction in risk of adult ALL (OR = 0.33; 95% CI, 0.15 to 0.73) and an individual with *MTHFR 1298CC* has a 14-fold decreased risk (OR = 0.07; 95% CI, 0.00 to 1.77). Franco et al. (80) also reported a similar result from childhood ALL. However, neither of the two major *MTHFR* polymorphisms has been observed to be related to myeloid leukemia risk, suggesting that differences in folate requirements or susceptibility to chromosomal damage may exist between myeloid and lymphoid cells. Although these observations suggest that the *MTHFR* polymorphism is important for leukemia risk, none of the studies to date has assessed the effect of interaction between folate and this gene on the risk of leukemia [81].

As for the relationship of MTHFR genotypes and cancer affecting other tissues, Lin et al. reported that individuals carrying the mutant *MTHFR* 677T allele either in hetero- or homozygosity (677CT or 677TT) with low dietary intake of folate had a significantly increased risk (3.51-fold) for bladder cancer compared to those individuals carrying the wild-type genotype and showing high dietary intake of folate [82]. Goodman et al. reported that women with either one or two *MTHFR* 677T mutant alleles and folate intake below the median had, respectively, two or three times higher risk for cervical squamous intraepithelial lesions, a precursor of cervical cancer, compared to those carrying the *MTHFR 677CC* wild-type genotype and having folate intakes above the median [83]. In a population-based case–control study [84] that demonstrated that the *MTHFR 677T* variant allele was associated with increased risk of breast cancer (*p* for trend = 0.03) compared to the *677TT* genotype, elevation of breast cancer risk was most pronounced among *677TT* women who consumed the lowest levels of dietary folate (OR = 1.83; 95% CI, 1.13 to 2.96) or total folate intake (OR = 1.71; 95% CI, 1.08 to 2.71) compared to *677CC* individuals with high folate intake. On the other hand, the *1298C* variant allele was inversely associated with breast cancer risk (*p* for trend = 0.03), and it was suggested that this finding was likely due to the linkage of this allele to the low risk of *677C* allele.

4.7 CONCLUSION

Epidemiological data, as well as animal studies, indicate that folate modulates the risk of cancer over a wide range of intakes, extending from deficient intake to levels several times above what is considered the basal requirement. Therefore, examining the mechanism(s) by which folate depletion enhances carcinogenesis is of absolute relevance, and will almost certainly reveal the mechanisms by which folate conveys protection when taken in supplemental quantities, as well. Most data in this regard refer to the effect of folate and the carcinogenetic process in the cancer of the colorectum, but findings from other studies propose that other tissues are also likely to be affected by the relationship with this nutrient. However, despite two decades of studies, the mechanisms that are responsible for mediating this effect have not been yet elucidated. In this chapter, we nevertheless considered it through the nutrient–gene interaction approach.

A common polymorphism in the *MTHFR gene (677C→T)*, which causes thermolability and reduced activity of MTHFR, is associated with a lower risk for development of colorectal cancer in individuals with adequate folate status. However, the protection conferred by the presence of the polymorphism is eliminated in those with low systemic folate status, and an even higher risk toward colorectal cancer is reported. This observation drew our attention to the interaction between folate and *MTHFR* gene in colorectal carcinogenesis. Subsequent studies on the interaction between folate and the polymorphism of *MTHFR* on both plasma homocysteine concentrations and genomic DNA methylation status provide the basis to investigate the mechanisms by which folate and *MTHFR* gene interaction affects carcinogenesis. Evidence for the beneficial effects of adequate folate status as well as altered folate coenzymatic forms' distribution by *MTHFR* polymorphism also enable cancer chemoprevention trials using folate.

In the future, studies regarding interactions between folate either combination of both polymorphisms in *MTHFR* gene or other polymorphic sites within genes in one-carbon metabolism [85], as well as interactions between folate and the *MTHFR* gene on DNA synthesis (thymidylate and purine synthesis), through which *MTHFR* *677TT* genotype has been regarded to have a protective effect on the risk of colorectal cancer, are needed.

ABBREVIATIONS

AdoHcy   *S*-adenosylhomocysteine
AdoMet   *S*-adenosylmethionine
ALL   acute lymphoblastic leukemia
BHMT   betaine homocysteine methyltransferase
CBS   cystathionine β-synthase
DHF   dihydrofolate
FAD   flavin adenine dinucleotide
MS   methionine synthase
MTHFR   methylenetetrahydrofolate reductase
SHMT   serine hydroxymethyltransferase
THF   tetrahydrofolate
tHcy   total plasma homocysteine

REFERENCES

1. Kim, Y.I., Folate and carcinogenesis: evidence, mechanisms, and implications, *J. Nutr. Biochem.,* 10, 66, 1999.
2. Heijmans, B.T., Boer, J.M., Suchiman, H.E., Cornelisse, C.J., Westendorp, R.G., Kromhout, D., Feskens, E.J., and Slagboom, P.E., A common variant of the methylenetetrahydrofolate reductase gene (1p36) is associated with an increased risk of cancer, *Cancer Res.,* 63, 1249, 2003.
3. Zhang, S.M., Willett, W.C., Selhub, J., Hunter, D.J., Giovannucci, E.L., Holmes, M.D., Colditz, G.A., and Hankinson, S.E., Plasma folate, vitamin B6, vitamin B12, homocysteine, and risk of breast cancer, *J. Natl. Cancer Inst.*, 95, 373, 2003.
4. Ziegler, R.G., Weinstein, S.J., and Fears, T.R., Nutritional and genetic inefficiencies in one-carbon metabolism and cervical cancer risk, *J. Nutr.,* 132 (Suppl. 8), 2345S, 2002.
5. Choi, S.W. and Mason, J.B., Folate status: effects on pathways of colorectal carcinogenesis, *J. Nutr.*, 132 (Suppl. 8), 2413S, 2002.
6. Cravo, M.L., Mason, J.B., Dayal, Y., Hutchinson, M., Smith, D., Selhub, J., and Rosenberg, I.H., Folate deficiency enhances the development of colonic neoplasia in dimethylhydrazine-treated rats, *Cancer Res.*, 52, 5002, 1992.
7. Kim, Y.I., Salomon, R.N., Graeme-Cook, F., Choi, S.W., Smith, D.E., Dallal, G.E., and Mason, J.B., Dietary folate protects against the development of macroscopic colonic neoplasia in a dose responsive manner in rats, *Gut,* 39, 732, 1996.
8. Song, J., Medline, A., Mason, J.B., Gallinger, S., and Kim, Y.I., Effects of dietary folate on intestinal tumorigenesis in the apcMin mouse, *Cancer Res.,* 60, 5434, 2000.
9. Ma, J., Stampfer, M.J., Giovannucci, E., Artigas, C., Hunter, D.J., Fuchs, C., Willett, W.C., Selhub, J., Hennekens, C.H., and Rozen, R., Methylenetetrahydrofolate reductase polymorphism, dietary interactions, and risk of colorectal cancer, *Cancer Res.,* 57, 1098, 1997.
10. Lashner, B.A., Heidenreich, P.A., Su, G.L., Kane, S.V., and Hanauer, S.B., Effect of folate supplementation on the incidence of dysplasia and cancer in chronic ulcerative colitis. A case-control study, *Gastroenterology,* 97, 255, 1989.
11. Lashner, B.A., Red blood cell folate is associated with the development of dysplasia and cancer in ulcerative colitis, *J. Cancer. Res. Clin. Oncol.,* 119, 549, 1993.
12. Benito, E., Stiggelbout, A., Bosch, F.X., Obrador, A., Kaldor, J., Mulet, M., and Munoz, N., Nutritional factors in colorectal cancer risk: a case-control study in Majorca, *Int. J. Cancer,* 49, 161, 1991.
13. Benito, E., Cabeza, E., Moreno, V., Obrador, A., and Bosch, F.X., Diet and colorectal adenomas: a case-control study in Majorca, *Int. J. Cancer,* 55, 213, 1993.
14. Freudenheim, J.L., Graham, S., Marshall, J.R., Haughey, B.P., Cholewinski, S., and Wilkinson, G., Folate intake and carcinogenesis of the colon and rectum, *Int. J. Epidemiol.,* 20, 368, 1991.
15. Paspatis, G.A., Kalafatis, E., Oros, L., Xourgias, V., Koutsioumpa, P., and Karamanolis, D.G., Folate status and adenomatous colonic polyps. A colonoscopically controlled study, *Dis. Colon Rectum,* 38, 64, 1995.
16. Giovannucci, E., Rimm E.B., Ascherio, A., Stampfer, M.J., Colditz, G.A., and Willett, W.C., Alcohol, low-methionine–low-folate diets, and risk of colon cancer in men, *J. Natl. Cancer Inst.*, 87, 265, 1995.
17. Giovannucci, E., Stampfer, M.J., Colditz, G.A., Rimm, E.B., Trichopoulos, D., Rosner, B.A., Speizer, F.E., and Willett, W.C., Folate, methionine, and alcohol intake and risk of colorectal adenoma, *J. Natl. Cancer Inst.*, 85, 875, 1993.

18. Choi, S.W. and Mason, J.B., Folate and carcinogenesis: an integrated scheme, *J. Nutr.,* 130, 129, 2000.
19. Kim, Y.I., Role of folate in colon cancer development and progression, *J. Nutr.,* 133 (11 Suppl. 1), 3731S, 2003.
20. Giovannucci, E., Stampfer, M.J., Colditz, G.A., Hunter, D.J., Fuchs, C., Rosner, B.A., Speizer, F.E., and Willett, W.C., Multivitamin use, folate, and colon cancer in women in the Nurses' Health Study, *Ann. Intern. Med.,* 129, 517, 1998.
21. Cravo, M., Fidalgo, P., Pereira, A.D., Gouveia-Oliveira, A., Chaves, P., Selhub, J., Mason, J.B., Mira, F.C., and Leitao, C.N., DNA methylation as an intermediate biomarker in colorectal cancer: modulation by folic acid supplementation, *Eur. J. Cancer Prev.* 3, 473, 1994.
22. Khosraviani, K., Weir, H.P., Hamilton, P., Moorehead, J., and Williamson, K., Effect of folate supplementation on mucosal cell proliferation in high risk patients for colon cancer, *Gut,* 51, 195, 2002.
23. MacKenzie, R.E., Biogenesis and interconversion of substituted tetrahydrofolates, in *Folate and Pterins,* Blakley, R.L. and Benkovic, S.J., Eds., Vol. 1, John Wiley & Sons, New York, 1984, pp. 255–306.
24. Shane, B., Folylpolyglutamate synthesis and role in the regulation of one-carbon metabolism, *Vitam. Horm.,* 45, 263, 1989.
25. Weissbach, H., and Taylor, R.T., Roles of vitamin B 12 and folic acid in methionine synthesis, *Vitam. Horm.,* 28, 415, 1970.
26. Miller, J.W., Nadeau, M.R., Smith, J., Smith, D., and Selhub, J., Folate-deficiency-induced homocysteinaemia in rats: disruption of S-adenosylmethionine's co-ordinate regulation of homocysteine metabolism, *Biochem. J.,* 298, 415, 1994.
27. Balaghi, M. and Wagner, C., DNA methylation in folate deficiency: use of CpG methylase, *Biochem. Biophys. Res. Commun.,* 193, 1184, 1993.
28. Jacob, R.A., Gretz, D.M., Taylor, P.C., James, S.J., Pogribny, I.P., Miller, B.J., Henning, S.M., and Swendseid, M.E., Moderate folate depletion increases plasma homocysteine and decreases lymphocyte DNA methylation in postmenopausal women, *J. Nutr.,* 128, 1204, 1998.
29. Blount, B.C. and Ames, B.N., Analysis of uracil in DNA by gas chromatography-mass spectrometry, *Anal. Biochem.,* 219, 195, 1994.
30. James, S.J., Basnakian, A.G., and Miller, B.J., In vitro folate deficiency induces deoxynucleotide pool imbalance, apoptosis, and mutagenesis in Chinese hamster ovary cells, *Cancer Res.,* 54, 5075, 1994.
31. Kunz, B.A., Mutagenesis and deoxyribonucleotide pool imbalance, *Mutat. Res.,* 200, 133, 1988.
32. Blount, B.C., Mack, M.M., Wehr, C.M., MacGregor, J.T., Hiatt, R.A., Wang, G., Wickramasinghe, S.N., Everson, R.B., and Ames, B.N., Folate deficiency causes uracil misincorporation into human DNA and chromosome breakage: implications for cancer and neuronal damage, *Proc. Natl. Acad. Sci. U.S.A.,* 94, 3290, 1997.
33. Melnyk, S., Pogribna, M., Miller, B.J., Basnakian, A.G., Pogribny, I.P., and James, S.J., Uracil misincorporation, DNA strand breaks, and gene amplification are associated with tumorigenic cell transformation in folate deficient/repleted Chinese hamster ovary cells, *Cancer Lett.,* 146, 35, 1999.
34. Dianov, G.L., Timchenko, T.V., Sinitsina, O.I., Kuzminov, A.V., Medvedev, O.A., and Salganik, R.I., Repair of uracil residues closely spaced on the opposite strands of plasmid DNA results in double-strand break and deletion formation, *Mol. Gen. Genet.,* 225, 448, 1991.
35. Reidy, J.A., Folate- and deoxyuridine-sensitive chromatid breakage may result from DNA repair during G2, *Mutat. Res.,* 192, 217, 1987.

36. Fenech, M., The role of folic acid and vitamin B12 in genomic stability of human cells, *Mutat. Res.*, 475, 57, 2001.
37. Moynahan, M.E. and Jasin, M., Loss of heterozygosity induced by a chromosomal double-strand break, *Proc. Natl. Acad. Sci. U.S.A.*, 94, 8988, 1997.
38. Choi, S.W., Friso, S., Dolnikowski, G.G., Bagley, P.J., Edmondson, A.N., Nadeau, M.R., Smith, D.E., and Mason, J.B., Biochemical and molecular indications that the elder rat colon is particularly susceptible to folate depletion, *J. Nutr.*, 133, 1206, 2003.
39. Selhub, J., Homocysteine metabolism, *Annu. Rev. Nutr.*, 19, 217, 1999.
40. Kang, S.S., Zhou, J., Wong, P.W., Kowalisyn. J., and Strokosch, G., Intermediate homocysteinemia: a thermolabile variant of methylenetetrahydrofolate reductase, *Am. J. Hum. Genet.*, 43, 414, 1988.
41. Frosst, P., Blom, H.J., Milos, R., Goyette, P., Sheppard, C.A., Matthews, R.G., Boers, G.J.H., denHeijer, M., Kluijtmans, L.A.J., van den Heuvel, L.P., and Rozen, R., A candidate genetic risk factor for vascular disease: a common mutation in methylene-tetrahydrofolate reductase, *Nat. Genet.*, 10, 111, 1995.
42. Ma, J., Stampfer, M.J., Hennekens, C.H., Frosst, P., Selhub, J., Horsford, J., Malinow, M.R., Willett, W.C., and Rozen, R., Methylenetetrahydrofolate reductase polymorphism, plasma folate, homocysteine, and risk of myocardial infarction in U.S. physicians, *Circulation*, 94, 2410, 1996.
43. Girelli, D., Friso, S., Trabetti, E., Olivieri, O., Russo, C., Pessotto, R., Faccini, G., Pignatti, P.F., Mazzucco, A., and Corrocher, R., Methylenetetrahydrofolate reductase C677T mutation, plasma homocysteine, and folate in subjects from northern Italy with or without angiographically documented severe coronary atherosclerotic disease: evidence for an important genetic-environmental interaction, *Blood*, 91, 4158, 1998.
44. Viel, A., Dall'Agnese, L., Simone, F., Canzonieri, V., Capozzi, E., Visentin, M.C., Valle, R., and Boiocchi, M., Loss of heterozygosity at the 5,10-methylenetetrahydro-folate reductase locus in human ovarian carcinomas, *Br. J. Cancer,* 75, 1105, 1997.
45. van der Put, N.M.J., Gabreels, F., Stevens, E.M.B., Smeitink, J.A.M., Trijbels, F.J.M., Eskes, T.K.A.B., van den Heuvel, L.P., and Blom, H.J., A second common mutation in the methylenetetrahydrofolate reductase gene: an additional risk factor for neural tube defects?, *Am. J. Hum. Genet.,* 62, 1044, 1998.
46. Yamada, K., Chen, Z., Rozen, R., and Matthews, R.G., Effects of common polymorphisms on the properties of recombinant human methylenetetrahydrofolate reductase, *Proc. Natl. Acad. Sci. U.S.A.,* 98, 14853, 2001.
47. Weisberg, I., Tran, P., Christensen, B., Sibani, S., and Rozen, R., A second genetic polymorphism in methylenetetrahydrofolate reductase (MTHFR) associated with decreased enzyme activity, *Mol. Genet. Metab.,* 64, 169, 1998.
48. Friso, S., Girelli, D., Trabetti, E., Stranieri, C., Olivieri, O., Tinazzi, E., Martinelli, N., Faccini, G., Pignatti, P.F., and Corrocher, R., A1298C methylenetetrahydrofolate reductase mutation and coronary artery disease: relationships with C677T polymorphism and homocysteine/folate metabolism, *Clin. Exp. Med.*, 2.7, 2002.
49. Chango, A., Boisson, F., Barbé, F., Quilliot, D., Droesch, S., Pfister, M., Fillon-Emery, N., Lambert, D., Frémont, S., Rosenblatt, D.S., and Nicolas, J.P., The effect of 677C→T and 1298A→C mutations on plasma homocysteine and 5,10-methylenetetra-hydrofolate reductase activity in healthy subjects, *Br. J. Nutr.*, 83, 593, 2000.
50. Friedman, G., Goldschmidt, N., Friedlander, Y., Ben-Yehuda, A., Selhub, J., Babaey, S., Mendel, M., Kidron, M., and Bar-On, H., A common mutation 1298 A→C in human methylenetetrahydrofolate reductase gene: association with plasma total homocysteine and folate concentrations, *J. Nutr.*, 129, 1656, 1999.

51. Guenther, B.D., Sheppard, C.A., Tran, P., Rozen, R., Matthews, R.G., and Ludwig, M.L., The structure and properties of methylenetetrahydrofolate reductase from *Escherichia coli* suggest how folate ameliorates human hyperhomocysteinemia, *Nat. Struct. Biol.*, 6, 359, 1999.

52. Isotalo, P.A., Wells, G.A., and Donnelly, J.G., Neonatal and fetal methylenetetrahydrofolate reductase genetic polymorphisms: an examination of C677T and A1298C mutations, *Am. J. Hum. Genet.*, 67, 986, 2000.

53. Ogino, S. and Wilson, R.B., Genotype and haplotype distributions of MTHFR677C>T and 1298A>C single nucleotide polymorphisms: a meta-analysis, *J. Hum. Genet.*, 48, 1, 2003.

54. Kim, Y.I., Methylenetetrahydrofolate reductase polymorphisms, folate, and cancer risk: a paradigm of gene-nutrient interactions in carcinogenesis, *Nutr. Rev.*, 58, 205, 2000.

55. Bagley, P.J. and Selhub, J., A common mutation in the methylenetetrahydrofolate reductase gene is associated with an accumulation of formylated tetrahydrofolates in red blood cells, *Proc. Natl. Acad. Sci. U.S.A.*, 95, 13217, 1998.

56. Stern, L.L., Mason, J.B., Selhub, J., and Choi, S.W., Genomic DNA hypomethylation, a characteristic of most cancers, is present peripheral leukocytes of individuals who are homozygous for the C677T polymorphism in the methylenetetrahydrofolate reductase gene, *Cancer Epidemiol. Biomarkers Prev.*, 9, 849, 2000.

57. Jacques, P.F., Bostom, A.G., Williams, R.R., Ellison, R.C., Eckfeldt, J.H., Rosenberg, I.H., Selhub, J., and Rozen, R., Relation between folate status, a common mutation in methylenetetrahydrofolate reductase, and plasma homocysteine concentrations, *Circulation*, 93, 7, 1996.

58. Girelli, D., Martinelli, N., Pizzolo, F., Friso, S., Olivieri, O., Stranieri, C., Trabetti, E., Faccini, G., Tinazzi, E., Pignatti, P.F., and Corrocher, R., The interaction between MTHFR 677 C→T genotype and folate status is a determinant of coronary atherosclerosis risk, *J. Nutr.*, 133, 1281, 2003.

59. Hustad, S., Ueland, P.M., Vollset, S.E., Zhang, Y., Bjorke-Monsen, A.L., and Schneede, J., Riboflavin as a determinant of plasma total homocysteine: effect modification by the methylenetetrahydrofolate reductase C677T polymorphism, *Clin. Chem.*, 46 (8 Pt. 1), 1065, 2000.

60. Lathrop Stern, L., Shane, B., Bagley, P.J., Nadeau, M., Shih, V., and Selhub, J., Combined marginal folate and riboflavin status affect homocysteine methylation in cultured immortalized lymphocytes from persons homozygous for the MTHFR C677T mutation, *J. Nutr.*, 133, 2716, 2003.

61. Friso, S., Choi, S.W., Girelli, D., Mason, J.B., Dolnikowski, G.G., Bagley, P.J., Olivieri, O., Jacques, P.F., Rosenberg, I.H., Corrocher, R., and Selhub, J., A common mutation in the 5, 10-methylenetetrahydrofolate reductase gene affects genomic DNA methylation through an interaction with folate status, *Proc. Natl. Acad. Sci. U.S.A.*, 99, 5606, 2002.

62. Friso, S. and Choi, S.W., Gene-nutrient interactions and DNA methylation, *J. Nutr.*, 132 (Suppl. 8), 2382S, 2002.

63. Friso, S., Girelli, D., Trabetti, E., Olivieri, O., Guarini, P., Pignatti, P.F., Corrocher, R., and Choi, S.W., The MTHFR 1298A>C polymorphism and genomic DNA methylation in human lymphocytes, *Cancer Epidemiol. Biomarkers Prev.*, 14, 938, 2005.

64. Bayline, S.B., Belinsky, S.A., and Herman, J.G., Aberrant methylation of gene promoters in cancer-concepts, misconcepts, and promise, *J. Natl. Cancer Inst.*, 92, 1460, 2000.

65. Tsujiuchi, T., Tsutsumi, M., Sasaki, Y., Takahama, M., and Konishi, Y., Hypomethylation of CpG sites and c-myc gene overexpression in hepatocellular carcinomas, but not hyperplastic nodules, induced by a choline-deficient L-amino acid-defined diet in rats, *Jpn. J. Cancer Res.*, 90, 909, 1999.

66. Pogribny, I.P., Miller, B.J., and James, S.J., Alterations in hepatic p53 gene methylation patterns during tumor progression with folate/methyl deficiency in the rat, *Cancer Lett.*, 115, 31, 1997.

67. Herman, J.G., Merlo, A., Mao, L., Lapidus, R.G., Issa, J.P., Davidson, N.E., Sidransky, D., and Baylin, S.B., Inactivation of the CDKN2/p16/MTS1 gene is frequently associated with aberrant DNA methylation in all common human cancers, *Cancer Res.*, 55, 4525, 1995.

68. Schroeder, M. and Mass, M.J., CpG methylation inactivates the transcriptional activity of the promoter of the human p53 tumor suppressor gene, *Biochem. Biophys. Res. Commun.*, 235, 403, 1997.

69. Hiltunen, M.O., Alhonen, L., Koistinaho, J., Myohanen, S., Paakkonen, M., Marin, S., Kosma, V.M., and Janne, J., Hypermethylation of the APC (adenomatous polyposis coli) gene promoter region in human colorectal carcinoma, *Int. J. Cancer,* 70, 644, 1997.

70. Jhaveri, M.S., Wagner, C., and Trepel, J.B., Impact of extracellular folate levels on global gene expression, *Mol. Pharmacol.*, 60, 1288, 2001.

71. Crott, J.W., Mashiyama, S.T., Ames, B.N., and Fenech, M., The effect of folic acid deficiency and MTHFR C677T polymorphism on chromosome damage in human lymphocytes in vitro, *Cancer Epidemiol. Biomarkers Prev.*, 10, 1089, 2001.

72. Narayanan, S., McConnell, J., Little, J., Sharp, L., Piyathilake, C.J., Powers, H., Basten, G., and Duthie, S.J., Associations between two common variants C677T and A1298C in the methylenetetrahydrofolate reductase gene and measures of folate metabolism and DNA stability (strand breaks, misincorporated uracil, and DNA methylation status) in human lymphocytes in vivo, *Cancer Epidemiol. Biomarkers Prev.*, 13, 1436, 2004.

73. Chen, J., Giovannucci, E., Kelsey, K., Rimm, E.B., Stampfer, M.J., Colditz, G.A., Spiegelman, D., Willett, W.C., and Hunter, D.J., A methylenetetrahydrofolate reductase polymorphism and the risk of colorectal cancer, *Cancer Res.*, 56, 4862, 1996.

74. Slattery, M.L., Potter, J.D., Samowitz, W., Schaffer, D., and Leppert, M., Methylenetetrahydrofolate reductase, diet, and risk of colon cancer, *Cancer Epidemiol. Biomarkers Prev.*, 8, 513, 1999.

75. Marugame, T., Tsuji, E., Kiyohara, C., Eguchi, H., Oda. T., Shinchi, K., and Kono, S., Relation of plasma folate and methylenetetrahydrofolate reductase C677T polymorphism to colorectal adenomas, *Int. J. Epidemiol.*, 32, 64, 2003.

76. Ulrich, C.M., Kampman, E., Bigler, J., Schwartz, S.M., Chen, C., Bostick, R., Fosdick, L., Beresford, S.A., Yasui, Y., and Potter, J.D., Colorectal adenomas and the C677T MTHFR polymorphism: evidence for gene-environment interaction?, *Cancer Epidemiol. Biomarkers Prev.*, 8, 659, 1999.

77. Chen, J., Ma, J., Stampfer, M.J., Palomeque, C., Selhub, J., and Hunter, D.J., Linkage disequilibrium between the $677C > T$ and $1298A > C$ polymorphisms in human methylenetetrahydrofolate reductase gene and their contributions to risk of colorectal cancer, *Pharmacogenetics*, 12, 339, 2002.

78. Keku, T., Millikan, R., Worley, K., Winkel, S., Eaton, A., Biscocho, L., Martin, C., and Sandler, R., 5,10-Methylenetetrahydrofolate reductase codon 677 and 1298 polymorphisms and colon cancer in African Americans and whites, *Cancer Epidemiol. Biomarkers Prev.*, 11, 1611, 2002.

79. Skibola, C.F., Smith, M.T., Kane, E., Roman, E., Rollinson, S., Cartwright, R.A., and Morgan, G., Polymorphisms in the methylenetetrahydrofolate reductase gene are associated with susceptibility to acute leukemia in adults, *Proc. Natl. Acad. Sci. U.S.A.*, 96, 12810, 1999.

80. Franco, R.F., Simoes, B.P., Tone, L.G., Gabellini, S.M., Zago, M.A., and Falcao, R.P., The methylenetetrahydrofolate reductase C677T gene polymorphism decreases the risk of childhood acute lymphocytic leukaemia, *Br. J. Haematol.*, 115, 616, 2001.

81. Robien, K. and Ulrich, C.M., 5,10-Methylenetetrahydrofolate reductase polymorphisms and leukemia risk: a HuGE minireview, *Am. J. Epidemiol.*, 157, 571, 2003.

82. Lin, J., Spitz, M.R., Wang, Y., Schabath, M.B., Gorlov, I.P., Hernandez, L.M., Pillow, P.C., Grossman, H.B., and Wu, X., Polymorphisms of folate metabolic genes and susceptibility to bladder cancer: a case-control study, *Carcinogenesis,* 25, 1639, 2004.

83. Goodman, M.T., McDuffie, K., Hernandez, B., Wilkens, L.R., Bertram, C.C., Killeen, J., Le Marchand, L., Selhub, J., Murphy, S., and Donlon, T.A., Association of methylenetetrahydrofolate reductase polymorphism C677T and dietary folate with the risk of cervical dysplasia, *Cancer Epidemiol. Biomarkers Prev.*, 10, 1275, 2001.

84. Chen, J., Gammon, M.D., Chan, W., Palomeque, C., Wetmur, J.G., Kabat, G.C., Teitelbaum, S.L., Britton, J.A., Terry, M.B., Neugut, A.I., and Santella, R.M., One-carbon metabolism, MTHFR polymorphisms, and risk of breast cancer, *Cancer Res.,* 65, 1606, 2005.

85. Friso, S. and Choi, S.W. Gene-nutrient interactions in one-carbon metabolism, *Curr. Drug Metab.,* 6, 37, 2005.

5 Genetic Variability in Folate-Mediated One-Carbon Metabolism and Cancer Risk

Cornelia M. Ulrich

CONTENTS

5.1 INTRODUCTION

Folate is an essential micronutrient in humans; its primary function is as a carrier of single-carbon units. These are used in multiple important biochemical reactions, including the biosynthesis of methionine, thymidine, purines, and glycine, and in the metabolism of serine, formate, and histidine (see also Chapter 4). Figure 5.1 illustrates the principal reactions of folate-mediated one-carbon metabolism (FOCM) in the cytosol, as well as the major transport mechanisms of folate into the cell.

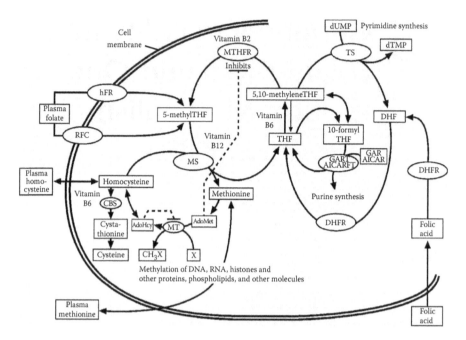

FIGURE 5.1 Overview of folate-mediated one-carbon metabolism (simplified), links to methylation reactions and nucleotide synthesis. **THF** = tetrahydrofolate; **CBS** = cystathionine β-synthase; **DHF** = dihydrofolate; **RFC** = reduced folate carrier; **hFR** = human folate receptor; **MTHFR** = 5,10-methylenetetrahydrofolate reductase; **DHFR** = dihydrofolate reductase; **GART** = glycinamide ribonucleotide transformylase; **AICARFT** = 5-amino-imidazole-4-carboxamide ribonucleotide transformylase; **AICAR** = 5-aminoimidazole-4-carboxamide ribonucleotide; **GAR** = glycinamide ribonucleotide; **SAM (AdoMet)** = S-adenosylmethionine; **SAH (AdoHcy)** = S-adenosylhomocysteine; **dUMP** = deoxyuridine monophosphate; **dTMP** = deoxythymidine monophosphate; **MS** = methionine synthase; **TS** = thymidylate synthase; **MT** = methyltransferases; **X** = a variety of substrates for methylation. (Modified from Ulrich, C.M., Robien, K., and Sparks, R. Pharmacogenetics and folate metabolism — a promising direction. *Pharmacogenomics*, 3: 299–313, 2002. With permission.)

As discussed in greater detail in Chapter 4, several lines of evidence link FOCM to cancer risk. These include experiments in animal models, as well as epidemiological studies investigating dietary intakes or biomarkers of folate status. Animal studies have shown that a methyl-group-deficient diet can enhance liver and colon carcinogenesis, possibly with different effects depending on the transformation state of the cell [1]. Epidemiological evidence is strongest with regard to an inverse association between folate status and colorectal neoplasia. Numerous studies on colorectal adenomas and several on colorectal cancer have quite consistently shown that high dietary folate intakes (or biomarkers of folate intake) are associated with a decreased risk [2–11]. With respect to other cancers, high dietary folate intakes or the biomarkers thereof have also been shown to be associated with a decreased risk of cervical cancer [12–14], esophageal or gastric cancer [15–17], breast cancer (especially in combination with low alcohol intakes) [18–22], and pancreatic cancer [23,24].

More recently, studies linking polymorphisms in FOCM to an altered risk of cancer provide evidence that this may be a causal relationship and is not just attributable to other factors that may correlate with a diet high in folate. This chapter provides an overview of genetic variability in FOCM beyond that due to the *MTHFR* gene (which has been discussed in Chapter 4) and epidemiological studies on cancer risk. Functioning of FOCM requires several nutrients as cofactors of various enzymes, specifically vitamin B_{12}, B_6, and B_2. Further, it is important to consider that folate metabolism represents a complex metabolic pathways with many feedback mechanisms and other regulatory processes that ensure its robustness [25,26]. Accordingly, one may hypothesize that multiple disturbances within the pathway or "stress" on the system are needed to result in phenotypic effects. Such "stress" could be present under low intakes of folate or other nutrients involved in FOCM. Indeed, genetic polymorphisms in *MTHFR* are most strongly associated with biomarkers, such as homocysteine concentrations, under a low folate status. This provides a rationale for investigating gene–gene and gene–nutrient interactions within this complex system.

5.1.1 Investigations of Genetic Variation in Epidemiological Studies

With the advent of the Human Genome Project, an immense amount of information on inherited human genetic variability has become available for research purposes. Studies on relationships between genetic susceptibility and disease are important in that they can (1) support a causal relationship between an environmental factor (e.g., folate) and disease end points, (2) help to understand whether certain individuals or population groups may benefit from higher or reduced intakes of specific nutrients, based on their genetic susceptibility, and (3) assist in elucidating biologic mechanisms linking specific biologic pathways to various disease end points.

Initial epidemiological studies have largely focused on specific "candidate polymorphisms" in proteins that appear critical in the biological pathway (e.g., folate metabolism) or have demonstrated functional relevance. However, this approach is limited in that it does not account for other genetic variants within the same biological pathway or for other genetic polymorphisms within the same gene. In the future it will become increasingly important to undertake comprehensive investigations covering genetic variability in a multitude of biologically interrelated proteins. This pathway approach has resulted in studies combining the investigations of several candidate polymorphisms within FOCM. However, a full integration of biological relationships into epidemiological data analysis can only be achieved if appropriate statistical methods are available and if sample sizes are sufficient to provide stable estimates for gene–gene and gene–environment interactions. Many of the studies reviewed here were limited in their sample sizes and thus reported that gene–gene or gene–nutrient interactions require confirmation in other study populations. Second, a candidate polymorphism approach does not account for additional genetic variation within the same gene or in adjacent genomic regions. The "functional impact" of polymorphisms is often not derived from experimental studies (e.g., knock-in experiments) but by association studies — for example, by measuring the relationship between a specific genotype and homocysteine concentrations. This type of evidence does not preclude that the "candidate polymorphism" is in reality not the causal variant; the cause may be yet another genetic polymorphism that is in linkage disequilibrium with the candidate polymorphism and may cause the observed associations. These concerns can be addressed by investigating gene-wide haplotypes or the combination of haplotypes (e.g., diplotypes), and method development is under-way for incorporating these approaches in epidemiological data analyses [27–30].

5.2 GENETIC VARIABILITY IN ONE-CARBON METABOLISM

Clearly, there is genetic variability in all proteins related to FOCM; resources such as the NIH dbSNP database provide an excellent avenue for exploring this genetic variability. However, many of these genetic polymorphisms, especially if they occur in intronic regions or do not result in an amino acid substitution, are unlikely to have functional impact on the activity or transcription of the protein. Thus, the following summaries of genetic variability focus on polymorphisms that are likely to have phenotypic effects, as indicated by biomarker measurements, or that have been implicated in studies with disease end points.

5.2.1 THYMIDYLATE SYNTHASE (*TS*)

A key substrate in folate metabolism, 5,10-methylene THF can be directed into one of three possible biosynthesis pathways: toward TS, purine synthesis, or via 5,10-methylenetetrahydrofolate reductase (MTHFR) toward methionine synthesis. TS catalyzes the transfer of a methyl group from 5,10-methyleneTHF to deoxyuridine monophosphate, creating deoxythymidine monophosphate and dihydrofolate. TS is also an important drug target for chemotherapeutic agents [21,31]. The 5′-UTR of the *TS* gene contains polymorphic *28-bp* tandem repeats, and these tandem repeat sequences function as a *cis*-acting transcriptional enhancer element [32]. Double and triple repeats occur most commonly; however, much rarer four and nine tandem repeats have also been observed, largely among populations of African descent [33]. The presence of the triple repeat results in approximately two- to fourfold greater gene expression compared to the double repeat [34,35]. The *3R/3R* genotype was found to be associated with reduced plasma folate and increased plasma homocysteine concentrations in individuals with low folate intake [36]. Further, a $G \rightarrow C$ polymorphism has been identified within the second repeat of *3R* alleles that alters the transcriptional activation of *TS* gene constructs bearing this genotype [37]. A third functionally relevant polymorphism, a *6-bp* deletion (*1494del6*), exists within the 3′-UTR of the *TS* gene [38], which has been associated with reduced mRNA stability [38].

5.2.2 METHIONINE SYNTHASE (*MTR*)

MTR catalyzes the methylation of homocysteine to methionine with simultaneous conversion of 5-methyl-tetrahydrofolate (5-methyl-THF) to tetrahydrofolate (THF). A variant in the *MTR* gene (*2756A* $\rightarrow$ *G*, Asp919Gly) [40] may affect plasma homocys-teine concentrations. For example, some studies [41,42], although not all [43–45], observed that homocysteine concentrations tend to decrease linearly across genotypes, with the *AA* genotype associated with the highest homocysteine concentrations.

5.2.3 METHIONINE SYNTHASE REDUCTASE (*MTRR*)

The enzyme methionine synthase reductase (MTRR) is responsible for the reductive methylation of the cobalamin cofactor of methionine synthase [40]. Individuals who lack this enzyme activity suffer from a variety of disorders of folate/cobalamin metabolism [46]. The functional impact of an *66A → G* (Ile22Met) polymorphism remains not well defined [45], although an association between this polymorphism and homocysteine concentrations has been reported [47,48]. A connection between the *66A → G* polymorphism and developmental defects has been proposed [47,49].

5.2.4 SERINE HYDROXYMETHYLTRANSFERASE (*SHMT*)

Serine hydroxymethyltransferase (SHMT) catalyzes the conversion of tetrahydro-folate to 5,10-methylenete THF in a reversible reaction that requires the cofactor pyridoxal-5-phosphate (vitamin B_6). As discussed previously, 5,10-methylene THF is a key substrate in folate metabolism that is directed toward thymidine synthesis, purine synthesis, or via MTHFR toward methionine synthesis. One primary regulatory mechanism within FOCM relates to the synthesis and use of 5,10-methylene THF. With increasing glycine concentrations, cytosolic SHMT (cSHMT) activity increases; thus, more 5,10-methylene THF is committed toward serine synthesis and less 5-methyl-THF is produced [50]. However, the role of cSHMT in FOCM is not clearly established because, in mammals, mitochondrial SHMT also contributes one-carbon units for the cytosolic metabolism [25,51–53].

For a *1420 C → T* polymorphism in the *cSHMT* gene (Leu474Phe), the average concentrations of red blood cell and plasma folate were elevated in individuals with the *T* allele compared to *CC* homozygotes [54]. cSHMT polymorphisms have been studied in relation to hematopoietic malignancies, as described below [55,56].

5.2.5 CYSTATHIONINE β-SYNTHASE (*CBS*)

CBS catalyzes the transsulfuration of homocysteine to cystathionine, and CBS deficiency results in classical homocysteinuria [57]. The reaction requires vitamin B_6 as a cofactor, thus providing a possible rationale for gene–nutrient interactions with respect to nutrients other than folate. Several polymorphisms that are in linkage disequilibrium (a *68-bp* insertion in exon 8, *699C → T, 1080C → T*, and *1985C → T*) have been described [58,59]. These variants may alter homocysteine levels [59,60], modify postmethionine-load homocysteine concentrations [61], and affect coronary artery disease risk [60]. A *31-bp* variable number tandem repeat that spans the exon 12–intron 12 boundary may also affect postmethionine-load homocysteine concentrations [62–64].

5.2.6 REDUCED FOLATE CARRIER (*RFC*)

RFC is responsible for the active transport of 5-methyl-THF from plasma to cytosol. A polymorphism in the *RFC* gene (*80 G → A*, Arg27His) may be associated with a greater carrier function or higher affinity for folate [65]. The variant *A* allele was found to be consistently and linearly associated with higher plasma folate concentrations compared to wild-type, although these differences were not statistically significant [65]. Further, plasma concentrations of methotrexate 24 to 48 h after administration were higher among children with the *AA* genotype, providing additional support for differential carrier activity among those with the variant allele [66].

5.2.7 OTHER GENES (*GGH, DHFR,* AND *TCII*)

Candidate polymorphisms have been described in virtually all proteins relevant to FOCM. To date, epidemiological studies of cancer risk have not yet covered enzymes responsible for polyglutamation or cleavage of γ-glutamyl groups or other key enzymes, such as those related to transcobalamin transport. Some of these candidate polymorphisms are briefly described here.

Intracellular folate concentrations are regulated to some extent by polyglutamation of folate molecules via folylpolyglutamyl synthase (FPGS) and cleavage of these glutamyl groups by γ-glutamyl hydrolase (GGH). Several variants have been reported in the *GGH* gene, *401C → T, 354G → T, 124T → G,* and *452C → T* [67,68], and some of these have been shown to enhance gene expression in hepatoma and breast cancer cells [67]. The polymorphism *452C → T* in exon 5 was found to be associated with GGH activity and to reduce GGH hydrolysis of long-chain methotrexate polyglutamates in leukemia patients treated with high-dose methotrexate [68].

Dihydrofolate reductase (DHFR) is essential for the entry of folic acid into the pathway. Whereas initial reports of several polymorphisms among Japanese could not be confirmed by our group [69], a *19-bp* deletion polymorphism within intron-1 of DHFR may increase risk of spina bifida [70].

Transcobalamin II (TCII) is a serum protein that transports vitamin B_{12} to tissues. As shown in Figure 5.1, vitamin B_{12} is an essential cofactor for the conversion of homocysteine to methionine by methionine synthase. Several variants of *TCII* have been reported, including *776C → G, 67A → G, 280 G → A, 1043 C → T,* and *1196 G → A* [71–73]. The *776C → G* polymorphism is the most common one studied. Studies regarding this polymorphism and either homocysteine or vitamin B_{12} concentrations have been inconsistent [71–81]. Perhaps more relevant are the two studies that found trends of increasing methylmalonic acid among those with the *776GG* genotype [74,75]. Several other variants of *TCII, 67A → G, 280 G → A, 1043 C → T,* and *1196 G → A,* have been reported which may be associated with homocysteine and vitamin B_{12} concentrations [72,73]. Considering the large number of polymorphisms within *TCII,* it will be critical to evaluate genetic variability within *TCII* in a comprehensive fashion.

5.3 GENETIC VARIABILITY IN ONE-CARBON METABOLISM AND CANCER RISK

Folate is essential for nucleotide synthesis and is thus critical for rapidly proliferating tissues. Chemotherapeutic agents, such as folate antagonists or thymidylate synthase inhibitors, reduce the availability of THF derivatives for DNA synthesis and reduce proliferation of neoplastic cells [21,82]. This rationale also explains why rapidly dividing tissues, such as the gastrointestinal tract and hematopoietic cells, are most susceptible to folate depletion and why they are the primary sites of antifolate chemo-therapeutic toxicity. The same pattern holds true for epidemiological studies — higher intakes of folate have shown to be inversely associated with cancers of the gastrointestinal tract (e.g., colon, stomach, and esophagus), and studies on genetic variability in folate metabolism and cancer risk have shown the most intriguing results for colon cancer and hematopoietic malignancies. In the following, an over-view of these findings is given.

5.3.1 COLORECTAL CANCER

Colorectal cancer is a major public health problem in the U.S. and confers a sub-stantial economic burden [83]. As this cancer is fairly common, several research groups have assembled large case–control or intermediate-sized prospective cohort studies. Whereas the case–control studies were generally substantially larger, pro-viding more statistical power for the evaluation of gene–gene or gene–nutrient interactions, they had to rely on questionnaire information for the assessment of dietary status because biomarkers such as serum folate may be affected by the presence of a tumor. This limitation is not given in prospective cohort investigations. Both case–control and prospective cohort studies have targeted associations with colorectal adenoma, an established precursor of colorectal cancer [84]. Studies of adenoma may be based on screening of the full colon by colonoscopy or the distal colon by sigmoidoscopy. The latter can result in misclassification of individuals as polyp free because a sigmoidoscopy does not detect polyps in the proximal colon. Studies of colorectal adenoma may be particularly relevant to FOCM in that genomic hypomethylation is considered an early stage in colorectal carcinogenesis, and thus folate may play a role earlier on during colorectal carcinogenesis [85]. Further, as reviewed by Kim [1] folate may protect against colon carcinogenesis early in the process, whereas higher intakes appear to foster the growth of existing premalignant lesions. Accordingly, one may expect that inverse associations between folate and colon carcinogenesis would be stronger for adenoma than for cancer risk.

Three published studies have investigated polymorphisms in TS and risk of colorectal neoplasia. The initial report by Ulrich et al., who used 510 cases and 604 polyp-free controls, showed little association between the *TS* gene promoter enhancer region (*TSER*) and *TS 1494del6* polymorphisms and the risk of colorectal adenoma [86]. However, a significant interaction between the *TSER* genotype and folate intake was observed: among individuals with *3R/3R* genotypes (corresponding to higher TS expression) folate intake > 440 µg/d (highest tertile) vs. ≤ 440 µg/d was associated with a twofold decreased risk, whereas among individuals with *2R/2R* genotypes high folate intake was associated with an 1.5-fold increased risk. Vitamin B_{12} showed a similar trend. However, a recent study by Chen et al. [87] did not confirm these interactions, yet reported a significant *TSER*–alcohol interaction: those with the *2R/2R* genotype were not at an elevated risk if they had high alcohol consumption, whereas those who were heterozygous or had the *3R/3R* genotype showed an increased risk. A prospective cohort study based on 270 cases of colorectal cancer and 454 controls showed a significantly decreased risk of colorectal cancer in those with lower TS expression (*TSER 2R/2R*) [102]. This risk reduction was consistent with results from the adenoma studies [86,87]. It has been hypothesized that reduced risks associated with *MTHFR 677TT* genotypes may be explained by a greater diversion of 5,10-methylene THF towards TS [88]. However, the findings on *TS* polymorphisms contradict this hypothesis and point toward purine synthesis as a possible mechanism linking FOCM to colorectal carcinogenesis [86]. As highlighted in the preceding text, there appear to be at least three genetic polymorphisms within the *TS* gene that affect gene expression or protein stability [34,37,38]. Accordingly, future studies should genotype all of these genetic variants and have sufficient sample sizes to accommodate the investigation of diplotype analyses.

A polymorphism in MTR [*2756A* → *G*, Asp919Gly) has been investigated by several groups [43,89–92]. This variant is less common, with a minor allele frequency of approximately 0.20; thus few studies have had sufficient sample sizes to investigate risks or gene–diet interactions associated with the homozygous variant genotype, which comprises about 3% of Caucasian populations. The Physician's Health Study and a study involving a very large Norwegian cohort of more than 2000 case–control pairs reported a substantially a decreased risk of colorectal cancer with the variant methionine synthase genotype (*MTR GG*) [43,92]. However, Le Marchand and colleagues did not observe any associations between this polymorphism and the risk of colorectal cancer (727 cases of Japanese, Caucasian, or Native Hawaiian origin with 727 ethnicity-matched controls were used in this study) [89]. Studies regarding colorectal adenoma are inconsistent, showing either an indication toward an increased risk [91] or reduced risk [90]. The variant genotype may reduce risk only in the presence of low alcohol intake [43,91] or high methionine intake [91]. Further, some interactions with *MTHFR* or *TS* have been suggested [89,91]. Unfortunately, the large Norwegian cohort does not have adequate specimens for nutritional biomarker measurements, except for homocysteine, which may be directly affected by methionine synthase genotypes rather than being an appropriate biomarker for folate status [92]. These inconsistencies may be related to limited statistical powers for investigations of gene–nutrient or gene–gene interactions. Thus, there is still need for a thorough evaluation of the risk of the methionine synthase variant and colorectal neoplasia under specific dietary conditions. Further, the direct phenotypic impact of the methionine synthase *2756G* → *A* has not been evaluated — it is unclear whether associations can really be ascribed to this genetic variant or whether it is in linkage disequilibrium with another polymorphism that has phenotypic effects. In addition to biochemical evaluations, haplotype studies, or studies including all common polymorphisms of methionine synthase will help resolve this question.

MTRR has been evaluated in only one case–control study of colorectal cancer, the study suggesting an increased risk among Caucasians but not other ethnicities [89]. Similarly, *cSHMT*, *CBS*, and polymorphisms in methylenetetrahydrofolate dehydrogenase, or glutamate carboxypeptidase have been investigated in only one study each, with no significant associations or gene–gene or gene–diet interactions detected [89,93]. However, sample sizes in these investigations were limited, especially with respect to the evaluation of gene–gene or gene–diet interactions.

5.3.2 Hematopoietic Malignancies

Findings regarding associations between *MTHFR* polymorphisms with several types of leukemia (reviewed in Reference 94) have spurred further investigation into genetic variability in folate-metabolizing enzymes and the risk of hematopoietic malignancies. The *TS* polymorphisms have been evaluated by Skibola et al., both with respect to the risks of adult lymphocytic leukemia (ALL) [55] and non-Hodgkin's lymphoma (NHL) [95]. They observed a significantly reduced risk of ALL among those with variant *2R* alleles in the *TSER* and a significant dose–response pattern [55]. The *1494del6* polymorphism was not investigated in this study. No differences in risk of NHL were seen related to the *TSER* variant. However, the deletion at the base pair *1494* conferred a reduced risk, and this was also apparent when several other polymorphisms that were in linkage disequilibrium with this variant were investigated. Skibola et al. also analyzed combinations of the *TSER* and *TS 1494del6* genotypes and saw that the associations with the *TSER* variant differed depending on the presence or absence of *TS 1494del6*. This significant interaction highlights the need for investigating genotypic variability at several functionally relevant loci within a gene by evaluating possible genotype combinations. Hishida et al. [56] analyzed the *TSER* polymorphism in relation to malignant lymphoma and observed that those who carried at least one variant *TS* 2 R allele were at increased risk. Further, the lymphoma risk was more pronounced among those with a *cSHMT* wild-type genotype (CC).

MTR polymorphisms and hematopoietic malignancies have been evaluated by four groups [95–98]. These studies were generally of insufficient sample size to provide stable risk estimates for the rare homozygous variant genotype. Nevertheless, a statistically significantly increased risk of malignant lymphoma was reported by Matsuo and colleagues [96,98]. One group reported no differences in the risk for ALL [55], whereas another study showed a reduced risk with the heterozygous and homozygous variant genotypes [97]. The latter group also investigated MTRR, but no significant associations were observed for either ALL or NHL.

There is initial evidence that variants in *cSHMT* (*1420C → T*) affect the risk of ALL [55], whereas no associations have been observed for NHL [95] Lastly, an initial investigation of the reduced folate carrier candidate polymorphism (*80G → A*) did not modify the risk of NHL [95].

In summary, these studies provide intriguing evidence that genetic variability in FOCM plays a role in the etiology of hematopoietic malignancies. Studies to date have been modest in sample size and highlight the need for larger investigations that provide sufficient statistical power for investigating rarer variants and gene–gene interactions.

5.3.3 Other Cancer Types

Some initial studies have investigated polymorphisms in folate-metabolizing proteins other than MTHFR and susceptibility to cancers of the bladder (MTR), esophagus or stomach (*TS 1494del*), or prostate (MTR and CBS) [99–101]. None of these reported significant findings. However, sample sizes were limited, and no interactions with dietary factors have been evaluated.

5.4 SUMMARY

As FOCM is essential for nucleotide synthesis and the provision of S-adenosylme-thionine (AdoMet) for methylation reactions, this biological pathway is highly relevant for cancer prevention. Studies on genetic variation in FOCM have just begun to investigate proteins other than MTHFR. There are many genetic polymorphisms, some with strong evidence for phenotypic impact *in vitro*. The epidemiological studies summarized in this chapter also show that these variants may also have *in vivo* effects on carcinogenic processes. Considering the complexities of the pathway, the multiplicity of genetic variability, and the many regulatory mechanisms, this area requires a comprehensive assessment of epidemiological associations with studies of sufficiently large sample sizes to take account of multiple polymorphisms. A complementary approach for understanding the pathway, effects of multiple genetic polymorphisms under various dietary conditions, and biological mechanisms linking FOCM to carcinogenesis may be mathematical modeling, which has yielded promising initial results [26].

ACKNOWLEDGMENT

I would like to thank Dr. Kim Robien and Alanna Boynton for their critical review of this chapter and my colleagues in folate-related research for their contributions during the past years.

REFERENCES

1. Kim, Y.I., Will mandatory folic acid fortification prevent or promote cancer? *Am J Clin Nutr,* 80: 1123–1128, 2004.
2. Benito, E., Obrador, A., Stiggelbout, A., Bosch, F.X., Mulet, M., Munoz, N., and Kaldor, J. A population-based case-control study of colorectal cancer in Majorca. I. Dietary factors. *Int J Cancer,* 45: 69–76, 1990.
3. Giovannucci, E., Rimm, E.B., Ascherio, A., Stampfer, M.J., Colditz, G.A., and Willett, W.C. Alcohol, low-methionine–low-folate diets, and risk of colon cancer in men. *J Natl Cancer Inst,* 87: 265–273, 1995.
4. Giovannucci, E., Stampfer, M.J., Colditz, G.A., Rimm, E.B., Trichopoulos, D., Rosner, B.A., Speizer, F.E., and Willett, W.C. Folate, methionine, and alcohol intake and risk of colorectal adenoma. *J Natl Cancer Inst,* 85: 875–884, 1993.
5. Boutron-Ruault, M.C., Senesse, P., Faivre, J., Couillault, C., and Belghiti, C. Folate and alcohol intakes: related or independent roles in the adenoma-carcinoma sequence? *Nutr Cancer,* 26: 337–346, 1996.
6. Freudenheim, J.L., Graham, S., Marshall, J.R., Haughey, B.P., Cholewinski, S., and Wilkinson, G. Folate intake and carcinogenesis of the colon and rectum. *Int J Epidemiol,* 20: 368–374, 1991.
7. Glynn, S.A., Albanes, D., Pietinen, P., Brown, C.C., Rautalahti, M., Tangrea, J.A., Gunter, E.W., Barrett, M.J., Virtamo, J., and Taylor, P.R. Colorectal cancer and folate status: a nested case-control study among male smokers. *Cancer Epidemiol Biomarkers Prev,* 5: 487–494, 1996.

8. Slattery, M.L., Schaffer, D., Edwards, S.L., Ma, K.N., and Potter, J.D. Are dietary factors involved in DNA methylation associated with colon cancer? *Nutr Cancer*, 28: 52–62, 1997.

9. Kato, I., Dnistrian, A.M., Schwartz, M., Toniolo, P., Koenig, K., Shore, R.E., Akhmed-khanov, A., Zeleniuch-Jacquotte, A., and Riboli, E. Serum folate, homocysteine and colorectal cancer risk in women: a nested case-control study. *Br J Cancer*, 79: 1917–1922, 1999.

10. Giovannucci, E. Epidemiologic studies of folate and colorectal neoplasia: a review. *J Nutr*, 132: 2350S–2355S, 2002.

11. Konings, E.J., Goldbohm, R.A., Brants, H.A., Saris, W.H., and van den Brandt, P.A. Intake of dietary folate vitamers and risk of colorectal carcinoma: results from the Netherlands cohort study. *Cancer*, 95: 1421–1433, 2002.

12. Weinstein, S.J., Ziegler, R.G., Frongillo, E.A., Jr., Colman, N., Sauberlich, H.E., Brinton, L.A., Hamman, R.F., Levine, R.S., Mallin, K., Stolley, P.D., and Bisogni, C.A. Low serum and red blood cell folate are moderately, but nonsignificantly associated with increased risk of invasive cervical cancer in U.S. women. *J Nutr*, 131: 2040–2048, 2001.

13. Alberg, A.J., Selhub, J., Shah, K.V., Viscidi, R.P., Comstock, G.W., and Helzlsouer, K.J. The risk of cervical cancer in relation to serum concentrations of folate, vitamin B12, and homocysteine. *Cancer Epidemiol Biomarkers Prev*, 9: 761–764, 2000.

14. Goodman, M.T., McDuffie, K., Hernandez, B., Wilkens, L.R., Bertram, C.C., Killeen, J., Le Marchand, L., Selhub, J., Murphy, S., and Donlon, T.A. Association of methylenetetrahydrofolate reductase polymorphism C677T and dietary folate with the risk of cervical dysplasia. *Cancer Epidemiol Biomarkers Prev*, 10: 1275–1280, 2001.

15. Zhang, Z.F., Kurtz, R.C., Yu, G.P., Sun, M., Gargon, N., Karpeh, M., Jr., Fein, J.S., and Harlap, S. Adenocarcinomas of the esophagus and gastric cardia: the role of diet. *Nutr Cancer*, 27: 298–309, 1997.

16. Mayne, S.T., Risch, H.A., Dubrow, R., Chow, W.H., Gammon, M.D., Vaughan, T.L., Farrow, D.C., Schoenberg, J.B., Stanford, J.L., Ahsan, H., West, A.B., Rotterdam, H., Blot, W.J., and Fraumeni, J.F., Jr. Nutrient intake and risk of subtypes of esophageal and gastric cancer. *Cancer Epidemiol Biomarkers Prev*, 10: 1055–1062, 2001.

17. Chen, H., Tucker, K.L., Graubard, B.I., Heineman, E.F., Markin, R.S., Potischman, N.A., Russell, R.M., Weisenburger, D.D., and Ward, M.H. Nutrient intakes and adenocarcinoma of the esophagus and distal stomach. *Nutr Cancer*, 42: 33–40, 2002.

18. Shrubsole, M.J., Jin, F., Dai, Q., Shu, X.O., Potter, J.D., Hebert, J.R., Gao, Y.T., and Zheng, W. Dietary folate intake and breast cancer risk: results from the Shanghai breast cancer study. *Cancer Res*, 61: 7136–7141, 2001.

19. Sellers, T.A., Kushi, L.H., Cerhan, J.R., Vierkant, R.A., Gapstur, S.M., Vachon, C.M., Olson, J.E., Therneau, T.M., and Folsom, A.R. Dietary folate intake, alcohol, and risk of breast cancer in a prospective study of postmenopausal women. *Epidemiology*, 12: 420–428, 2001.

20. Rohan, T.E., Jain, M.G., Howe, G.R., and Miller, A.B. Dietary folate consumption and breast cancer risk. *J Natl Cancer Inst*, 92: 266–269, 2000.

21. Ulrich, C.M., Robien, K., and Sparks, R. Pharmacogenetics and folate metabolism — a promising direction. *Pharmacogenomics*, 3: 299–313, 2002.

22. Sellers, T.A., Vierkant, R.A., Cerhan, J.R., Gapstur, S.M., Vachon, C.M., Olson, J.E., Pankratz, V.S., Kushi, L.H., and Folsom, A.R. Interaction of dietary folate intake, alcohol, and risk of hormone receptor-defined breast cancer in a prospective study of postmenopausal women. *Cancer Epidemiol Biomarkers Prev*, 11: 1104–1107, 2002.

23. Stolzenberg-Solomon, R.Z., Albanes, D., Nieto, F.J., Hartman, T.J., Tangrea, J.A., Rautalahti, M., Sehlub, J., Virtamo, J., and Taylor, P.R. Pancreatic cancer risk and nutrition-related methyl-group availability indicators in male smokers. *J Natl Cancer Inst*, 91: 535–541, 1999.

24. Stolzenberg-Solomon, R.Z., Pietinen, P., Barrett, M.J., Taylor, P.R., Virtamo, J., and Albanes, D. Dietary and other methyl-group availability factors and pancreatic cancer risk in a cohort of male smokers. *Am J Epidemiol*, 153: 680–687, 2001.

25. Wagner, C. Biochemical role of folate in cellular metabolism, in *Folate in Health and Disease*. New York: Marcel Dekker, 1995.

26. Nijhout, H.F., Reed, M.C., Budu, P., and Ulrich, C.M. A mathematical model of the folate cycle: new insights into folate homeostasis. *J Biol Chem*, 279: 55008–55016, 2004.

27. Dawson, E., Abecasis, G.R., Bumpstead, S., Chen, Y., Hunt, S., Beare, D.M., Pabial, J., Dibling, T., Tinsley, E., Kirby, S., Carter, D., Papaspyridonos, M., Livingstone, S., Ganske, R., Lohmussaar, E., Zernant, J., Tonisson, N., Remm, M., Magi, R., Puurand, T., Vilo, J., Kurg, A., Rice, K., Deloukas, P., Mott, R., Metspalu, A., Bentley, D.R., Cardon, L.R., and Dunham, I. A first-generation linkage disequilibrium map of human chromosome 22. *Nature*, 418: 544–548, 2002.

28. Johnson, G.C., Esposito, L., Barratt, B.J., Smith, A.N., Heward, J., Di Genova, G., Ueda, H., Cordell, H.J., Eaves, I.A., Dudbridge, F., Twells, R.C., Payne, F., Hughes, W., Nutland, S., Stevens, H., Carr, P., Tuomilehto-Wolf, E., Tuomilehto, J., Gough, S.C., Clayton, D.G., and Todd, J.A. Haplotype tagging for the identification of common disease genes. *Nat Genet*, 29: 233–237, 2001.

29. Patil, N., Berno, A.J., Hinds, D.A., Barrett, W.A., Doshi, J.M., Hacker, C.R., Kautzer, C.R., Lee, D.H., Marjoribanks, C., McDonough, D.P., Nguyen, B.T., Norris, M.C., Sheehan, J.B., Shen, N., Stern, D., Stokowski, R.P., Thomas, D.J., Trulson, M.O., Vyas, K.R., Frazer, K.A., Fodor, S.P., and Cox, D.R. Blocks of limited haplotype diversity revealed by high-resolution scanning of human chromosome 21. *Science*, 294: 1719–1723, 2001.

30. Gabriel, S.B., Schaffner, S.F., Nguyen, H., Moore, J.M., Roy, J., Blumenstiel, B., Higgins, J., DeFelice, M., Lochner, A., Faggart, M., Liu-Cordero, S.N., Rotimi, C., Adeyemo, A., Cooper, R., Ward, R., Lander, E.S., Daly, M.J., and Altshuler, D. The structure of haplotype blocks in the human genome. *Science*, 296: 2225–2229, 2002.

31. Ulrich, C.M., Robien, K., and McLeod, H.L. Cancer pharmacogenetics: polymorphisms, pathways and beyond. *Nat Rev Cancer*, 3: 912–920, 2003.

32. Kaneda, S., Takeishi, K., Ayusawa, D., Shimizu, K., Seno, T., and Altman, S. Role in translation of a triple tandemly repeated sequence in the 5-untranslated region of human thymidylate synthase mRNA. *Nucleic Acids Res*, 15: 1259–1270, 1987.

33. Marsh, S., Ameyaw, M.M., Githang'a, J., Indalo, A., Ofori-Adjei, D., and McLeod, H.L. Novel thymidylate synthase enhancer region alleles in African populations. *Hum Mutation*, 16: 528, 2000.

34. Horie, N., Aiba, H., Oguro, K., Hojo, H., and Takeishi, K. Functional analysis and DNA polymorphism of the tandemly repeated sequences in the 5-terminal regulatory region of the human gene for thymidylate synthase. *Cell Struct Function*, 20: 191–197, 1995.

35. Pullarkat, S.T., Stoehlmacher, J., Ghaderi, V., Xiong, Y.-P., Ingles, S.A., Sherrod, A., Warren, R., Tsao-Wei, D., Groshen, S., and Lenz, H.-J. Thymidylate synthase gene polymorphism determines response and toxicity of 5-FU chemotherapy. *Pharmacogenomics J*, 1: 65–70, 2001.

36. Trinh, B.N., Ong, C.-N., Coetzee, G.A., Yu, M.C., and Laird, P.W. Thymidylate synthase: a novel genetic determinant of plasma homocysteine and folate levels. *Hum Genet*, 111: 299–302, 2002.

37. Mandola, M.V., Stoehlmacher, J., Muller-Weeks, S., Cesarone, G., Yu, M.C., Lenz, H.J., and Ladner, R.D. A novel single nucleotide polymorphism within the 5 tandem repeat polymorphism of the thymidylate synthase gene abolishes USF-1 binding and alters transcriptional activity. *Cancer Res*, 63: 2898–2904, 2003.

38. Ulrich, C., Bigler, J., Velicer, C., Greene, E., Farin, F., and Potter, J. Searching expressed sequence tag databases: discovery and confirmation of a common polymorphism in the thymidylate synthase gene. *Cancer Epidemiol Biomarkers Prev*, 9: 1381–1385, 2000.

39. Mandola, M.V., Stoehlmacher, J., Zhang, W., Groshen, S., Yu, M.C., Iqbal, S., Lenz, H.J., and Ladner, R.D. A 6 bp polymorphism in the thymidylate synthase gene causes message instability and is associated with decreased intratumoral TS mRNA levels. *Pharmacogenetics*, 14: 319–327, 2004.

40. Leclerc, D., Wilson, A., Dumas, R., Gafuik, C., Song, D., Watkins, D., Heng, H.H., Rommens, J.M., Scherer, S.W., Rosenblatt, D.S., and Gravel, R.A. Cloning and mapping of a cDNA for methionine synthase reductase, a flavoprotein defective in patients with homocystinuria. *Proc Natl Acad Sci USA*, 95: 3059–3064, 1998.

41. Chen, J., Stampfer, M.J., Ma, J., Selhub, J., Malinow, M.R., Hennekens, C.H., and Hunter, D.J. Influence of a methionine synthase (D919G) polymorphism on plasma homocysteine and folate levels and relation to risk of myocardial infarction. *Atherosclerosis*, 154: 667–672, 2001.

42. Harmon, D., Shields, D., Woodside, J., McMaster, D., Yarnell, J., Young, I., Peng, K., Shane, B., Evans, A., and Whitehead, A. Methionine synthase D919G polymorphism is a significant but modest determinant of circulating homocysteine concentrations. *Genet Epidemiol*, 17: 298–309, 1999.

43. Ma, J., Stampfer, M.J., Christensen, B., Giovannucci, E., Hunter, D.J., Chen, J., Willett, W.C., Selhub, J., Hennekens, C.H., Gravel, R., and Rozen, R. A polymorphism of the methionine synthase gene: association with plasma folate, vitamin B12, homocyst(e)ine, and colorectal cancer risk. *Cancer Epidemiol Biomarkers Prev*, 8: 825–829, 1999.

44. van der Put, N.M., van der Molen, E.F., Kluijtmans, L.A., Heil, S.G., Trijbels, J.M., Eskes, T.K., Van Oppenraaij-Emmerzaal, D., Banerjee, R., and Blom, H.J. Sequence analysis of the coding region of human methionine synthase: relevance to hyperhomocysteinaemia in neural-tube defects and vascular disease. *QJM*, 90: 511–517, 1997.

45. Jacques, P.F., Bostom, A.G., Selhub, J., Rich, S., Curtis Ellison, R., Eckfeldt, J.H., Gravel, R.A., and Rozen, R. Effects of polymorphisms of methionine synthase and methionine synthase reductase on total plasma homocysteine in the NHLBI Family Heart Study. *Atherosclerosis*, 166: 49–55, 2003.

46. Watkins, D. and Rosenblatt, D.S. Functional methionine synthase deficiency (cblE and cblG): clinical and biochemical heterogeneity. *Am J Med Genet*, 34: 427–434, 1989.

47. Wilson, A., Platt, R., Wu, Q., Leclerc, D., Christensen, B., Yang, H., Gravel, R.A., and Rozen, R. A common variant in methionine synthase reductase combined with low cobalamin (vitamin B12) increases risk for spina bifida. *Mol Genet Metab*, 67: 317–323, 1999.

48. Gaughan, D.J., Kluijtmans, L.A., Barbaux, S., McMaster, D., Young, I.S., Yarnell, J.W., Evans, A., and Whitehead, A.S. The methionine synthase reductase (MTRR) A66G polymorphism is a novel genetic determinant of plasma homocysteine concentrations. *Atherosclerosis*, 157: 451–456, 2001.

49. O'Leary, V.B., Parle-McDermott, A., Molloy, A.M., Kirke, P.N., Johnson, Z., Conley, M., Scott, J.M., and Mills, J.L. MTRR and MTHFR polymorphism: link to Down syndrome? *Am J Med Genet*, 107: 151–155, 2002.

50. Herbig, K., Chiang, E.P., Lee, L.R., Hills, J., Shane, B., and Stover, P.J. Cytoplasmic serine hydroxymethyltransferase mediates competition between folate-dependent deoxyribonucleotide and S-adenosylmethionine biosyntheses. *J Biol Chem*, 277: 38381–38389, 2002.

51. Garrow, T.A., Brenner, A.A., Whitehead, V.M., Chen, X.N., Duncan, R.G., Korenberg, J.R., and Shane, B. Cloning of human cDNAs encoding mitochondrial and cytosolic serine hydroxymethyltransferases and chromosomal localization. *J Biol Chem*, 268: 11910–11916, 1993.

52. Liu, X., Szebenyi, D.M., Anguera, M.C., Thiel, D.J., and Stover, P.J. Lack of catalytic activity of a murine mRNA cytoplasmic serine hydroxymethyltransferase splice variant: evidence against alternative splicing as a regulatory mechanism. *Biochemistry*, 40: 4932–4939, 2001.

53. Stover, P.J., Chen, L.H., Suh, J.R., Stover, D.M., Keyomarsi, K., and Shane, B. Molecular cloning, characterization, and regulation of the human mitochondrial serine hydroxymethyltransferase gene. *J Biol Chem*, 272: 1842–1848, 1997.

54. Heil, S.G., Van der Put, N.M., Waas, E.T., den Heijer, M., Trijbels, F.J., and Blom, H.J. Is mutated serine hydroxymethyltransferase (SHMT) involved in the etiology of neural tube defects? *Mol Genet Metab*, 73: 164–172, 2001.

55. Skibola, C.F., Smith, M.T., Hubbard, A., Shane, B., Roberts, A.C., Law, G.R., Rollinson, S., Roman, E., Cartwright, R.A., and Morgan, G.J. Polymorphisms in the thymidylate synthase and serine hydroxymethyltransferase genes and risk of adult acute lymphocytic leukemia. *Blood*, 99: 3786–3791, 2002.

56. Hishida, A., Matsuo, K., Hamajima, N., Ito, H., Ogura, M., Kagami, Y., Taji, H., Morishima, Y., Emi, N., and Tajima, K. Associations between polymorphisms in the thymidylate synthase and serine hydroxymethyltransferase genes and susceptibility to malignant lymphoma. *Haematologica*, 88: 159–166, 2003.

57. Mudd, S.H., Levy, H.L., and Skovby, F. Disorders of transsulfuration, in Scriver, C.R., Beaudet, A.L., Sly, W.S., and Valle, D., Eds., *The Metabolic and Molecular Basis of Inherited Disease*. New York: McGraw-Hill, 1995, pp. 1279–1327.

58. Kraus, J.P., Oliveriusova, J., Sokolova, J., Kraus, E., Vlcek, C., de Franchis, R., Maclean, K.N., Bao, L., Bukovsk, Patterson, D., Paces, V., Ansorge, W., and Kozich, V. The human cystathionine beta-synthase (CBS) gene: complete sequence, alternative splicing, and polymorphisms. *Genomics*, 52: 312–324, 1998.

59. De Stefano, V., Dekou, V., Nicaud, V., Chasse, J.F., London, J., Stansbie, D., Humphries, S.E., and Gudnason, V. Linkage disequilibrium at the cystathionine beta synthase (CBS) locus and the association between genetic variation at the CBS locus and plasma levels of homocysteine. The Ears II Group. European Atherosclerosis Research Study. *Ann Hum Genet*, 62: 481–490, 1998.

60. Kruger, W.D., Evans, A.A., Wang, L., Malinow, M.R., Duell, P.B., Anderson, P.H., Block, P.C., Hess, D.L., Graf, E.E., and Upson, B. Polymorphisms in the CBS gene associated with decreased risk of coronary artery disease and increased responsiveness to total homocysteine lowering by folic acid. *Mol Genet Metab*, 70: 53–60, 2000.

61. Aras, O., Hanson, N.Q., Yang, F., and Tsai, M.Y. Influence of 699C→T and 1080C→T polymorphisms of the cystathionine beta-synthase gene on plasma homocysteine levels. *Clin Genet*, 58: 455–459, 2000.

62. Sebastio, G., Sperandeo, M.P., Panico, M., de Franchis, R., Kraus, J.P., and Andria, G. The molecular basis of homocystinuria due to cystathionine beta-synthase deficiency in Italian families, and report of four novel mutations. *Am J Hum Genet*, 56: 1324–1333, 1995.

63. Lievers, K.J., Kluijtmans, L.A., Heil, S.G., Boers, G.H., Verhoef, P., van Oppenraay-Emmerzaal, D., den Heijer, M., Trijbels, F.J., and Blom, H.J. A 31 bp VNTR in the cystathionine beta-synthase (CBS) gene is associated with reduced CBS activity and elevated post-load homocysteine levels. *Eur J Hum Genet*, 9: 583–589, 2001.

64. Yang, F., Hanson, N.Q., Schwichtenberg, K., and Tsai, M.Y. Variable number tandem repeat in exon/intron border of the cystathionine beta-synthase gene: a single nucleotide substitution in the second repeat prevents multiple alternate splicing. *Am J Med Genet*, 95: 385–390, 2000.

65. Chango, A., Emery-Fillon, N., de Courcy, G.P., Lambert, D., Pfister, M., Rosenblatt, D.S., and Nicolas, J.P. A polymorphism (80G→A) in the reduced folate carrier gene and its associations with folate status and homocysteinemia. *Mol Genet Metab*, 70: 310–315, 2000.

66. Laverdiere, C., Chiasson, S., Costea, I., Moghrabi, A., and Krajinovic, M. Polymorphism G80A in the reduced folate carrier gene and its relationship to methotrexate plasma levels and outcome of childhood acute lymphoblastic leukemia. *Blood*, 100: 3832–3834, 2002.

67. Chave, K.J., Ryan, T.J., Chmura, S.E., and Galivan, J. Identification of single nucleotide polymorphisms in the human gamma-glutamyl hydrolase gene and characterization of promoter polymorphisms. *Gene*, 319: 167–175, 2003.

68. Cheng, Q., Wu, B., Kager, L., Panetta, J.C., Zheng, J., Pui, C.H., Relling, M.V., and Evans, W.E. A substrate specific functional polymorphism of human gamma-glutamyl hydrolase alters catalytic activity and methotrexate polyglutamate accumulation in acute lymphoblastic leukaemia cells. *Pharmacogenetics*, 14: 557–567, 2004.

69. Goto, Y., Yue, L., Yokoi, A., Nishimura, R., Uehara, T., Koizumi, S., and Saikawa, Y. A novel single-nucleotide polymorphism in the 3-untranslated region of the human dihydrofolate reductase gene with enhanced expression. *Clin Cancer Res*, 7: 1952–1956, 2001.

70. Johnson, W.G., Stenroos, E.S., Spychala, J.R., Chatkupt, S., Ming, S.X., and Buyske, S. New 19 bp deletion polymorphism in intron-1 of dihydrofolate reductase (DHFR): a risk factor for spina bifida acting in mothers during pregnancy? *Am J Med Genet*, 124A: 339–345, 2004.

71. Afman, L.A., Van Der Put, N.M., Thomas, C.M., Trijbels, J.M., and Blom, H.J. Reduced vitamin B12 binding by transcobalamin II increases the risk of neural tube defects. *QJM*, 94: 159–166, 2001.

72. Afman, L.A., Lievers, K.J., van der Put, N.M., Trijbels, F.J., and Blom, H.J. Single nucleotide polymorphisms in the transcobalamin gene: relationship with transcobalamin concentrations and risk for neural tube defects. *Eur J Hum Genet*, 10: 433–438, 2002.

73. Lievers, K.J., Afman, L.A., Kluijtmans, L.A., Boers, G.H., Verhoef, P., den Heijer, M., Trijbels, F.J., and Blom, H.J. Polymorphisms in the transcobalamin gene: association with plasma homocysteine in healthy individuals and vascular disease patients. *Clin Chem*, 48: 1383–1389, 2002.

74. Geisel, J., Hubner, U., Bodis, M., Schorr, H., Knapp, J.P., Obeid, R., and Herrmann, W. The role of genetic factors in the development of hyperhomocysteinemia. *Clin Chem Lab Med*, 41: 1427–1434, 2003.

75. Miller, J.W., Ramos, M.I., Garrod, M.G., Flynn, M.A., and Green, R. Transcobalamin II 775G > C polymorphism and indices of vitamin B12 status in healthy older adults. *Blood*, 100: 718–720, 2002.

76. Zetterberg, H., Nexo, E., Regland, B., Minthon, L., Boson, R., Palmer, M., Rymo, L., and Blennow, K. The transcobalamin (TC) codon 259 genetic polymorphism influences holo-TC concentration in cerebrospinal fluid from patients with Alzheimer disease. *Clin Chem*, 49: 1195–1198, 2003.

77. Zetterberg, H., Coppola, A., D'Angelo, A., Palmer, M., Rymo, L., and Blennow, K. No association between the MTHFR A1298C and transcobalamin C776G genetic polymorphisms and hyperhomocysteinemia in thrombotic disease. *Thromb Res*, 108: 127–131, 2002.

78. Winkelmayer, W.C., Skoupy, S., Eberle, C., Fodinger, M., and Sunder-Plassmann, G. Effects of TCN2 776C > G on vitamin B, folate, and total homocysteine levels in kidney transplant patients. *Kidney Int*, 65: 1877–1881, 2004.

79. Wans, S., Schuttler, K., Jakubiczka, S., Muller, A., Luley, C., and Dierkes, J. Analysis of the transcobalamin II 776C > G (259P > R) single nucleotide polymorphism by denaturing HPLC in healthy elderly: associations with cobalamin, homocysteine and holo-transcobalamin II. *Clin Chem Lab Med*, 41: 1532–1536, 2003.

80. Fodinger, M., Veitl, M., Skoupy, S., Wojcik, J., Rohrer, C., Hagen, W., Puttinger, H., Hauser, A.C., Vychytil, A., and Sunder-Plassmann, G. Effect of TCN2 776C > G on vitamin B12 cellular availability in end-stage renal disease patients. *Kidney Int*, 64: 1095–1100, 2003.

81. Anello, G., Gueant-Rodriguez, R.M., Bosco, P., Gueant, J.L., Romano, A., Namour, B., Spada, R., Caraci, F., Pourie, G., Daval, J.L., and Ferri, R. Homocysteine and methylenetetrahydrofolate reductase polymorphism in Alzheimer's disease. *Neuroreport*, 15: 859–861, 2004.

82. Chu, E. and Allegra, C. Antifolates, in Chabner, B. and Longo, D., Eds., *Cancer Chemotherapy and Biotherapy*, Philadelphia: Lippincott-Raven, 1996, pp. 109–148.

83. Sandler, R.S., Everhart, J.E., Donowitz, M., Adams, E., Cronin, K., Goodman, C., Gemmen, E., Shah, S., Avdic, A., and Rubin, R. The burden of selected digestive diseases in the United States. *Gastroenterology*, 122: 1500–1511, 2002.

84. Winawer, S.J., Zauber, A.G., Ho, M.N., MJ, O.B., Gottlieb, L.S., Sternberg, S.S., Waye, J.D., Schapiro, M., Bond, J.H., Panish, J.F., Ackroyd, F., Shike, M., Kurtz, R.C., Hornsby-Lewis, L., Gerdes, H., Stewart, E.T., and The National Polyp Study Workgroup. Prevention of colorectal cancer by colonoscopic polypectomy. The National Polyp Study Workgroup, *N Engl J Med*, 329: 1977–1981, 1993.

85. Fearon, E.R., and Vogelstein, B. A genetic model for colorectal tumorigenesis. *Cell*, 61: 759–767, 1990.

86. Ulrich, C.M., Bigler, J., Bostick, R., Fosdick, L., and Potter, J.D. Thymidylate synthase promoter polymorphism, interaction with folate intake, and risk of colorectal adenomas. *Cancer Res*, 62: 3361–3364, 2002.

87. Chen, J., Kyte, C., Chan, W., Wetmur, J.G., Fuchs, C.S., and Giovannucci, E. Polymorphism in the thymidylate synthase promoter enhancer region and risk of colorectal adenomas. *Cancer Epidemiol Biomarkers Prev*, 13: 2247–2250, 2004.

88. Choi, S.W. and Mason, J.B. Folate and carcinogenesis: an integrated scheme. *J Nutr*, 130: 129–132, 2000.

89. Le Marchand, L., Donlon, T., Hankin, J.H., Kolonel, L.N., Wilkens, L.R., and Seifried, A. B-vitamin intake, metabolic genes, and colorectal cancer risk (United States). *Cancer Causes Control*, 13: 239–248, 2002.

90. Chen, J., Giovannucci, E., Hankinson, S.E., Ma, J., Willett, W.C., Spiegelman, D., Kelsey, K.T., and Hunter, D.J. A prospective study of methylenetetrahydrofolate reductase and methionine synthase gene polymorphisms, and risk of colorectal adenoma. *Carcinogenesis*, 19: 2129–2132, 1998.

91. Goode, E.L., Potter, J.D., Bigler, J., and Ulrich, C.M. Methionine synthase D919G polymorphism, folate metabolism, and colorectal adenoma risk. *Cancer Epidemiol Biomarkers Prev*, 13: 157–162, 2004.

92. Ulvik, A., Vollset, S.E., Hansen, S., Gislefoss, R., Jellum, E., and Ueland, P.M. Colorectal cancer and the methylenetetrahydrofolate reductase 677C→T and methionine synthase 2756A→G polymorphisms: a study of 2,168 case-control pairs from the JANUS Cohort. *Cancer Epidemiol Biomarkers Prev*, 13: 2175–2180, 2004.

93. Chen, J., Kyte, C., Valcin, M., Chan, W., Wetmur, J.G., Selhub, J., Hunter, D.J., and Ma, J. Polymorphisms in the one-carbon metabolic pathway, plasma folate levels and colorectal cancer in a prospective study. *Int J Cancer*, 110: 617–620, 2004.

94. Robien, K. and Ulrich, C.M. 5,10-methylenetetrahydrofolate reductase polymorphisms and leukemia risk. *Am J Epidemiol*, 157: 571–582, 2003.

95. Skibola, C.F., Forrest, M.S., Coppede, F., Agana, L., Hubbard, A., Smith, M.T., Bracci, P.M., and Holly, E.A. Polymorphisms and haplotypes in folate-metabolizing genes and risk of non-Hodgkin lymphoma. *Blood*, 104: 2155–2162, 2004.

96. Matsuo, K., Hamajima, N., Suzuki, R., Ogura, M., Kagami, Y., Taji, H., Yasue, T., Mueller, N.E., Nakamura, S., Seto, M., Morishima, Y., and Tajima, K. Methylenetetrahydrofolate reductase (MTHFR) gene polymorphisms and reduced risk of malignant lymphoma. *Am J Hematol*, 77: 351–357, 2004.

97. Gemmati, D., Ongaro, A., Scapoli, G.L., Della Porta, M., Tognazzo, S., Serino, M.L., Di Bona, E., Rodeghiero, F., Gilli, G., Reverberi, R., Caruso, A., Pasello, M., Pellati, A., and De Mattei, M. Common gene polymorphisms in the metabolic folate and methylation pathway and the risk of acute lymphoblastic leukemia and non-Hodgkin's lymphoma in adults. *Cancer Epidemiol Biomarkers Prev*, 13: 787–94, 2004.

98. Matsuo, K., Suzuki, R., Hamajima, N., Ogura, M., Kagami, Y., Taji, H., Kondoh, E., Maeda, S., Asakura, S., Kaba, S., Nakamura, S., Seto, M., Morishima, Y., and Tajima, K. Association between polymorphisms of folate- and methionine-metabolizing enzymes and susceptibility to malignant lymphoma. *Blood,* 97: 3205–3209, 2001.

99. Lin, J., Spitz, M.R., Wang, Y., Schabath, M.B., Gorlov, I.P., Hernandez, L.M., Pillow, P.C., Grossman, H.B., and Wu, X. Polymorphisms of folate metabolic genes and susceptibility to bladder cancer: a case-control study. *Carcinogenesis,* 25: 1639–1647, 2004.

100. Gao, C.M., Takezaki, T., Wu, J.Z., Liu, Y.T., Ding, J.H., Li, S.P., Su, P., Hu, X., Kai, H.T., Li, Z.Y., Matsuo, K., Hamajima, N., Sugimura, H., and Tajima, K. Polymorphisms in thymidylate synthase and methylenetetrahydrofolate reductase genes and the susceptibility to esophageal and stomach cancer with smoking. *Asian Pac J Cancer Prev*, 5: 133–138, 2004.

101. Kimura, F., Franke, K.H., Steinhoff, C., Golka, K., Roemer, H.C., Anastasiadis, A.G., and Schulz, W.A. Methyl group metabolism gene polymorphisms and susceptibility to prostatic carcinoma. *Prostate*, 45: 225–231, 2000.

102. Chen, J., Hunter, D.J., Stampfer, M.J., Kyte, C., Chan, W., Wetmur, J.G., Mosig, R., Selhub, J., and Ma, J. Polymorphisms in the thymidylate synthase promoter enhancer region modifies the risk and survival of colorectal cancer. *Cancer Epidemiol. Biomarkers Prev.,* 12: 958–962, 2003.

6 S-Adenosylmethionine and Methionine Adenosyltransferase Genes

José M. Mato, M. Luz Martínez-Chantar, and Shelly C. Lu

CONTENTS

6.1 ADOMET METABOLISM

S-Adenosylmethionine (AdoMet, also abbreviated as SAMe or SAM) was discovered by Giulio Cantoni about 50 years ago; however, the story of AdoMet begins in 1890 with Whilhelm His when he fed pyridine to dogs and isolated *N*-methylpyridine from their urine. His work emphasized the need to demonstrate both the origin of the methyl group as well as the mechanism for its addition to pyridine (reviewed by Finkelstein, [1]). Both issues were addressed by Vincent du Vigneaud who, during the late 1930s, demonstrated that the sulfur atom of methionine was converted to cysteine through the "transsulfuration" pathway and discovered the "transmethylation" pathway, that is, the exchange of methyl groups between methionine, choline, betaine, and creatine. In 1951, Cantoni showed that a liver homogenate supplemented with ATP and methionine converted nicotinamide to N-methylnicotinamide. Two years later, he established that methionine and ATP reacted to form a product that he originally called *active methionine*, capable of transferring its methyl group to nicotinamide or guanidoacetic acid to form N-methylmethionine or creatine in the absence of ATP which, after determination of its structure, he called AdoMet. Subsequently, Cantoni and his colleagues discovered the enzyme that synthesizes AdoMet, methionine adenosyltransferase (MAT); S-adenosylhomocysteine (AdoHcy), the product of transmethylation reactions; and AdoHcy-hydrolase, the enzyme that converts AdoHcy into adenosine and homocysteine (Hcy). At about the same time, Bennett discovered that folate and vitamin B_{12} could replace choline as a source of methyl groups in rats maintained on diets containing Hcy in place of methionine, a finding that led to the discovery of methionine synthase (MS). In 1961, Tabor demonstrated that the propylamino moiety of AdoMet is converted via a series of enzymatic steps to spermidine and spermine. In the biosynthesis of polyamines, 5'-deoxy-5'-methylthioadenosine (MTA) was identified as an end product. Thus, by the beginning of the Sixties, Laster's group could finally provide an integrated view, similar to that depicted in Figure 6.1, combining the transmethylation and transsulfuration pathways with polyamine synthesis, known as the methionine cycle.

The crucial role of the liver in the regulation of blood methionine concentration was first established by Kinsell et al. [2], who showed a marked impairment of methionine metabolism in patients with liver cirrhosis. Later work, mainly by Finkelstein and Mudd, demonstrated that under normal conditions, both in humans and rats, about 85% of all transmethylation reactions and approximately 50% of all methionine metabolism occur in the liver [3,4].

6.2 *MAT* GENES AND THEIR REGULATION

In mammals, there are three distinct enzymes that synthesize AdoMet: MATI, MATII, and MATIII. MATI and MATIII are the gene products of *MAT1A*, whereas MATII is the gene product of *MAT2A* (reviewed by Kotb et al. [5]). In adults, *MAT1A* is expressed exclusively in the liver and pancreas, whereas *MAT2A* is expressed in all tissues including the liver. In fetal rat liver, *MAT1A* expression increases progressively from day 20 of gestation, increases tenfold immediately after birth, and reaches a peak at 10 d of age, decreasing slightly by adulthood. Conversely, *MAT2A* expression decreases after birth, increases threefold in the newborn and decreases further in postnatal life, reaching a minimum in the adult liver (about 5% of *MAT1A*). Due to differences in the regulatory and kinetic properties of various MATs, MATII cannot maintain the same high levels of AdoMet as compared to the combination of MATI and MATIII (reviewed by Mato et al. [6]). Consequently, a switch in *MAT*

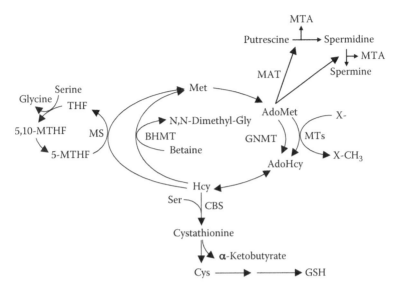

FIGURE 6.1 Hepatic AdoMet metabolism. *S*-adenosylmethionine (AdoMet) is generated from methionine (Met) in a reaction catalyzed by methionine adenosyltransferase (MAT). AdoMet is the principal biological methyl donor and a precursor for polyamine synthesis. In the polyamine synthesis pathway, AdoMet is decarboxylated and the remaining propylamino moiety attached to its sulfonium ion is donated to putrescine to form spermidine and methyl-thioadenosine (MTA) and to spermidine to form spermine and a second molecule of MTA. In transmethylation, AdoMet donates its methyl group to a large variety of acceptor molecules in reactions catalyzed by dozens of methyltransferase (MTs), the most abundant in the liver being glycine-*N*-methyltransferase (GNMT). *S*-adenosylhomocysteine (AdoHcy) is generated as a product of transmethylation and is hydrolyzed to form homocysteine (Hcy) and adenosine through a reversible reaction catalyzed by AdoHcy hydrolase. AdoHcy is a potent competitive inhibitor of methylation reactions and prompt removal of adenosine and Hcy is required to prevent accumulation of AdoHcy. Hcy can be remethylated to form methionine by two enzymes: methionine synthase (MS) and betaine homocysteine methyltransferase (BHMT). In the liver, Hcy can also undergo the transsulfuration pathway to form cysteine (a precursor of GSH) via a two-step enzymatic process catalyzed by cystathionine β-synthetase (CBS) and cystathionase. In tissues other than the liver, kidney, and pancreas, cystathionine is not converted to GSH owing to the lack of expression of one or more enzymes of the transsulfuration pathway. All mammalian tissues express MAT and MS, whereas BHMT expression is limited to the liver.

gene expression can affect the steady state hepatic AdoMet content. Thus, in *MAT1A* knockout mice, despite a significant increase in *MAT2A* expression, the liver content of AdoMet is reduced about threefold from birth, when the switch from *MAT2A* to *MAT1A* takes place in wild-type mice [7].

MATII has the lowest K_m for methionine but is tightly regulated by AdoMet with an IC_{50} of 60 μmol/l, which is close to the normal intracellular hepatic AdoMet concentration [5]. In contrast, AdoMet has a minimal inhibitory effect on MATI and stimulates MATIII [5]. Thus, the AdoMet content in cells that express only the

MATII isoform is relatively unaffected by fluctuations in methionine availability because of the negative feedback inhibition, whereas the rate of AdoMet synthesis and AdoMet content increases with increasing methionine availability in cells that express mostly MATI and MATIII [6]. The liver also contains glycine N-methyl-transferase (GNMT), a liver-specific enzyme accounting for about 1% of the cytosolic protein in this organ, which shows positive cooperativity for AdoMet and whose main function is to remove excess AdoMet synthesized during methionine load [8]. In this way, when the liver synthesizes large amounts of AdoMet, the excess of this molecule is not used to hypermethylate nucleic acid or proteins or to synthesize of polyamines, which may be detrimental to the liver [9], but is converted rapidly to AdoHcy by GNMT (Figure 6.1). MATII is regulated by a MAT β subunit that associates with the enzyme, lowers its K_m for methionine, and renders the enzyme more susceptible to feedback inhibition by AdoMet [10]. Accordingly, an increase in the concentration of the MAT β subunit leads to a reduction in the cellular content of AdoMet [11]. MATI and MATIII, but not MATII, are regulated by nitric oxide (NO) and hydroxyl radical. It has been demonstrated, both *in vitro* and *in vivo*, that NO reversibly inhibits MAT I/III activity through S-nitrosylation of a cysteine residue (C121) situated in a flexible loop at the entrance of the active site of the enzyme [12–15]. The inactivation of MATI and MATIII by NO and hydroxyl radical is reversed by physiological (millimolar) concentrations of glutathione (GSH). Consistently, and because the half-life of AdoMet in the liver is only of about 2 to 5 min [3], conditions that lead to an increase in NO, such as hypoxia, liver regeneration, and cytokines, induce a transient reduction in hepatic AdoMet content [6].

The liver-restricted expression of *MAT1A* is not mediated by the action of tissue-specific factors but by the hypermethylation of two promoter CpG sites. It has been found that *MAT1A* promoter is hypermethylated in extrahepatic tissues and fetal liver but unmethylated in adult liver, in which the gene is actively transcribed [16,17]. The degree of acetylation of histones associated with *MAT1A* promoter, which is critical to maintain a decondensed and active state of the chromatin, is markedly higher in the liver than in the kidney [16,17]. In HepG2, a human-derived hepatoma cell line, in which the expression of *MAT1A* is undetectable, *MAT1A* promoter is hypermethylated, and the treatment of these cells with demethylating agents or histone deacetylase inhibitors results in the induction of *MAT1A* gene expression [16]. In livers from patients with cirrhosis, independently of the etiology (alcohol, hepatitis B, and hepatitis C), *MAT1A* expression is also reduced, *MAT1A* promoter hypermethylated [18], and MAT activity diminished [19].

In the liver, the expression of *MAT1A* and *MAT2A* is regulated by the cellular AdoMet content. Thus, in hepatocytes in culture, there is a switch in *MAT* gene expression; *MAT2A* expression is induced, and *MAT1A* mRNA levels decrease [20]. Both effects are prevented by the addition of AdoMet to the culture medium [20]. Moreover, the addition of hepatocyte growth factor (HGF, a potent mitogen for hepatocytes that plays a key role in liver regeneration) [21] to culture hepatocytes markedly stimulates *MAT2A* expression through a process that is blocked by AdoMet [22]. The mechanism by which AdoMet exerts these effects on *MAT1A* and *MAT2A* expression is not well known.

6.3 ADOMET REGULATION OF HEPATOCYTE GROWTH

Why is hepatocyte AdoMet content under such tight control? In HuH-7, a human-derived hepatoma cell line, cells differing only in the type of *MAT* gene that is expressed, *MAT2A* expression is associated with more rapid growth, whereas the opposite is observed for *MAT1A* [23,24]. Cells expressing *MAT2A* had lower AdoMet content than cells expressing *MAT1A*, and treatment of HuH-7 cells with AdoMet led to reduced cell growth [24]. Similarly, transfection with the MAT β subunit reduced AdoMet content and stimulated DNA synthesis in HuH-7 cells, whereas downregulation of the MAT β subunit in HepG2 cells increased AdoMet content and diminished DNA synthesis [25]. These data suggested, for the first time, that cellular AdoMet content is related to the growth status of the hepatocytes. Additionally, whereas in *MAT1A* knockout mice, a chronic hepatic AdoMet deficiency leads to hyperplasia and malignant transformation (see Section 6.5), a transient fall in hepatic AdoMet content precedes liver regeneration after 2/3 partial hepatectomy (PH) [26,27] and is necessary for normal regeneration to occur [27–29]. Accordingly, the addition of AdoMet to culture hepatocytes has been found to markedly inhibit the mitogenic activity of HGF [20]. How AdoMet regulates hepatocyte growth is unclear, but because AdoMet blocks HGF-induced cyclin D1 and D2 expression and DNA synthesis without affecting HGF-induced ERK (extracellular signal-regulated protein kinase) phosphorylation [20], the MAPK signaling pathway is probably not the target.

Recently, it has been shown that HGF stimulates the transport from the nucleus to the cytosol of HuR, an RNA-binding protein that increases the half-life of cell cycle genes such as cyclin A, via activation of AMP-activated protein kinase (AMPK) through a process blocked by AdoMet (Martínez-Chantar, M. L. and Mato, J. M., unpublished data). Consistently, in *MAT1A* knockout mice in which hepatic AdoMet is depleted, AMPK is activated, and the transport of HuR from the nucleus to the cytosol is stimulated (Martínez-Chantar, M. L. and Mato, J. M., unpublished data). These results identify not only a previously unknown mechanism by which hepatocytes respond to HGF but also a novel mechanism by which AdoMet may regulate liver growth *in vivo*.

Culture hepatocytes from *MAT1A* knockout mice do not respond to the mitogenic effect of HGF despite having a higher baseline DNA synthesis, which is consistent with a heightened proliferative state observed *in vivo* in these knockouts [27]. Likewise, liver regeneration following 2/3 PH is markedly impaired in *MAT1A* knockout mice, indicating that whereas a transient decrease in AdoMet content is essential for normal liver growth, a chronic AdoMet deficiency induces desensitization to mitogenic signals [27]. How a chronic deficiency in hepatic AdoMet leads to a loss of response to mitogenic signals is still unclear. Livers from *MAT1A* knockout mice have higher baseline expression of proliferating cell nuclear antigen (PCNA) and cyclin D1, and the c-Jun-N-terminal kinase (JNK) and ERK, two upstream signaling pathways involved in hepatic cell proliferation, are also more activated in the knockouts, whereas the nuclear factor κB (NFκB) and signal transducer and activator of transcription-3 (STAT-3), the other two signaling pathways involved in cell cycle progression, are similar to those of wild-type mice [27]. The abnormal regulation at baseline in the knockouts of these, and probably other, signaling pathways involved in cell cycle progression may be the reason for the impaired responsiveness to mitogenic signals and liver regeneration in AdoMet-deficient mice. This situation is reminiscent of the abnormal liver regeneration in obese *ob/ob* mice, in which impaired liver regeneration is also associated with abnormal regulation of signaling pathways involved in cell proliferation [30].

There are two critical steps in liver regeneration: the transition of the quiescent hepatocyte into the cell cycle (priming) and the progression beyond the restriction point in the G_1 phase of the cell cycle [31]. Priming is believed to be largely attributed to TNF-α and IL-6, which then activate several signal transduction pathways, including NFκB, JNK, and STAT-3 in early G_1 phase [31,32]. Whereas priming is largely under the control of cytokines, progression in the G_1 phase and beyond the restriction point is believed to be controlled by growth factors such as HGF and transforming growth factor α (TGFα), as well as cyclin D1 [32]. The early priming events seem to be intact in *MAT1A* knockout mice and therefore independent of hepatic AdoMet content. Thus, both TNF-α and IL-6 responses in the knockouts are similar to those in wild-type mice. This is consistent with the early induction of NFκB, c-Jun, and STAT-3 [27]. *MAT2A* and *iNOS*, two genes that have been shown to be essential for liver regeneration [31,32], are also similarly induced in both types of mice. Intact iNOS response also suggests that NFκB signaling is not impaired in knockout mice. However, whereas AdoMet content fell in wild-type mice following 2/3 PH owing to the NO-dependent inactivation of MAT I/III, AdoMet levels remained unchanged in the knockout livers because of the inability of NO to decrease MAT II activity in *MAT1A* knockout mice [27]. Consequently, whereas the blocking effect that AdoMet exerts on the mitogenic activity of HGF (see the preceding text) is released in wild-type mice by the action of NO, in knockout mice the mitogenic response beyond this point progresses in a desynchronized and erratic way. Thus, following 2/3 PH, ERK phosphorylation fell in the knockout mice, and cyclin D1 failed to increase [27]. These findings have direct relevance to human liver cirrhosis, a condition with a risk of developing spontaneous liver neoplasms, in which *MAT1A* is often silenced and hepatic AdoMet content reduced [18,19].

6.4 ADOMET REGULATION OF HEPATOCYTE APOPTOSIS

6.4.1 DIFFERENTIAL EFFECT IN NORMAL VS. CANCEROUS HEPATOCYTES

AdoMet not only regulates hepatocyte's growth, it also regulates hepatocyte's death response. AdoMet is widely known as a hepatoprotective agent in both experimental models of liver injury as well as in patients with various forms of liver disease [6]. However, AdoMet has also been shown to be chemopreventive. It prevented the development of liver cancer in experimental hepatocarcinogenesis [33,34]. Interestingly, the chemopreventive effect of AdoMet can be mimicked by its metabolite 5-deoxy-5-methylthioadenosine (MTA), which is neither a methyl donor nor a precursor of GSH [29]. How can AdoMet be hepatoprotective and also chemopreventive? Recent work on the differential effect of AdoMet on apoptosis in normal vs. cancerous liver cells provided some clues [35,36].

Apoptosis has been implicated to be a major pathogenetic factor in the development of liver injury under different pathological conditions that are palliated by AdoMet treatment. These results have prompted the examination of the effect of AdoMet on apoptosis. In this work, okadaic acid has been used to induce apoptosis in primary cultures of rat hepatocytes. AdoMet prevented okadaic acid-induced apoptosis in a dose-dependent fashion. This was accompanied by the inhibition of mitochondrial cytochrome c release, a central event in the apoptotic pathway [37], and one of the downstream effects, namely, poly(ADP-ribose) polymerase cleavage [35]. Facilitation of methylation reactions and increase in cellular GSH levels are two major mechanisms often proposed for the hepatoprotective effect of AdoMet [38]. However, the ability of AdoMet to prevent okadaic-acid-induced apoptosis in rat hepatocytes is independent of GSH synthesis as treatment with propargylglycine, which blocks the conversion of AdoMet to GSH precursor cysteine [4], did not prevent its protective effect [35]. The antiapoptotic effect of AdoMet is also independent of its role as a methyl donor because the antiapoptotic effect can be mimicked by MTA. MTA can be derived from AdoMet spontaneously (nonenzymatic hydrolysis) and as a product of AdoMet metabolism in the polyamine pathway [4,39]. MTA is not a methyl donor (in fact, it inhibits methylation), and it does not contribute to GSH synthesis [40]. Others have also found MTA to be hepatoprotective and have suggested that the beneficial effects of AdoMet in liver damage could be attributed in part to its conversion to MTA [29,39]. In favor of this hypothesis is the recent finding that MTA has potent antiinflammatory and protective action in a rodent model of lipopolysaccharide-induced lethality [41]. Taken together, these observations emphasize previously unrecognized actions of AdoMet that are independent of methylation and GSH synthesis and the possibility that MTA may mediate some of its effects.

Although AdoMet and MTA protected against apoptosis in normal rat hepatocytes, they induced apoptosis in human liver cancer cell lines HepG2 and HuH-7 as well as rat liver cancer cell line H4IIE. Thus, AdoMet and MTA exert a differential effect on apoptosis in normal vs. cancerous hepatocytes. This differential effect is not due to the fact that primary hepatocytes are quiescent whereas cell lines display enhanced proliferation, because AdoMet and MTA exhibited a similar antiapoptotic effect on proliferating hepatocytes treated with hepatocyte growth factor [35]. Interestingly, the chemopreventive action of AdoMet in an *in vivo* model of chemical hepatocarcinogenesis in rats was accompanied by an increase of apoptotic bodies in atypical nodules and hepatocellular carcinoma (HCC) foci [34,42]. The present results suggest that this *in vivo* effect of AdoMet could be partially mediated through a direct action of this molecule on the neoplastic cell.

6.4.2 ADOMET-INDUCED SELECTIVE UPREGULATION OF BCL-X$_S$ IN HEPG2 CELLS

The influence of AdoMet and MTA on Bcl-2 family members has been recently investigated [36]. The rationale for this is that (1) AdoMet- and MTA-induced apoptosis in HepG2 and Huh-7 cells is accompanied by the release of cytochrome c, implicating the involvement of mitochondria in apoptosis [35,37], and (2) Bcl-2 family members are known to modulate apoptosis at the mitochondrial level [43]. Using microarray analysis, it has been found that Bcl-x is upregulated in HepG2 cells in response to AdoMet treatment. Bcl-x is alternatively spliced to produce two major distinct mRNAs and variant proteins, Bcl-x$_L$ and Bcl-x$_S$, that have antagonistic functions [43–45]. Whereas the larger Bcl-x$_L$ is antiapoptotic, the shorter Bcl-x$_S$ is proapoptotic [44]. In terms of a critical ratio for apoptosis, Minn and coworkers demonstrated that only one molecule of Bcl-x$_S$ per four molecules of Bcl-x$_L$ was necessary to overcome the Bcl-x$_L$ survival mechanism [46]. AdoMet and MTA have been found to selectively upregulate Bcl-x$_S$ in a time- and dose-dependent fashion with the effective dose of MTA lower than that of AdoMet, suggesting that the effect of AdoMet may be mediated in part by MTA. Known determinants of Bcl-x variant expression include alternative splicing and promoter usage [47,48]. Specifically, Chalfant et al. demonstrated the ability of ceramide to differentially induce Bcl-x$_S$ through activation of alternative splicing [47], and promoter usage has been demonstrated to influence Bcl-x isoform expression in the mouse gene [48]. These potential mechanisms that are known to influence the expression of Bcl-x variants have also been explored.

Similar to the mouse gene, the human Bcl-x gene also has multiple transcription start sites [36]. In control HepG2 cells, there are three promoters in the Bcl-x gene that yield only Bcl-x$_L$ mRNA. AdoMet and MTA treatment did not affect promoter usage, but whereas promoter 1 yielded only Bcl-x$_L$, the other two promoters yielded both Bcl-x$_L$ and Bcl-x$_S$, with Bcl-x$_S$ the predominant mRNA species. Thus, the mechanism of increased Bcl-x$_S$ expression is via increased alternative splicing of promoters 2 and 3 [36].

Pre-mRNA splicing is a critical step in gene expression for metazoans [49]. Whereas the small nuclear ribonuclear particles (snRNPs) are important determinants for splice site recognition and catalysis, non-snRNP protein splicing factors are essential in establishing and stabilizing interactions necessary for splicing [49,50]. SR proteins are a family of highly conserved non-snRNP factors that are vital to constitutive and regulated splicing [49–52]. The function of SR proteins is regulated by phosphorylation. Phosphorylation of SR proteins is required for spliceosome formation, whereas dephosphorylation is required for progression of the splicing reaction [50]. SR proteins are specific substrates of protein phosphatase 1 (PP1), and PP1 has been shown to regulate alternative splicing [47]. Consistent with an important role of PP1 in AdoMet- and MTA-induced activation of alternative splicing of the Bcl-x gene calyculin A, an inhibitor of both PP1 and protein phosphatase 2A (PP2A), as well as tautomycin, a selective inhibitor of PP1, blocked the induction of Bcl-x$_S$ by AdoMet and MTA, but okadaic acid, an inhibitor of PP2A, had no effect. Furthermore, AdoMet and MTA treatment of HepG2 cells led to dephosphorylation of SR proteins, which was prevented by calyculin A, but not okadaic acid. These results suggest that dephosphorylation of SR proteins occurred as a result of increased PP1 activity. This was subsequently confirmed as AdoMet and MTA treatment of HepG2 cells led to increased steady state mRNA and protein levels of PP1 catalytic subunit [36].

Increased PP1 activity can result in multiple consequences, one being SR protein dephosphorylation. This in turn can activate alternative splicing of multiple genes, Bcl-x being one example. When the dephosphorylation is blocked by calyculin A, apoptosis is prevented. These findings support the conclusion that the trigger for the apoptotic cascade in HepG2 cells by AdoMet or MTA is increased PP1 and its activity, because its inhibition prevents all the downstream steps. PP1 in turn dephosphorylates the SR proteins, resulting in the formation of the alternate variant Bcl-x$_S$ and apoptosis. This sequence of events is supported by the fact that induction of PP1 and SR protein dephosphorylation preceded Bcl-x$_S$ induction [36]. Bcl-x$_S$ induction is one of many downstream targets of PP1; more work will be necessary to identify other targets that can also contribute to apoptosis.

Although AdoMet and MTA induced the expression of PP1 catalytic subunit and Bcl-x$_S$ in HepG2 cells, they have no effect in primary mouse hepatocytes. This lack of effect in primary hepatocytes may be a major factor in the differential response of liver cancer cell lines and primary hepatocytes to AdoMet- and MTA-induced apoptosis [35].

The ability of AdoMet and MTA to modulate alternative splicing through changes in SR protein phosphorylation is a highly novel biological action of these agents, which has not been previously described. The fact that AdoMet and MTA can modulate the state of phosphorylation further widens the impact these agents have on cellular function. However, this action depends on whether the hepatocyte is normal or cancerous. Future studies elucidating the molecular mechanism of this differential response will be important in understanding how AdoMet and MTA exert opposite effects on apoptosis in normal vs. cancerous hepatocytes.

6.5 CONSEQUENCES OF CHRONIC HEPATIC ADOMET DEFICIENCY — THE *MAT1A* KNOCKOUT MOUSE MODEL

6.5.1 PHENOTYPE OF THE *MAT1A* NULL MICE

In all forms of cirrhosis examined thus far, hepatic MAT activity is markedly lower because of both decreased *MAT1A* expression and inactivation of the MAT I/III isoenzymes [6]. Decreased *MAT1A* expression also occurs in precirrhotic stage of alcoholic hepatitis [53]. This would lead to chronic hepatic AdoMet deficiency that can impact a wide array of cellular processes. To examine the biological consequence of chronic hepatic AdoMet deficiency, a *MAT1A* knockout mouse model has been developed [7]. This model has provided important insights regarding the importance of *MAT1A* in systemic methionine metabolism and AdoMet in liver health and disease.

In the normal adult animal, *MAT1A* is expressed predominantly in the liver [6]. As to the question of why the liver expresses *MAT1A* when all other tissues express *MAT2A*, a teleological explanation may be that the liver needs to express the MAT isoforms that can handle methionine excess. The expression of *MAT2A* would not allow that to occur because the MAT II isoenzyme is under tight negative feedback regulation by AdoMet [6] (see Section 6.2). However, by expressing predominantly *MAT1A*, AdoMet biosynthesis in the liver can be inhibited by oxidative stress, which occurs commonly in liver injury. This is because of the presence of a critical cysteine residue in MAT I/III, but not in MAT II, which can be covalently modified by nitric oxide and hydroxyl radical, leading to enzyme inactivation [6]. As mentioned earlier, *MAT* expression correlates with the growth and differentiation of hepatocytes [23,24,26,54]. Specifically, *MAT1A* expression correlates with high cellular AdoMet level, normal differentiated phenotype, and slow growth, whereas *MAT2A* expression correlates with lower AdoMet level, rapid growth, and dedifferentiation [24,26,54]. The *MAT1A* knockout mouse has allowed the examination of the role of *MAT1A* on hepatic AdoMet level, liver differentiation, and response to injury.

MAT1A knockout mice have markedly increased serum methionine levels and reduced hepatic AdoMet and GSH levels [7]. This confirms the importance of *MAT1A* in methionine catabolism and the influence of *MAT* expression on hepatic AdoMet level. *MAT1A* knockout mice display a phenotype resembling that observed in liver injury or stress with a vast array of growth genes, dedifferentiation genes, and acute phase response genes (such as PCNA, α-fetoprotein, and orosomucoid) upregulated [7]. Although histologically normal, 3-month-old *MAT1A* knockout mice have hepatic hyperplasia; develop massive fatty liver, following a choline-deficient diet for 6 d (Figure 6.2); and at 8 months of age, develop spontaneous nonalcoholic steatohepatitis (NASH) on a normal diet [7] (Figure 6.2). It has been shown that when rats and mice are fed a diet deficient in lipotropes (choline, methionine, folate, and vitamin B_{12}), the liver develops steatosis within a few days [55]. If the deficient diet continues, the liver develops NASH, fibrosis, and cirrhosis, some animals

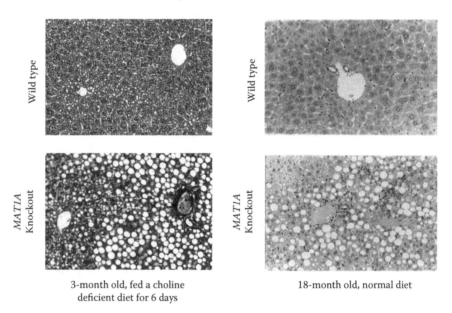

3-month old, fed a choline
deficient diet for 6 days

18-month old, normal diet

FIGURE 6.2 Liver histology of *MAT1A* knockout mice. Three-month-old *MAT1A* knockout mice developed massive fatty liver when fed a choline-deficient diet for 6 d (left panels) and 8-month-old knockout mice developed spontaneous steatohepatitis (right panels).

ultimately developing HCC [56]. Deficiency in lipotropes is well known to cause a decrease in hepatic levels of AdoMet and an increase in AdoHcy content [28,57]. Data from *MAT1A* knockout mice would suggest that lipotrope deficiency exerts its pathogenic effect in the liver through a decreased availability of AdoMet. Furthermore, these results suggest that the deficiency in MAT activity observed in human liver cirrhosis may contribute to the pathogenesis and progression of the disease.

6.5.2 Genomics of *MAT1A* Knockout Mice

A genomic approach has been used to gain insight into the molecular mechanism of the effect of chronic hepatic AdoMet deficiency in which liver gene expression from 3-month-old wild-type and *MAT1A* knockout mice were compared using the Affymetrix murine U74A array. Genes with a twofold or higher expression change were classified according to the biological process category or first subcategory in which they are involved, following the criteria of the Gene Ontology Consortium [58]. Most genes that were upregulated in the *MAT1A* knockout mouse liver clustered into four biological processes: cell communication, cell growth and/or maintenance, cell death, and development. Most genes that were downregulated in the *MAT1A* knockout mouse were involved in metabolism. For a complete list of genes, see Tables I and II of the paper published by Martínez-Chantar et al. [59].

Some of the genes identified in these clusters have been previously implicated in hepatocyte differentiation and proliferation (i.e., α-fetoprotein, *MAT2A*, PCNA). Likewise, altered gene expression was observed in a variety of genes known to be involved in acute phase response and oxidative stress (i.e., orosomucoid, lipopolysaccharide-binding protein, and Fas-antigen were upregulated, whereas mitochondrial ribosomal protein S12, CYP4A10, and CYP4A14 were downregulated in *MAT1A* knockout mice). In addition, the expression of numerous genes involved in lipid and carbohydrate metabolism was altered in *MAT1A* knockout mice liver [59]. Consistent with this abnormal expression of genes involved in lipid and carbohydrate metabolism, *MAT1A* knockout mice had elevated hepatic triglyceride levels and hyperglycemia although the circulating levels of insulin were normal.

Because cytochrome P450 2E1 (CYP2E1) is upregulated in conditions associated with steatohepatitis, such as NASH, diabetes, obesity, and alcoholic liver disease [60–62], the hypothesis that CYP2E1 is also increased in *MAT1A* knockout mouse has also been tested. Indeed, liver *CYP2E1* mRNA and CYP2E1 activity were increased in 3-month-old *MAT1A* knockout mice as compared to wild-type animals. Furthermore, diallyl sulfide (DAS), an effective inhibitor of CYP2E1 [63], lowered the hepatic CYP2E1 activity in both groups of mice to comparable levels [59].

To see if increased CYP2E1 activity in the *MAT1A* knockout mice would predispose these animals to liver injury, the toxicity of CCl4, a hepatotoxic molecule that is biotransformed by CYP2E1, has also been determined. Indeed, liver injury was much more severe in *MAT1A* knockout mice than in wild-type animals, and DAS treatment prevented CCl_4-induced liver injury in both groups of mice [59]. In addition, the serum concentration of malondialdehyde, a measure of lipid peroxidation, was higher in *MAT1A* knockout mice at baseline and following CCl_4 treatment as compared to wild-type mice. This suggests the *MAT1A* knockout mice have increased baseline oxidative stress, perhaps contributed by increased CYP2E1 activity. This also predisposes them to liver injury caused by hepatotoxic agents that are biotransformed by CYP2E1. How chronic hepatic AdoMet deficiency leads to increased CYP2E1 expression is unclear and needs to be investigated.

6.5.3 Proteomics of *MAT1A* Knockout Mice

A proteomic approach has also been used to gain insight into the molecular mechanism of the effect of chronic hepatic AdoMet deficiency on liver function. This is important because there is often discordance between the expression of genes and proteins. The study by Santamaría et al. [64] illustrates this point. In this study, the differential protein expression in the *MAT1A* knockout mouse liver from the time of birth to the development of NASH at 8 months has been examined in order to identify potential targets responsible for the development of NASH. One hundred and seventeen protein spots, differentially expressed during the development of NASH, were selected and identified by peptide mass fingerprinting. However, most of these differentially expressed proteins were not maintained during the development of NASH. Only 12 proteins were found to be differentially expressed from birth to onset of NASH at 8 months. Interestingly, 4 of the 12 proteins (prohibitin 1, cytochrome C oxidase I and II, and ATPase β subunit) have known roles in mitochondrial function. Western blot analysis confirmed that the protein levels of prohibitin 1 and cytochrome C oxidase I and II were reduced, whereas the protein level of ATPase β subunit was increased. Importantly, reduced prohibitin 1 and cytochrome C oxidase II protein levels occurred most likely owing to posttranslational mechanisms as the mRNA levels remained unchanged. Thus, adopting only a genomic approach would have missed this. Increased ATPase β subunit occurred at the pretranslational level as the mRNA level was also increased. Reduced prohibitin 1 protein level can potentially explain the downregulation of cytochrome C oxidase. Prohibitin 1 is the product of a nuclear gene that is targeted to the inner mitochondrial membrane [65]. Prohibitin 1 has been proposed to be a chaperone-like protein that participates in the correct folding and assembly of some of the components of the mitochondrial respiratory chain [66,67]. A deficiency in prohibitin 1 may impair the native and functional organization of respiratory proteins that are subsequently degraded by mitochondrial proteases, compromising mitochondrial functionality [66,67]. Consistent with this hypothesis, the mitochondrial inner membrane potential was reduced by 40% in the *MAT1A* knockout mice, indicating impairment in mitochondrial function [64]. Prohibitin 1 protein levels fell in primary cultures of rat hepatocytes cultured in the absence of methionine. This fall can be prevented if the medium is supplemented with AdoMet. Furthermore, if the conversion of methionine to AdoMet is blocked, prohibitin 1 level also fell [64]. Collectively, these results demonstrate that AdoMet can regulate the protein level of prohibitin 1 in hepatocytes. How this occurs is unknown and requires further study. Finally, it has also been found that the protein levels of prohibitin 1 and cytochrome C oxidase are reduced in *ob/ob* mice and obese patients who are at risk of NASH. This further strengthens the relevance of prohibitin 1 in steatohepatitis and as a novel target of AdoMet. In addition to its being a mitochondrial chaperon protein, prohibitin has been proposed recently to be a tumor suppressor factor [68]. This can also contribute to the predisposition to HCC in the *MAT1A* knockout mouse model (see text following).

6.5.4 LIVER CANCER IN *MAT1A* KNOCKOUT MICE

Lipotrope deficiency is well known to result in AdoMet deficiency and HCC formation [56]. Three-month-old *MAT1A* knockout mice have hepatic hyperplasia, an early event during the neoplastic process, and express genes that favor increased growth. Previous studies have also shown that *MAT1A* expression is associated with a normal differentiated liver phenotype, whereas *MAT2A* expression is associated with rapid liver growth and dedifferentiation [6]. In the *MAT1A* knockout mouse, hepatic *MAT2A* expression is induced to compensate for the loss of *MAT1A* [7]. Consistently, the hypothesis has been tested that chronic hepatic AdoMet deficiency may increase the risk of HCC. Indeed, the majority of *MAT1A* knockout mice developed HCC by 18 months [59], and all have HCC by 20 months [Lu, S.C. and Mato, J.M., unpublished observation]. The molecular mechanisms of hepatocarcinogenesis in this model remain to be defined, but recent work has shown that decreased AdoMet can lead to increased transport from the nucleus to the cytosol of HuR, an RNA-binding protein that increases the half-life of cell cycle genes such as cyclin A (see Section 6.3), and decreased expression of tumor suppressor such as prohibitin 1. Other mechanisms are likely to be involved and require further investigation.

The fact that *MAT1A* knockout mice have chronic hepatic AdoMet depletion and develop spontaneous NASH and HCC [7,59] strongly suggests that AdoMet deficiency may be a key component of the mechanism by which lipotrope deficiency causes hepatic lesions. Genomic and proteomic experiments using liver from *MAT1A* knockout mice [7,59,64] indicate that AdoMet regulates the expression of a diverse set of genes, including many metabolic genes that were abnormal in the knockout mice long before the appearance of any histological lesion. This surprising result suggests that reduced AdoMet levels may cause liver injury and cancer through perturbation of multiple metabolic pathways in the cell, a possibility that makes *MAT1A* knockout mice especially useful for system biologists to study metabolic networks and their physiological function.

6.6 CONCLUSIONS AND FUTURE DIRECTIONS

Since Cantoni discovered MAT and AdoMet in the 1950s [69], we have come a long way in understanding the function and regulation of this essential cellular enzyme and its product AdoMet. The type of MAT expressed by the liver has important implications in regard to the steady-state AdoMet level and the phenotype. *MAT1A* expression correlates with high AdoMet level and a differentiated liver phenotype, whereas *MAT2A* expression correlates with lower AdoMet level and rapid growth and dedifferentiation of the liver. Further, recent findings define a critical role for *MAT1A* and AdoMet in maintaining normal hepatic function and in the pathogenesis of NASH and hepatic malignant transformation. Based on these recent findings, we envision the following scenario for hepatocytes: a normal level of AdoMet favors the differentiated state of hepatocytes, blocks apoptosis, and prevents cell proliferation. A fall in the concentration of AdoMet facilitates liver regeneration, and if this conditions persists, predisposes the liver to injury, steatohepatitis and, finally, to the development of HCC. The physiopathological relevance of this observation is obvious, because the development of HCC is a common complication of liver cirrhosis, a condition in which the synthesis of AdoMet is markedly impaired. Recent work also demonstrated highly novel actions of AdoMet through modulation of the state of protein phosphorylation. Thus, AdoMet should not be viewed only as a methyl donor and a precursor of GSH anymore but also as an intracellular signal that controls essential hepatic functions such as growth and differentiation as well as the sensitivity to liver injury and apoptosis. Figure 6.3 summarizes our current understanding of the role of AdoMet in the regulation of liver function. Future investigations elucidating the mechanisms of AdoMet's growth and death modulatory effects in normal vs. cancerous hepatocytes, as well as defining other proteins affected by phosphorylation will provide important insights into how AdoMet impacts cellular functions. Whether AdoMet and MTA act through the same signaling pathway is also of importance. Ultimately, a better understanding of *MAT* genes regulation and modulation of liver function by AdoMet may lead to development of strategies to treat and prevent complications of liver disease and cancer.

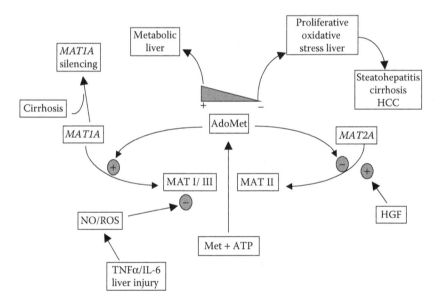

FIGURE 6.3 AdoMet regulation of liver function. Under normal condition, the high hepatic AdoMet level is maintained by two main mechanisms: (1) high expression of *MAT1A*, which can be further stimulated by AdoMet; and (2) the high capacity of MAT I/III to convert dietary methionine into AdoMet. AdoMet actually downregulates *MAT2A* expression and inhibits MAT II activity, so the contribution of this enzyme to the net synthesis of hepatic AdoMet is small. Under pathological conditions such as liver injury caused by hepatotoxins or partial

ACKNOWLEDGMENTS

This work was supported by NIH grants DK51719 (to SC Lu), AA12677, AA13847, and AT-1576 (to SC Lu and JM Mato), and Plan Nacional de I+D (SAF2002-00168 to JM Mato).

ABBREVIATIONS

AdoHcy	*S*-adenosylhomocysteine
AdoMet	*S*-adenosylmethionine
AMPK	AMP-activated protein kinase
CYP2E1	cytochrome P450 2E1
DAS	diallyl sulfide
ERK	extracellular signal-regulated protein kinase
GNMT	glycine *N*-methyltransferase
GSH	glutathione
HCC	hepatocellular carcinoma
HGF	hepatocyte growth factor
Hcy	homocysteine
JNK	c-Jun-N-terminal kinase
MAT	methionine adenosyltransferase
MS	methionine synthase
MTA	5-deoxy-5-methylthioadensoine
NASH	nonalcoholic steatohepatitis
NFκB	nuclear factor κB
NO	nitric oxide
PCNA	proliferating cell nuclear antigen
PH	partial hepatectomy

FIGURE 6.3 (continued) hepatectomy, a cellular response is initiated that involves a vast number of growth factors and cytokines (such as HGF, TNF, and IL-6) and the generation of oxidative stress (NO and ROS). NO and ROS can inactivate MAT I/III and lower the hepatic AdoMet content. This reduction in AdoMet content releases the inhibitory effect it has on *MAT2A* expression and MAT II activity (which is not inactivated by NO or ROS). As a consequence, a new, lower steady-state level of AdoMet is reached. The reduced content of hepatic AdoMet also releases the inhibitory effect that this molecule exerts on the proliferative activity of HGF, allowing it to induce *MAT2A* expression and facilitate liver regeneration. With restoration of the original liver mass, the inhibitory effect that NO and ROS exert on MAT I/III is released, *MAT1A* expression is induced, AdoMet content returns to its original value, and *MAT2A* expression is again downregulated. However, if the conditions leading to oxidative stress persist (e.g., chronic exposure to alcohol and viral hepatitis), hepatic AdoMet levels remain persistently low and this may predispose the liver to further injury, development of steatohepatitis, cirrhosis, and ultimately, HCC. In cirrhosis, *MAT1A* expression is progressively silenced by a mechanism that involves methylation of the *MAT1A* promoter and its association with hypoacetylated histones.

PP1   protein phosphatase 1
PP2A   protein phosphatase 2A
snRNPS   small nuclear ribonuclear particles
STAT-3   signal transducer and activator of transcription-3
TGFα   transforming growth factor α
WT   wild type

REFERENCES

1. Finkelstein, J.D., Homocysteine: a history in progress, *Nutr Rev,* 58, 193, 2000.
2. Kinsell, L.W. et al., Rate of disappearance from plasma of intravenously administered methionine in patients with liver damage, *Science,* 106, 589, 1947.
3. Mudd, S.H. and Poole, J.R. Labile methyl balances for normal humans of various dietary regimens, *Metabolism,* 24, 721, 1975.
4. Finkelstein, J.D., Methionine metabolism in mammals, *J Nutr Biochem,* 1, 228, 1990.
5. Kotb, M. et al., Consensus nomenclature for the mammalian methionine adenosyltransferase genes and gene products, *Trends Genet,* 13, 51, 1997.
6. Mato, J.M. et al., S-Adenosylmethionine: a control switch that regulates liver function, *FASEB J,* 16, 15, 2002.
7. Lu, S.C. et al., Methionine adenosyltransferase 1A knockout mice are predisposed to liver injury and exhibit increased expression of genes involved in proliferation, *Proc Natl Acad Sci USA,* 98, 5560, 2001.
8. Wagner, C. et al., Glycine N-methyltransferase: structure and function, in *Methionine Metabolism: Molecular and Clinical Implication,* Mato, J.M. and Caballero, A., Eds., CSIC, Madrid, pp. 35–48, 1998.
9. Mudd, S.H. et al., Glycine N-methyltransferase deficiency: a novel inborn error causing persistent isolated hypermethioninemia, *J Inherit Metab Dis,* 24, 448, 2001.
10. Halim, A.B. et al., Expression and functional interaction of the catalytic and regulatory subunits of human methionine adenosyltransferase in mammalian cells, *J Biol Chem,* 274, 29720, 1999.
11. LeGros, H.M. et al., Cloning, expression, and functional characterization of the b regulatory subunit of human methionine adenosyltransferase (MAT II), *J Biol Chem,* 275, 2359, 2000.
12. Avila, M.A. et al., Regulation of rat liver S-adenosylmethionine synthetase during septic shock: role of nitric oxide, *Hepatology,* 25, 391, 1997.
13. Ruiz, F. et al., Nitric oxide inactivates rat hepatic methionine adenosyltransferase in vivo by S-nitrosylation, *Hepatology,* 28, 1051, 1998.
14. Corrales, F.J., Ruiz, F.A., and Mato, J.M., In vivo regulation by glutathione of methionine adenosyltransferase S-nitrosylation, *J Hepatol,* 31, 887, 1999.
15. Pérez-Mato, I. et al., Methionine adenosyltransferase S-nitrosylation is regulated by the basic and acidic amino acids surrounding the target thiol, *J Biol Chem,* 274, 17075, 1999.
16. Torres, L. et al. Liver-specific methionine adenosyltransferase MAT1A gene expression is associated with a specific pattern of promoter methylation and histone acetylation: implications for MAT1A silencing during transformation, *FASEB J,* 14, 95, 2000.
17. Torres, L. et al., DNA methylation and histone acetylation of rat methionine adenosyltransferase 1A and 2A genes is tissue specific, *Int J Biochem Cell Biol,* 32, 397, 2000.

18. Avila, M.A. et al., Reduced mRNA abundance of the main enzymes involved in methionine metabolism in human liver cirrhosis and hepatocellular carcinoma, *J Hepatol,* 33, 907, 2000.

19. Martín-Duce, A. et al., S-Adenosylmethionine synthetase and phospholipid methyltransferase are inhibited in human cirrhosis, *Hepatology,* 8, 65, 1988.

20. García-Trevijano, E.R. et al., NO sensitizes rat hepatocytes to hepatocyte growth factor-induced proliferation through the modulation of S-adenosylmethionine levels, *Gastroenterology,* 122, 135, 2002.

21. Michalopoulos, G.K. and DeFrances, M.C., Liver regeneration, *Science,* 276, 60, 1997.

22. Latasa, M.U. et al., Hepatocyte growth factor induces MAT2A expression and histone acetylation in rat hepatocytes: role in liver regeneration, *FASEB J,* 15, 1248, 2001.

23. Cai, J. et al., Changes in S-adenosylmethionine synthetase in human liver cancer: molecular characterization and significance, *Hepatology,* 24, 1090, 1996.

24. Cai, J. et al., Differential expression of methionine adenosyltransferase genes influences the rate of growth of human hepatocellular carcinoma cells, *Cancer Res,* 58, 1444, 1998.

25. Martínez-Chantar, M.L. et al., Methionine Adenosyltransferase II β subunit gene expression provides a proliferative advantage in human hepatoma, *Gastroenterology,* 124, 940, 2003.

26. Huang, Z.Z. et al., Changes in methionine adenosyltransferase during liver regeneration in the rat, *Am J Physiol,* 38, G14, 1998.

27. Chen, L. et al., Impaired liver regeneration in mice lacking methionine adenosyltransferase 1A, *FASEB J,* 18, 914, 2004.

28. Shivapurkar, N. and Poirier, L.A., Tissue levels of S-adenosylmethionine and S-adenosylhomocysteine in rats fed methyl-defricient, amino acid-defined diets for one to five weeks, *Carcinogenesis,* 4, 1051, 1983.

29. Pascale, R.M. et al., Comparative effects of L-methionine, S-adenosyl-L-methionine and 5-methylthioadenosine on the growth of preneoplastic lesions and DNA methylation in rat liver during the early stages of hepatocarcinogenesi, *Anticancer Res,* 11, 1617, 1991.

30. Yang, S.Q. et al., Disrupted signaling and inhibited regeneration in obese mice with fatty livers: implications for nonalcoholic fatty liver disease pathophysiology, *Hepatology,* 34, 694, 2001.

31. Fausto, N., Liver regeneration, *J Hepatol,* 32, 19, 2000.

32. Talarmin, H. et al., The mitogen-activated protein kinase kinase/extracellular signal-regulated kinase cascade activation is a key signaling pathway involved in the regulation of G_1 phase progression in proliferating hepatocytes, *Mol Cell Biol,* 19, 6003, 1999.

33. Pascale, R.M. et al., Chemoprevention of rat liver carcinogenesis by S-adenosyl-L-methionine: a long-term study, *Cancer Res,* 52, 4979, 1992.

34. Pascale, R.M. et al., Chemoprevention by S-adenosyl-L-methionine of rat liver carcinogenesis initiated by 1,2-dimethylhydrazine and promoted by orotic acid, *Carcinogenesis,* 16, 427, 1995.

35. Ansorena, E. et al., S-adenosylmethionine and methylthioadenosine are anti-apoptotic in cultured rat hepatocytes but pro-apoptotic in human hepatoma cells, *Hepatology,* 35, 274, 2002.

36. Yang, H.P. et al., S-Adenosylmethionine and its metabolite induce apoptosis in HepG2 cells: role of protein phosphatase 1 and Bcl-x_S, *Hepatology,* 40, 221, 2004.

37. Bossy-Wetzel, E., Newmeyer, D.D., and Green, D.R., Mitochondrial cytochrome *c* release in apoptosis occurs upstream of DEVD-specific caspase activation and independently of mitochondrial transmembrane depolarization, *EMBO J,* 17, 37, 1994.

38. Mato, J.M. et al., S-adenosylmethionine synthesis: molecular mechanisms and clinical implications, *Pharmacol Ther,* 73, 265, 1997.

39. Simile, M.M. et al., 5′-Methylthioadenosine administration prevents lipid peroxidation and fibrogenesis induced in rat liver by carbon-tetrachloride intoxication. *J Hepatol,* 34, 386, 2001.

40. Dante, R., Arnaud, M., and Niveleau, A., Effects of 5′-deoxy-5′-methylthioadenosine on the metabolism of S-adenosyl methionine, *Biochem Biophys Res Commun,* 114, 214, 1983.

41. Hevia H. et al., 5-Methylthioadenosine modulates the inflammatory response to endotoxin in mice and in rat hepatocytes, *Hepatology,* 39, 1088, 2004.

42. Garcea, R. et al., Inhibition of promotion and persistent nodule growth by S-adenosyl-L-methionine in rat liver carcinogenesis: role of remodeling and apoptosis, *Cancer Res,* 49, 1850, 1989.

43. Borner, C., The Bcl-2 protein family: sensors and checkpoints for life-or-death decisions, *Mol Immunol,* 9, 615, 2003.

44. Boise, L.H. et al., Bcl-x, a bcl-2-related gene that functions as a dominant regulator of apoptotic cell death, *Cell,* 74, 597, 1993.

45. Grillot, D. A.M. et al., Genomic organization, promoter region analysis, and chromosome localization of the mouse bcl-x gene, *J Immunol,* 158, 4750, 1997.

46. Minn, A.J., Boise, L.H., and Thompson, C.B., Bcl-x_S antagonizes the protective effects of Bcl-x_L, *J Biol Chem,* 271, 6306, 1996.

47. Chalfant, C.E. et al., *De novo* ceramide regulates the alternative splicing of caspase 9 and Bcl-x in A549 lung adenocarcinoma cells, *J Biol Chem,* 277, 12587, 2002.

48. Pecci, A. et al., Promoter choice influences alternative splicing and determines the balance of isoforms expressed from the mouse bcl-X gene, *J Biol Chem,* 276, 21062, 2001.

49. Sciabica, K.S., Dai, Q.J., and Sandri-Goldin, R.M., ICP27 interacts with SRPK1 to mediate HSV splicing inhibition by altering SR protein phosphorylation, *EMBO J,* 22, 1608, 2003.

50. Misteli, T., RNA splicing: what has phosphorylation got to do with it? *Curr Biol,* 9, R198, 1999.

51. Pilch, B. et al., Specific inhibition of serine- and arginine-rich splicing factors phosphorylation, spliceosome assembly, and splicing by the antitumor drug NB-506, *Cancer Res,* 61, 6876, 2001.

52. Graveley, B.R. and Maniatis, T., Arginine/serine-rich domains of SR proteins can function as activators of pre-mRNA splicing, *Mol Cell,* 1, 765, 1998.

53. Lee, T.D. et al., Abnormal hepatic methionine and GSH metabolism in patients with alcoholic hepatitis, *Alcoholism: Clin Exp Res,* 28, 173, 2004.

54. Huang, Z.Z. et al., Differential effect of thioacetamide on hepatic methionine adenosyltransferase expression, *Hepatology,* 29, 1471, 1999.

55. Best, C.H., Hershey, J.M., and Huntsman, C., The effect of lecithin on fat deposition in the liver of the normal rat, *J Physiol,* 75, 56, 1932.

56. Newberne, P.M., Lipotropic factors and oncogenesis, *Adv Exp Med Biol,* 206, 223, 1986.

57. Cook, R.J., Horne, D.W., and Wagner, C., Effect of dietary methyl group deficiency on one-carbon metabolism in rats, *J Nutr,* 119, 612, 1989.

58. Ashburner, M. et al., Gene ontology: tool for the unification of biology. The Gene Ontology Consortium, *Nat Genet,* 25, 25, 2000.
59. Martínez-Chantar, M.L. et al., Spontaneous oxidative stress and liver tumors in mice lacking methionine adenosyltransaferase 1A, *FASEB J,* 16, 1292, 2002.
60. Weltman, M.D., Farrell, G.C., and Liddle, C., Increased hepatocyte CYP2E1 expression in a rat nutritional model of hepatic steatosis with inflammation, *Gastroenterology,* 111, 1645, 1996.
61. Leclercq, I.A. et al., CYP2E1 and CYP4A as microsomal catalysts of lipid peroxides in murine nonalcoholic steatohepatitis, *J Clin Invest,* 105, 1067, 2000.
62. Robertson, G., Leclercq, I., and Farrell, G.C., Nonalcoholic steatosis and steatohepatitis II. Cytochrome P-450 enzymes and oxidative stress, *Am J Physiol,* 281, G1135, 2001.
63. Chen, L. et al., Relationship between cytochrome P450 2E1 and acetone catabolism in rats as studied with diallyl sulfide as an inhibitor, *Biochem Pharmacol,* 48, 2199, 1994.
64. Santamaría, E. et al., Functional proteomics of non-alcoholic steatohepatitis: mitochondrial proteins as targets of S-adenosylmethionine, *Proc Natl Acad Sci USA,* 100, 3065, 2003.
65. Ikonen, E. et al., Prohibitin, an antiproliferative protein, is localized to mitochondria, *FEBS Lett,* 358, 273, 1995.
66. Nijtmans, L.G. et al., Prohibitins act as a membrane-bound chaperone for the stabilization of mitochondrial proteins, *EMBO J,* 19, 2444, 2000.
67. Nijtmans, L.G. et al., The mitochondrial PHB complex: roles in mitochondrial respiratory complex assembly, aging and degenerative disease, *Cell Mol Life Sci,* 59, 143, 2002.
68. Wang, S. et al., Prohibitin co-localizes with Rb in the nucleus and recruits N-CoR and HDAC1 for transcriptional repression, *Oncogene,* 21, 8388, 2002.
69. Cantoni, G.L., S-adenosylmethionine: a new intermediate formed enzymatically from L-methionine and adenosine triphosphate, *J Biol Chem,* 204, 403, 1953.

7 Effects of Carotenoid Supplementation on Signal Transduction Pathways: Significance in Lung Cancer Prevention

Xiang-Dong Wang and Stacey King

CONTENTS

7.1   INTRODUCTION

There are six major carotenoids (β-carotene, α-carotene, lycopene, cryptoxanthin, lutein, and zeaxanthin) that can be found routinely in human plasma and tissues. Of these, provitamin A carotenoids (β-carotene, α-carotene, and β-cryptoxanthin) and nonprovitamin A carotenoid (lycopene) have been studied for their potential chemoprotective roles in cancers. These carotenoids are lipophilic plant pigments with polyisoprenoid structures, typically containing a series of conjugated double bonds in the central chain of the molecule, which makes them susceptible to oxidation, isomerization from *trans* to *cis* forms, and formation of potentially beneficial or harmful metabolites (Figure 7.1). This is of physiological relevance in humans, because these provitamin A carotenoids are subject to either central cleavage by carotene-15,15′-monooxygenase [1–4], forming retinal, which further can be oxidized into retinoic acid, or excentric cleavage by β-carotene-9′,10′-monooxytenase [5,6], yielding β-apo-carotenals of varying lengths, which may be converted to retinoic acid by a process comparable to β-oxidation [7,8]. Lycopene, as a nonprovitamin A

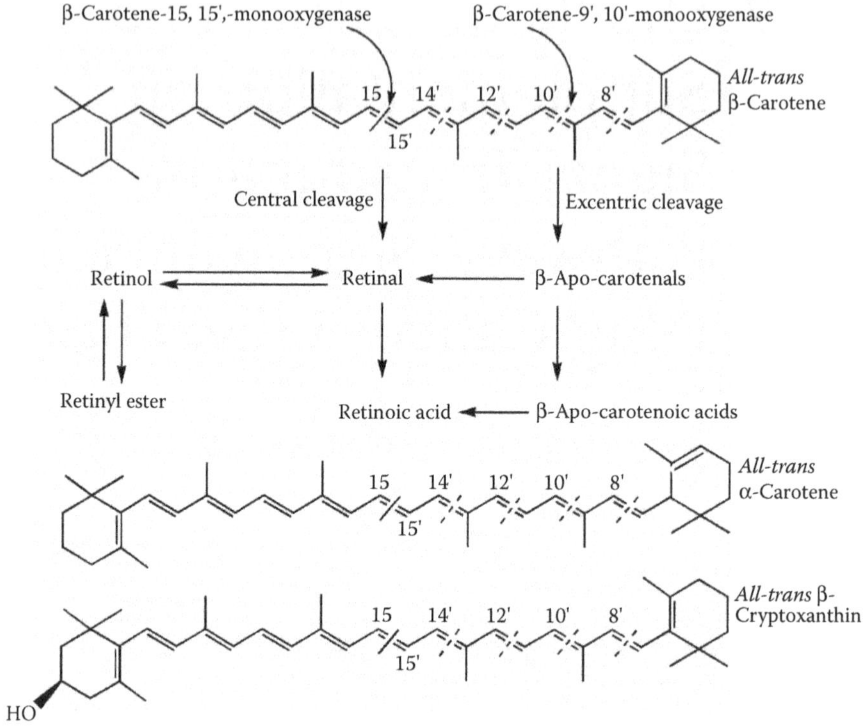

FIGURE 7.1 Chemical structures and metabolism of provitamin A carotenoids. (Adapted from Wang, X.D., Carotenoid oxidative/degradative products and their biological activities, in Krinsky, N.I., Mayneand, S.T., Sies, H., Eds., *Carotenoids in Health and Disease*, Marcel Dekker, New York, pp. 313–335, 2004.)

carotenoid may have a similar metabolic pathway, although the exact mechanisms are still poorly understood [5,9].

To better understand the potential function of carotenoids in the chemoprevention of cancer, greater knowledge of carotenoid dose effects and genetic signaling pathways is necessary [10]. Despite the fact that clinical intervention trials conducted to determine the chemoprotective effect of β-carotene on the incidence of lung cancer in smokers found either a no-protective effect or a negative effect [11–14], supporting evidence of a protective role of fruits and vegetables rich in carotenoids in cancer prevention continues to be reported in human epidemiological and intervention studies [15–18]. Recent studies show strong inverse correlations between lung cancer and dietary intake or plasma levels of β-cryptoxanthin [19,20]. A prospective cohort study exploring the question of whether combinations of dietary carotenoid and other antioxidants (vitamins C and E) affect lung cancer morbidity and mortality in male smokers, has shown that men with the highest antioxidant index scores had a significantly lower (16%) risk of lung cancer than men with the lowest scores [21]. Numerous animal and tissue culture studies have also shown that carotenoids block certain carcinogenic processes and inhibit specific tumor cell growth [22–25].

The role of carotenoids in carcinogenesis is more intricate than originally thought. In all cases, dosage effects are of particular importance due to the impact of oxidation on these carotenoids and the potential for beneficial effects of small quantities or harmful effects of large quantities of the resulting metabolic products (Figure 7.2) [26]. Recent studies using appropriate *in vitro* cell experiments and/or animal models have provided potential molecular mechanisms regarding protective (or harmful) effects of carotenoids in a dose-dependent manner. Whereas the initial impetus for studying the benefits of carotenoids in lung cancer was their antioxidant capacity, carotenoids are now recognized to act through other mechanisms, such as a number of biological functions that are mediated via their oxidative metabolites. Carotenoids, in particular, are now being examined for their roles in cancer prevention through their effects on signal transduction pathways. In this chapter, we will focus on understanding the dosage effects of carotenoid on several important molecular targets and signaling pathways, and the significance of these changes in lung cancer prevention. The three main signal transduction pathways discussed are (1) the retinoid signaling pathway, (2) the mitogen-activated protein kinase (MAPK) pathway, and (3) the insulin-like growth factor 1 (IGF-1) signal transduction pathway.

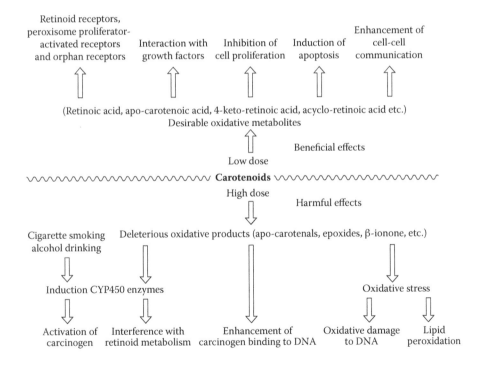

FIGURE 7.2 Simplified schematic illustration of possible mechanisms of carotenoids and their oxidative metabolites and their beneficial and detrimental effects on human health. (Adapted from Wang, X.D., Carotenoid oxidative/degradative products and their biological activities, in Krinsky, N.I., Mayneand, S.T., Sies, H., Eds., *Carotenoids in Health and Disease*, Marcel Dekker, New York, pp. 313–335, 2004.)

The interactions between these signaling pathways and carotenoids will be discussed in this chapter.

7.2 EFFECTS OF CAROTENOID SUPPLEMENTATION ON RETINOID SIGNALING PATHWAY

Retinoids, the most biologically active oxidative products from provitamin A carotenoids, play an important role in several critical life processes. Considerable evidence demonstrates that retinoids may be effective in the prevention and treatment of a variety of human chronic diseases, including cancer [27,28]. The mechanism by which retinoids are able to elicit these effects resides in their ability to regulate gene expression at specific target sites within the body. Both retinoic acid receptor (RARα, RARβ, and RARγ) and retinoid X receptor (RXRα, RXRβ, and RXRγ) function as transcription factors and regulate gene expression by binding as dimeric complexes to the retinoic acid response element (RARE) and the retinoid X response element (RXRE), which are located in the 5′ promoter region of susceptible genes [29]. All-*trans* retinoic acid binds and transactivates both RAR and RXR, whereas 9-*cis*-retinoic acid binds and transactivates only the RXR. Provitamin A carotenoids, such as β-carotene and its excentric cleavage metabolites, can serve as direct precursors for the all-*trans*- and 9-*cis*-retinoic acids [30,31]. Therefore, the molecular mode of action of provitamin A carotenoids can be mediated by retinoic acid, whereby subsequent binding of retinoid receptor dimers to RAREs in target gene promoters transcriptionally activates a series of genes with distinct antiproliferative or proapoptotic activity, thus eliminating cells with irreparable alterations in the genome or killing neoplastic cells.

It has been demonstrated that the upregulation of retinoid receptor expression and function by provitamin A carotenoids may play a role in mediating the growth inhibitory effects of retinoids in animals [32] and cells [33]. Both *in vivo* and *in vitro* studies indicate that RARβ2 expression is frequently reduced in various cancer cells and tissues [27,34,35]. We have observed that the downregulation of RARβ by smoke-borne carcinogens was completely reversed by treatments with either β-carotene or apo-14′-carotenoic acid in normal bronchial epithelium cells [33]. This could be due to the conversion of β-carotene and apo-carotenoic acid to retinoic acid, as RARβ can be induced by retinoic acid. This is supported by our further observation that the transactivation of the RARβ2 promoter by β-apo-14′-carotenoic acid appears to occur, in large part, via metabolism to all-*trans*-retinoic acid, the most potent RAR ligand [33].

On the other hand, the downregulation of retinoid receptors (loss of, or low expression of specific RARs and RXRs, e.g., RARβ) can interfere with retinoid signal transduction and result in enhanced cell proliferation and potentially malignant transformation. Retinoid receptors can also be functionally downregulated due to a lack of the ligand, retinoic acid. This may be seen in cases of cigarette smoking and excessive alcohol drinking, resulting in higher cytochrome P450 enzymes and breakdown of retinoic acid [36,37]. Previous studies in ferrets, which exhibit lung function highly analogous to humans, have shown that high-dose β-carotene supplementation (equivalent to an intake of 30 mg of β-carotene/d/70-kg human, considered a pharmacological dose) and/or cigarette smoke exposure decrease levels of retinoic acid and RARβ protein but increase cell proliferation in lung tissue and levels of c-Jun and cyclin D1 proteins [22,38]. Other isoforms of RAR, RARα, and RARγ were not affected. Further studies by Liu et al. [37] demonstrated that diminished levels of retinoic acid in the lungs of ferrets after either smoke exposure or high-dose β-carotene supplementation or both are partly caused by enhancement of retinoic acid catabolism via induction of cytochrome P450 (CYPs). When using retinoic acid as the substrate, the formation of the polar metabolites, 18-hydroxy-retinoic acid and 4-oxo-retinoic acid, increased 6- to 10-fold after incubation with smoke-exposed and/or high-dose β-carotene-supplemented ferret lung microsomes as compared to the controls [37]. This enhancement of microsomal retinoic acid catabolism can be inhibited by liarozole, a nonspecific inhibitor for CYPs. These studies provide possible explanations for enhanced lung carcinogenesis with pharmacological dose β-carotene supplementation in cigarette smokers. Paolini et al. [39] showed a significant increase in several cytochrome P450 enzymes (CYP1A1/2, CYP2A1, CYP2B1, and CYP3A1/2) in the lungs of rats supplemented with very high doses of β-carotene (500 mg per kg body weight). Therefore, induction of CYPs by either β-carotene oxidative cleavage products or by cigarette smoke has two possible detrimental actions in the lung tissue that enhance carcinogenesis: (1) bioactivation of carcinogens and (2) destruction of retinoic acid.

In contrast to the animals receiving high-dose β-carotene supplementation, neither the level of retinoic acid nor the expression of RARβ in the lung was affected in animals treated with low-dose β-carotene (equivalent to an intake of 6 mg of β-carotene/d/70-kg human, a physiological dose) as compared to the control group. In fact, compared to the smoke-exposed group, low-dose β-carotene supplementation in the smoke-exposed group resulted in a significantly smaller decrease of lung retinoic acid levels [22]. This supports the possibility that β-carotene, when given at a low dose, could act to supply adequate retinoic acid to the lung tissue of smoke-exposed ferrets. In a recent research using a ferret as a lung cancer model, Kim et al. [40] demonstrated that the combination of three major antioxidants (β-carotene, α-tocopherol, and ascorbic acid) provides a protection against lung carcinogenesis by maintaining normal levels of retinoic acid, which is lower in the smoke-exposed animals. This study indicates that this combination of nutrients would be an effective chemopreventive strategy against lung cancer in smokers.

As the beneficial and harmful effects of carotenoids could be due to their metabolites or decomposition products [10], the quantities of these metabolites should be considered. Excentric cleavage products of β-carotene may be formed in small quantities in cells to increase the retinoic acid level by their conversion into retinoic acid at physiological concentrations; conversely, excessive quantities of excentric cleavage products may be formed in the cell (e.g., due to supplementation with high-dose β-carotene in the highly oxidative conditions of the lung) which enhance catabolism of retinoic acid by their induction of cytochrome P450 enzymes at high concentrations [37]. It should be noted that excentric cleavage products, which may be formed in excess in cancerous lung tissue, have not been shown to competitively bind to RARβ at physiologically relevant levels [41]. In a previous study by Prakash et al. [33], the intracellular concentration of β-carotene of the cells was 3% (~ 0.9 µmol/l) of the β-carotene concentration (30 µmol/l) added to the cell medium. This intracellular concentration of β-carotene is slightly higher than the normal plasma levels in the U.S. adults aged ≥ 19 yr (0.4 µmol/l), but much less than the serum levels in the intervention groups (6 µmol/l) in the Alpha-Tocopherol, Beta-Carotene Cancer Prevention Study (ATBC Study), which resulted in procarcinogenic effects. Therefore, the experimental conditions in this study were more relevant to physiological effects achieved through dietary sources, that is, β-apo-14′-carotenoic acid, an excentric cleavage metabolite of β-carotene, can prevent the reduction of RARβ caused by benzo[a]pyrene and induce transcriptional activity of the RARβ2 promoter by its conversion into retinoic acid, providing more evidence to support the possibility that β-carotene or its metabolites, when given at low doses, could act to supply adequate retinoic acid to induce RARβ.

The effects of other carotenoids, such as cryptoxanthin, on the retinoid signaling pathway have yet to be elucidated but may have similar interactions with cleavage enzymes based on dose and the oxidative conditions of the lungs. Accumulating evidence suggests that RARβ2 and RARβ4 have contrasting biological effects (tumor suppressor and tumor promoter) in human carcinogenesis [35]. In addition, RXRs may function not only as heterodimeric partners of other nuclear receptors but also as active transducers of tumor suppressive signals [28]. It will be interesting to investigate whether the biological activity of carotenoids or their metabolites are mediated through interaction with RARs, RXRs, PPAR, or other orphan receptors.

The dosages of β-carotene used in the ATBC and CARET (Beta-Carotene and Retinol Efficacy Trial) studies were 20 to 30 mg/d for 2 to 8 yr, and these doses are 10- to 15-fold higher than the average intake (2 mg) of β-carotene in the typical American diet. Such a pharmacological dose of β-carotene in humans could result in the accumulation of relatively high β-carotene levels in the lung tissue, especially after long periods of supplementation, potentially leading to a decrease in lung retinoic acid concentration via induction of CYP enzymes [37]. Recent β-carotene intervention studies in humans indicate that β-carotene may prevent gastric carcinogenesis and oral precancerous lesions [17,18]. Unlike lung tissue, which has a slow turnover, the elimination of β-carotene in epithelial cells via sloughing of the gastrointestinal lining can prevent accumulation of excessive β-carotene in oral and gastric mucosa, thus reducing the risk of metabolite buildup. This hypothesis was also supported by a recent animal study which reported that both dietary and topical β-carotene prevents skin carcinoma formation in mice and induces retinoic acid receptor expression, while failing to act as a tumor promoter in the two-stage model of skin tumorigenesis [32]. In addition, the pro- or anticarcinogenic response to β-carotene supplementation reported in the human intervention trials and animal studies may be related to the stability of β-carotene and its metabolites depending on different environments of those organs. This is particularly related to the lungs of smokers, having a high oxidative stress by low antioxidant levels, such as vitamins E and C. A recent study by Liu et al. [42] has shown that the β-carotene in presence of α-tocopherol and ascorbic acid prevented the reduction of lung concentrations of β-carotene and retinoic acid in a smoke-exposed group of ferrets and increased the production of retinoic acid from β-carotene in the postnuclear fractions of lung tissues.

7.3 EFFECTS OF CAROTENOID SUPPLEMENTATION ON MAPK PATHWAY

Jun N-terminal kinase (JNK), extracellular-signal-regulated protein kinase (ERK), and p38 mitogen-activated protein kinase belong to the MAPK family that are activated by phosphorylation in response to many extracellular stimuli and environmental stress (e.g., smoke exposure) and may play an important role in carcinogenesis [43,44]. JNK was shown to phosphorylate c-Jun on sites Ser-63 and Ser-73, increase AP-1 transcription activity and, eventually, mediate cell proliferation and apoptosis [43,44]. ERK induced c-Jun through phosphorylation and activation of AP-1 component ATF1 at Ser63 [45]. Wang et al. [38] observed that AP-1 (c-Jun and c-Fos) expression was upregulated in the lungs of the high-dose β-carotene-supplemented ferrets with smoke exposure, as compared to control animals. These overexpressions of AP-1 were positively associated with squamous metaplasia in the lungs of the high-dose β-carotene-supplemented animals with smoke exposure [22].

MAPK phosphatases (MKPs), a family of dual-specificity protein phosphatases, can dephosphorylate both phospho-threonine and phosphor-tyrosine residues to inactivate JNK, ERK, and p38, both *in vitro* and *in vivo* [46–48]. It has been shown that phosphorylated-JNK, phosphorylated-ERK, and phosphorylated-p38 are preferred substrates for MKP-1 *in vivo* among isomers of MKPs [47,48]. Lee et al. [49,50] provided evidence that all-*trans*-retinoic acid suppresses JNK activity by inhibiting JNK phosphorylation and inducing MKP-1. It has been reported that c-Jun is required for progression through the G1 phase of the cell cycle by a mechanism that involves direct transcriptional control of the *cyclin D1* gene [51]. It is conceivable that the overexpression of c-Jun induced by cigarette smoke or chronic excess β-carotene intake may cause abnormal cell cycle regulation, driving cells into a premature S phase, which may result in an aberrant mitotic process, thereby causing cell proliferation and promoting carcinogenesis (Figure 7.3). This hypothesis is supported by a recent observation that smoke exposure, high-dose β-carotene, and their combination activated the phosphorylation of JNK and p38 but significantly reduced lung MKP-1 protein levels [52]. In contrast, low-dose β-carotene attenuated smoke-induced JNK phosphorylation by preventing downregulation of MKP-1 due to smoke exposure [52]. These data suggest a potential biological explanation for previous observations that the overexpression of total c-Jun induced by smoke exposure, high-dose β-carotene, or their combination increased cyclin D1 and proliferating cell nuclear antigen levels in ferrets after 6 months of treatment [22].

Srinivas et al. [53] showed that stress-induced increases in MAPK kinase 4 (MKK4) levels caused subsequent activation of JNK. This resulted in ligand-independent decreased stability of RARα through phosphorylation of Thr-181, Ser-445, and Ser-461, conjugation with ubiquitin ligases E1, E2, and E3, and degradation by the proteasomal pathway. Whereas there is considerable support for a role of RARβ as a tumor suppressor gene, the function of RARα in carcinogenesis is not well

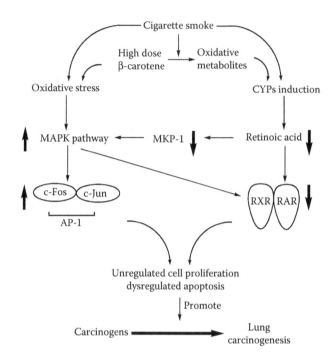

FIGURE 7.3 Simplified schematic illustration of possible molecular mechanisms of cigarette smoke and high-dose β-carotene supplementation on lung cell proliferation and carcinogenesis. (Adapted from Wang, X.D., Mechanistic understanding of potential adverse effects of beta-carotene supplementation, in Eisenbrand, G., Ed., *Functional Food: Safety Aspects,* Wiley-Vch., Weinheim, pp. 313–319, 2004.)

defined, although it does activate the RARE of RARβ, suggesting a possible accessory role for RARα in RARβ expression [54]. Recent results show that decreased expression of all RAR and RXR receptor subtypes is a frequent event in nonsmall-cell lung cancer [55]. Widely coregulated downregulation of expression of all retinoid subclasses suggests a fundamental dysregulation of the retinoid pathway in this cancer [55]. Further examination of carotenoid dosage on the stability and degradation of RARs, through JNK-mediated pathways, should be considered for future studies (Figure 7.3).

7.4 EFFECTS OF CAROTENOID SUPPLEMENTATION ON IGF-1 SIGNAL TRANSDUCTION PATHWAY

IGFs are recognized for their mitogenic ability to stimulate proliferation, differentiation, and apoptosis in cells [56]. Abnormal IGF-1 signaling has been implicated in the proliferation of cancer cells, whereas circulating IGF-binding proteins may limit IGF-1-stimulated cell growth by sequestering mitogenic IGF peptides in plasma. Numerous prospective studies have linked high IGF-1 levels with cancer [57], and a case–control analysis by Yu et al. [58] found that high IGF-1 levels and low IGF binding protein-3 (IGFBP-3) levels were associated with lung cancer. A subsequent case–control study [59] utilizing the placebo group from the CARET cohort, however, generated inconclusive results, indicating that age, length of time since cessation of smoking, and amount of smoke exposure may affect IGF-1 and IGFBP-3 levels differently.

The binding of IGF-1 to its receptor, IGF-1R, produces carcinogenic effects through two upregulated signaling mechanisms — the phosphatidylinositol 3′-kinase (PI3K)/Akt/protein kinase B (PKB) pathway and the Ras/Raf/mitogen-activated protein kinase (MAPK) pathway (Figure 7.4). Activation of these pathways results in inhibition of apoptosis through phosphorylation of BAD (on residue Ser 136 via the PI3K/Akt/PKB pathway or on residues Ser 112 and Ser 155 via the MAPK pathway). Additionally, stimulation of the cell cycle through activator protein 1 (AP-1)

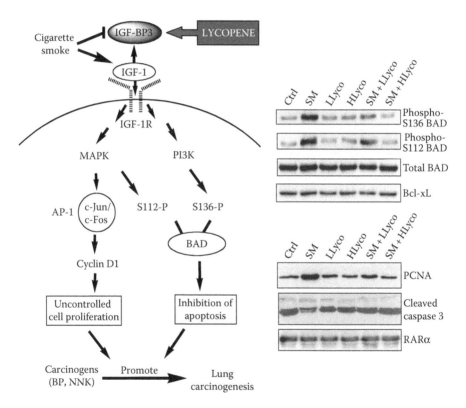

FIGURE 7.4 IGF binding protein-3 (IGFBP-3) regulates bioactivity of IGF-1 by sequestering IGF-1 away from its receptor in the extracellular milieu, thereby inhibiting the mitogenic and antiapoptotic action of IGF-1 and reducing cancer risk. One hypothesis is that lycopene or lycopene metabolites exert their protective effects against smoke-induced lung carcinogenesis through upregulating IGFBP-3, interrupting the signal transduction pathway of IGF-1, downregulating phosphorylation of BAD, promoting apoptosis, and inhibiting cell proliferation, thereby preventing lung carcinogenesis. (Adapted from Wang, X.D., Biological activity of lycopene against smoke-induced lung lesions: targeting the IGF-I/IGFBP-3 signal transduction pathway, in Packer, L., Kraemer, K., Obermuller-Jevicand, U., Sies, H., Eds., *Carotenoids and Retinoids: Molecular Aspects and Health Issues*. AOCS Press, Champaign, IL, pp. 168–181, 2005.)

occurs as a result of induction of MAPK activation. IGFBP-3 is a powerful inhibitor of both the signal transduction pathways by binding circulating IGF-1 [60], thereby inhibiting carcinogenesis (Figure 7.4). In patients with stage I nonsmall-cell lung cancer, IGFBP-3 is frequently downregulated, and lower levels correlate with disease-specific survival probability [61,62]. In addition, number of cigarettes smoked per day or pack-year history of smoking is negatively associated with IGFBP-3 plasma levels [63], further supporting its chemoprotective role in lung cancer.

At the cellular level, the mechanisms of action of IGF-1 and IGF-1R, have been examined in lung carcinomas by Pavelic et al. [64]. A correlation between increased expression (at mRNA and protein levels) for IGF-1 and IGF-1R and decreased apoptosis were found in large-cell carcinomas and adenocarcinomas. Squamous carcinoma cells treated with IGF-1 increased telomerase activity. The opposite was observed when the cells were treated with alphaIR3, which inhibits the activity of IGF-1 receptors, indicating that disruption of the IGF/IGF receptors axis is involved in lung cancer formation. Frankel et al. [65] using an IGF-1 transgenic mouse model expressed human IGF-1 in alveolar type II cells, demonstrated that increased expression of human IGF-1A in alveolar air spaces does not affect the development of pulmonary fibrosis but promotes premalignant changes in the alveolar epithelium.

Lycopene, commonly derived from tomatoes and tomato products, is notable for its strong antioxidant capacity; its physical quenching rate constant for singlet oxygen is almost double that of β-carotene. Other beneficial effects of lycopene include improved gap junction communication, inhibition of neoplastic transformation, and suppression of growth-factor-stimulated cell proliferation. In epidemiological studies, high carotenoid intake through diets rich in fruits and vegetables was found to be negatively associated with the risk of lung cancer, whereas lycopene, in particular, appeared to be beneficial [66,67]. The association between dietary lycopene and reduced lung cancer risk was found to be stronger than that observed for total fruit and vegetable intake [16,68]. An animal study by Kim et al. [69] showed a decreased incidence of lung tumors in B6C3F1 mice supplemented with lycopene. The inhibitory effect of lycopene on cell proliferation is supported by increasing evidence of upregulation of IGFBP-3, which interrupts the signaling of free IGF-1. The plasma ratio of IGF-1 to IGFBP-3 may be more accurate as a marker for increased risk of development of lung cancer and other cancers than absolute plasma levels of either protein.

Liu et al. [24] examined the effects of high- and low-dose lycopene supplementation on plasma levels of IGF-1 and IGFBP-3 in cigarette smoke-exposed and nonexposed ferrets, as well as histopathological changes, proliferating cellular nuclear antigen (PCNA) expression, BAD phosphorylation, and caspase 3 cleavage (apoptosis). The low dose of lycopene was 1.1 mg/(kg/d), equivalent to 15 mg/d in humans; the high-dose group was supplemented with 4.3 mg/(kg/d), equivalent to 60 mg/d in humans and achievable through a diet rich in fruits and vegetables. The average human intake of lycopene in the U.S. is 9.4 ± 0.3 mg/d. Whereas there were no differences in plasma IGF-1 levels between the groups, in the nonsmoke-exposed group, the ratio of IGF-1/IGFBP-3 was lower in ferrets supplemented with either a low dose or a high dose of lycopene and reached significance for the high-dose group. In ferrets exposed to cigarette smoke, the ratio of IGF-1 to IGFBP-3 was significantly higher than both the nonsmoke-exposed group and the smoke-exposed ferrets supplemented with lycopene at either a high or a low dose. In addition, the lung tissue of smoke-exposed ferrets exhibited decreased proportions of all-*trans*-lycopene and higher levels of 13-*cis*-lycopene and 9-*cis*-lycopene isomers. Smoke exposure increased PCNA expression by threefold and decreased cleaved caspase 3 by 74%; normal levels of PCNA and cleaved caspase 3 were restored with both low and high supplementation of lycopene. Levels of total BAD and Bcl-x_L did not differ among groups, although smoke exposure increased BAD phosphorylation fourfold at Ser-112 and 3.4-fold at Ser-136; both low and high doses of lycopene appeared to block this effect in smoke-exposed ferrets and resulted in similar levels of phosphorylated BAD, total BAD, and Bcl-s_L compared to nonsmoke-exposed ferrets. Contrary to the negative effects seen with high-dose β-carotene supplementation in combination with smoke exposure, in this study, both low- and high-dose lycopene were beneficial. This may be due to lower accumulation of lycopene in the lung tissue. In this study, the concentration of lycopene in the lungs was 1.2 μmol/kg after supplementation with 60 mg/d, whereas previous studies with β-carotene supplementation at 30 mg/d resulted in β-carotene accumulation in the lungs of 26 μmol/kg. The differences in accumulation of the different carotenoids may be partially responsible for the beneficial vs. deleterious effects in each study [70].

7.5 CONCLUSION

Understanding of the actions of carotenoids at molecular levels is critically needed for future human studies involving carotenoids for prevention of lung cancer and cancers at other tissue sites. Whereas the original hypothesis prompting the ATBC and CARET intervention trials was that β-carotene exerts beneficial effects through antioxidant activity, the harmful effects of high dosage led to further animal studies showing that the free-radical-rich environment of smokers' lungs decreased stability of the β-carotene molecule, depending on the presence of vitamins E and C. In addition, recent studies indicate that the beneficial vs. detrimental effects of carotenoids are related to the carotenoid dose administered *in vivo* and the accumulation of carotenoids and their metabolites or decomposition products in the lung, as well as to their effects on several important cellular signaling pathways and molecular targets (RARβ, MAPK, and IGFBP-3). β-Carotene at low doses or its excentric cleavage products can transactivate the RARβ2 promoter, primarily via conversion to retinoic acid, and prevent the reduction of RARβ caused by benzo[*a*]pyrene, a carcinogen from cigarette smoke, in normal human bronchial epithelial cells. Low-dose β-carotene supplementation with or without other antioxidants inhibits tobacco smoke-induced phosphorylation of JNK, ERK, and p38 MAPK by increasing MKP-1 and retinoic acid levels in the lung tissues, thereby preventing the formation of smoke-induced precancerous lesions. Lycopene supplementation protects against smoke-induced lung carcinogenesis by upregulating IGFBP-3, a molecular target that interrupts the signal transduction pathway of IGF-1, thereby lowering the risk of lung cancer. Furthermore, the oxidative cleavage products of β-carotene formed in large quantities in the cell due to supplementation with high-dose β-carotene in the highly oxidative conditions of the smoke-exposed lung enhance catabolism of retinoic acid by their induction of cytochrome P450 enzymes. These lower retinoic acid levels then enhance smoke-induced phosphorylation of MAPK, and downregulate MKP-1 expression, thereby promoting lung carcinogenesis. Lastly, β-carotene combined with other antioxidants (ascorbic acid and α-tocopherol) would be an effective chemopreventive strategy against lung cancer in smokers.

REFERENCES

1. von Lintig, J. and Vogt, K., Filling the gap in vitamin A research, molecular identification of an enzyme cleaving beta-carotene to retinal, *J Biol Chem,* 275, 11915–11920, 2000.
2. von Lintig, J. and Wyss, A., Molecular analysis of vitamin A formation: cloning and characterization of beta-carotene 15,15′-dioxygenases, *Arch Biochem Biophys,* 385, 47–52, 2001.
3. Wyss, A., Wirtz, G., Woggon, W., Brugger, R., Wyss, M., Friedlein, A., Bachmann, H., and Hunziker, W., Cloning and expression of beta, beta-carotene 15,15′-dioxygenase, *Biochem Biophys Res Commun,* 271, 334–336, 2000.
4. Wyss, A., Wirtz, G.M., Woggon, W.D., Brugger, R., Wyss, M., Friedlein, A., Riss, G., Bachmann, H., and Hunziker, W., Expression pattern and localization of beta, beta-carotene 15,15′-dioxygenase in different tissues, *Biochem J,* 354, 521–529, 2001.
5. Kiefer, C., Hessel, S., Lampert, J.M., Vogt, K., Lederer, M.O., Breithaupt, D.E., and von Lintig, J., Identification and characterization of a mammalian enzyme catalyzing the asymmetric oxidative cleavage of provitamin A, *J Biol Chem,* 276, 14110–14116, 2001.
6. Hu, K., Liu, C., Russell, R.M., and Wang, X.D., Cigarette smoke exposure upregulates carotene excentric cleaving enzyme, carotene-9′,10′-monooxygenase, in the lungs of ferrets with or without lycopene supplementation, *Cancer Epidemiol Biomarkers Prev,* 11, 1196s, 2003.
7. Wang, X.D., Krinsky, N.I., Tang, G.W., and Russell, R.M., Retinoic acid can be produced from excentric cleavage of beta-carotene in human intestinal mucosa, *Arch Biochem Biophys,* 293, 298–304, 1992.
8. Wang, X.D., Russell, R.M., Liu, C., Stickel, F., Smith, D.E., and Krinsky, N.I., Beta-oxidation in rabbit liver in vitro and in the perfused ferret liver contributes to retinoic acid biosynthesis from beta-apocarotenoic acids, *J Biol Chem,* 271, 26490–26498, 1996.
9. dos Anjos Ferreira, A.L., Yeum, K.J., Russell, R.M., Krinsky, N.I., and Tang, G., Enzymatic and oxidative metabolites of lycopene, *J Nutr Biochem,* 15, 493–502, 2004.
10. Wang, X.D., Carotenoid oxidative/degradative products and their biological activities, in Krinsky, N.I., Mayneand, S.T., Sies, H., Eds., *Carotenoids in Health and Disease,* Marcel Dekker, New York. pp. 313–335, 2004.
11. The Alpha-Tocopherol, Beta Carotene Cancer Prevention Study Group, The effect of vitamin E and beta carotene on the incidence of lung cancer and other cancers in male smokers, *N Engl J Med,* 330, 1029–1035, 1994.
12. Albanes, D., Heinonen, O.P., Taylor, P.R., Virtamo, J., Edwards, B.K., Rautalahti, M., Hartman, A.M., Palmgren, J., Freedman, L.S., Haapakoski, J., Barrett, M.J., Pietinen, P., Malila, N., Tala, E., Liippo, K., Salomaa, E.R., Tangrea, J.A., Teppo, L., Askin, F.B., Taskinen, E., Erozan, Y., Greenwald, P., and Huttunen, J.K., Alpha-tocopherol and beta-carotene supplements and lung cancer incidence in the alpha-tocopherol, beta-carotene cancer prevention study: effects of base-line characteristics and study compliance, *J Natl Cancer Inst,* 88, 1560–1570, 1996.

13. Omenn, G.S., Goodman, G., Thornquist, M., Grizzle, J., Rosenstock, L., Barnhart, S., Balmes, J., Cherniack, M.G., Cullen, M.R., Glass, A., and et al., The beta-carotene and retinol efficacy trial (CARET) for chemoprevention of lung cancer in high risk populations: smokers and asbestos-exposed workers, *Cancer Res,* 54, 2038S–2043S, 1994.

14. Hennekens, C.H., Buring, J.E., Manson, J.E., Stampfer, M., Rosner, B., Cook, N.R., Belanger, C., LaMotte, F., Gaziano, J.M., Ridker, P.M., Willett, W., and Peto, R., Lack of effect of long-term supplementation with beta carotene on the incidence of malignant neoplasms and cardiovascular disease, *N Engl J Med,* 334, 1145–1149, 1996.

15. Feskanich, D., Ziegler, R.G., Michaud, D.S., Giovannucci, E.L., Speizer, F.E., Willett, W.C., and Colditz, G.A., Prospective study of fruit and vegetable consumption and risk of lung cancer among men and women, *J Natl Cancer Inst,* 92, 1812–1823, 2000.

16. Michaud, D.S., Feskanich, D., Rimm, E.B., Colditz, G.A., Speizer, F.E., Willett, W.C., and Giovannucci, E., Intake of specific carotenoids and risk of lung cancer in 2 prospective U.S. cohorts, *Am J Clin Nutr,* 72, 990–997, 2000.

17. Mayne, S.T., Cartmel, B., Baum, M., Shor-Posner, G., Fallon, B.G., Briskin, K., Bean, J., Zheng, T., Cooper, D., Friedman, C., and Goodwin, W.J., Jr., Randomized trial of supplemental beta-carotene to prevent second head and neck cancer, *Cancer Res,* 61, 1457–1463, 2001.

18. Correa, P., Fontham, E.T., Bravo, J.C., Bravo, L.E., Ruiz, B., Zarama, G., Realpe, J.L., Malcom, G.T., Li, D., Johnson, W.D., and Mera, R., Chemoprevention of gastric dysplasia: randomized trial of antioxidant supplements and anti-helicobacter pylori therapy, *J Natl Cancer Inst,* 92, 1881–1888, 2000.

19. Yuan, J.M., Ross, R.K., Chu, X.D., Gao, Y.T., and Yu, M.C., Prediagnostic levels of serum beta-cryptoxanthin and retinol predict smoking-related lung cancer risk in Shanghai, China, *Cancer Epidemiol Biomarkers Prev,* 10, 767–773, 2001.

20. Mannisto, S., Smith-Warner, S.A., Spiegelman, D., Albanes, D., Anderson, K., van den Brandt, P.A., Cerhan, J.R., Colditz, G., Feskanich, D., Freudenheim, J.L., Giovannucci, E., Goldbohm, R.A., Graham, S., Miller, A.B., Rohan, T.E., Virtamo, J., Willett, W.C., and Hunter, D.J., Dietary carotenoids and risk of lung cancer in a pooled analysis of seven cohort studies, *Cancer Epidemiol Biomarkers Prev,* 13, 40–48, 2004.

21. Wright, M.E., Mayne, S.T., Stolzenberg-Solomon, R.Z., Li, Z., Pietinen, P., Taylor, P.R., Virtamo, J., and Albanes, D., Development of a comprehensive dietary antioxidant index and application to lung cancer risk in a cohort of male smokers, *Am J Epidemiol,* 160, 68–76, 2004.

22. Liu, C., Wang, X.D., Bronson, R.T., Smith, D.E., Krinsky, N.I., and Russell, R.M., Effects of physiological versus pharmacological beta-carotene supplementation on cell proliferation and histopathological changes in the lungs of cigarette smoke-exposed ferrets, *Carcinogenesis,* 21, 2245–2253, 2000.

23. Witschi, H., Carcinogenic activity of cigarette smoke gas phase and its modulation by beta-carotene and N-acetylcysteine, *Toxicol Sci,* 84, 81–87, 2005.

24. Liu, C., Lian, F., Smith, D.E., Russell, R.M., and Wang, X.D., Lycopene supplementation inhibits lung squamous metaplasia and induces apoptosis via up-regulating insulin-like growth factor-binding protein 3 in cigarette smoke-exposed ferrets, *Cancer Res,* 63, 3138–3144, 2003.

25. Palozza, P., Serini, S., Torsello, A., Boninsegna, A., Covacci, V., Maggiano, N., Ranelletti, F.O., Wolf, F.I., and Calviello, G., Regulation of cell cycle progression and apoptosis by beta-carotene in undifferentiated and differentiated HL-60 leukemia cells: possible involvement of a redox mechanism, *Int J Cancer,* 97, 593–600, 2002.

26. Wang, X.D., Mechanistic understanding of potential adverse effects of beta-carotene supplementation, in Eisenbrand, G., Ed., *Functional Food: Safety Aspects*, Wiley-Vch, Weinheim, pp. 313–319, 2004

27. Lippman, S.M. and Lotan, R., Advances in the development of retinoids as chemopreventive agents, *J Nutr,* 130, 479S–482S, 2000.

28. Altucci, L. and Gronemeyer, H., The promise of retinoids to fight against cancer, *Nat Rev Cancer,* 1, 181–193, 2001.

29. Soprano, D.R., Qin, P., and Soprano, K.J., Retinoic acid receptors and cancers, *Annu Rev Nutr,* 24, 201–221, 2004.

30. Napoli, J.L. and Race, K.R., Biogenesis of retinoic acid from beta-carotene: differences between the metabolism of beta-carotene and retinal, *J Biol Chem,* 263, 17372–17377, 1988.

31. Wang, X.-D., Krinsky, N.I., Benotti, P.N., and Russell, R.M., Biosynthesis of 9-*cis*-retinoic acid from 9-*cis*-b-carotene in human intestinal mucosa *in vitro*, *Arch Biochem Biophys,* 313, 150–155, 1994.

32. Ponnamperuma, R.M., Shimizu, Y., Kirchhof, S.M., and De Luca, L.M., Beta-carotene fails to act as a tumor promoter, induces RAR expression, and prevents carcinoma formation in a two-stage model of skin carcinogenesis in male Sencar mice, *Nutr Cancer,* 37, 82–88, 2000.

33. Prakash, P., Liu, C., Hu, K.Q., Krinsky, N.I., Russell, R.M., and Wang, X.D., Beta-carotene and beta-apo-14′-carotenoic acid prevent the reduction of retinoic acid receptor beta in benzo[a]pyrene-treated normal human bronchial epithelial cells, *J Nutr,* 134, 667–673, 2004.

34. Xu, X.C., Detection of altered retinoic acid receptor expression in tissue sections using in situ hybridization, *Histol Histopathol,* 16, 205–212, 2001.

35. Xu, X.C., Lee, J.J., Wu, T.T., Hoque, A., Ajani, J.A., and Lippman, S.M., Increased retinoic acid receptor-beta4 correlates in vivo with reduced retinoic acid receptor-beta2 in esophageal squamous cell carcinoma, *Cancer Epidemiol Biomarkers Prev,* 14, 826–829, 2005.

36. Liu, C., Russell, R.M., Seitz, H.K., and Wang, X.D., Ethanol enhances retinoic acid metabolism into polar metabolites in rat liver via induction of cytochrome P4502E1, *Gastroenterology,* 120, 179–189, 2001.

37. Liu, C., Russell, R.M., and Wang, X.D., Exposing ferrets to cigarette smoke and a pharmacological dose of beta-carotene supplementation enhance in vitro retinoic acid catabolism in lungs via induction of cytochrome P450 enzymes, *J Nutr,* 133, 173–179, 2003.

38. Wang, X.D., Liu, C., Bronson, R.T., Smith, D.E., Krinsky, N.I., and Russell, R.M., Retinoid signaling and activator protein-1 expression in ferrets given beta-carotene supplements and exposed to tobacco smoke, *J Natl Cancer Inst,* 91, 60–66, 1999.

39. Paolini, M., Cantelli-Forti, G., Perocco, P., Pedulli, G.F., Abdel-Rahman, S.Z., and Legator, M.S., Co-carcinogenic effect of beta-carotene, *Nature,* 398, 760–761, 1999.

40. Kim, Y., Chongviriyaphan, N., Liu, C., Russell, R.M., and Wang, X.D., Combined antioxidant β-carotene, α-tocopherol and ascorbic acid) supplementation increases the levels of lung retinoic acid and inhibits the activation of mitogen-activated protein kinase in the ferret lung cancer model, *Carcinogenesis,* (in press).

41. Tibaduiza, E.C., Fleet, J.C., Russell, R.M., and Krinsky, N.I., Excentric cleavage products of beta-carotene inhibit estrogen receptor positive and negative breast tumor cell growth in vitro and inhibit activator protein-1-mediated transcriptional activation, *J Nutr,* 132, 1368–1375, 2002.

42. Liu, C., Russell, R.M., and Wang, X.D., Alpha-tocopherol and ascorbic acid decrease the production of beta-apo-carotenals and increase the formation of retinoids from beta-carotene in the lung tissues of cigarette smoke-exposed ferrets in vitro, *J Nutr,* 134, 426–430, 2004.

43. Davis, R.J., Signal transduction by the JNK group of MAP kinases, *Cell,* 103, 239–252, 2000.

44. Karin, M., Liu, Z., and Zandi, E., AP-1 function and regulation, *Curr Opin Cell Biol,* 9, 240–246, 1997.

45. Gupta, P. and Prywes, R., ATF1 phosphorylation by the ERK MAPK pathway is required for epidermal growth factor-induced c-jun expression, *J Biol Chem,* 277, 50550–50556, 2002.

46. Sun, H., Charles, C.H., Lau, L.F., and Tonks, N.K., MKP-1 (3CH134), an immediate early gene product, is a dual specificity phosphatase that dephosphorylates MAP kinase in vivo, *Cell,* 75, 487–493, 1993.

47. Liu, Y., Gorospe, M., Yang, C., and Holbrook, N.J., Role of mitogen-activated protein kinase phosphatase during the cellular response to genotoxic stress. Inhibition of c-Jun N-terminal kinase activity and AP-1-dependent gene activation, *J Biol Chem,* 270, 8377–8380, 1995.

48. Slack, D.N., Seternes, O.M., Gabrielsen, M., and Keyse, S.M., Distinct binding determinants for ERK2/p38alpha and JNK map kinases mediate catalytic activation and substrate selectivity of map kinase phosphatase-1, *J Biol Chem,* 276, 16491–16500, 2001.

49. Lee, H.Y., Walsh, G.L., Dawson, M.I., Hong, W.K., and Kurie, J.M., All-trans-retinoic acid inhibits Jun N-terminal kinase-dependent signaling pathways, *J Biol Chem,* 273, 7066–7071, 1998.

50. Lee, H.Y., Sueoka, N., Hong, W.K., Mangelsdorf, D.J., Claret, F.X., and Kurie, J.M., All-trans-retinoic acid inhibits Jun N-terminal kinase by increasing dual-specificity phosphatase activity, *Mol Cell Biol,* 19, 1973–1980, 1999.

51. Wisdom, R., Johnson, R.S., and Moore, C., c-Jun regulates cell cycle progression and apoptosis by distinct mechanisms, *Embo J,* 18, 188–197, 1999.

52. Liu, C., Russell, R.M., and Wang, X.D., Low dose beta-carotene supplementation of ferrets attenuates smoke-induced lung phosphorylation of JNK, p38 MAPK, and p53 proteins, *J Nutr,* 134, 2705–2710, 2004.

53. Srinivas, H., Juroske, D.M., Kalyankrishna, S., Cody, D.D., Price, R.E., Xu, X.C., Narayanan, R., Weigel, N.L., and Kurie, J.M., c-Jun N-terminal kinase contributes to aberrant retinoid signaling in lung cancer cells by phosphorylating and inducing proteasomal degradation of retinoic acid receptor alpha, *Mol Cell Biol, 25,* 1054–1069, 2005.

54. Inui, N., Sasaki, S., Suda, T., Chida, K., and Nakamura, H., The loss of retinoic acid receptor alpha, beta and alcohol dehydrogenase3 expression in non-small cell lung cancer, *Respirology,* 8, 302–309, 2003.

55. Brabender, J., Metzger, R., Salonga, D., Danenberg, K.D., Danenberg, P.V., Holscher, A.H., and Schneider, P.M., Comprehensive expression analysis of retinoic acid receptors and retinoid X receptors in non-small cell lung cancer: implications for tumor development and prognosis, *Carcinogenesis,* 26, 525–530, 2005.

56. Yu, H. and Rohan, T., Role of the insulin-like growth factor family in cancer development and progression, *J Natl Cancer Inst,* 92, 1472–1489, 2000.

57. Giovannucci, E., Insulin-like growth factor-I and binding protein-3 and risk of cancer, *Horm Res,* 51 (Suppl. 3), 34–41, 1999.

58. Yu, H., Spitz, M.R., Mistry, J., Gu, J., Hong, W.K., and Wu, X., Plasma levels of insulin-like growth factor-I and lung cancer risk: a case-control analysis, *J Natl Cancer Inst,* 91, 151–156, 1999.

59. Spitz, M.R., Barnett, M.J., Goodman, G.E., Thornquist, M.D., Wu, X., and Pollak, M., Serum insulin-like growth factor (IGF) and IGF-binding protein levels and risk of lung cancer: a case-control study nested in the beta-Carotene and Retinol Efficacy Trial Cohort, *Cancer Epidemiol Biomarkers Prev,* 11, 1413–1418, 2002.

60. Lee, H.Y., Chun, K.H., Liu, B., Wiehle, S.A., Cristiano, R.J., Hong, W.K., Cohen, P., and Kurie, J.M., Insulin-like growth factor binding protein-3 inhibits the growth of non-small cell lung cancer, *Cancer Res,* 62, 3530–3537, 2002.

61. Chang, Y.S., Kong, G., Sun, S., Liu, D., El-Naggar, A.K., Khuri, F.R., Hong, W.K., Lee, H.Y., and Gong, K., Clinical significance of insulin-like growth factor-binding protein-3 expression in stage I non-small cell lung cancer, *Clin Cancer Res,* 8, 3796–3802, 2002.

62. Chang, Y.S., Wang, L., Liu, D., Mao, L., Hong, W.K., Khuri, F.R., and Lee, H.Y., Correlation between insulin-like growth factor-binding protein-3 promoter methylation and prognosis of patients with stage I non-small cell lung cancer, *Clin Cancer Res,* 8, 3669–3675, 2002.

63. Kaklamani, V.G., Linos, A., Kaklamani, E., Markaki, I., and Mantzoros, C., Age, sex, and smoking are predictors of circulating insulin-like growth factor 1 and insulin-like growth factor-binding protein 3, *J Clin Oncol,* 17, 813–817, 1999.

64. Pavelic, J., Krizanac, S., Kapitanovic, S., Pavelic, L., Samarzija, M., Pavicic, F., Spaventi, S., Jakopovic, M., Herceg-Ivanovi, Z., and Pavelic, K., The consequences of insulin-like growth factors/receptors dysfunction in lung cancer, *Am J Respir Cell Mol Biol,* 32, 65–71, 2005.

65. Frankel, S.K., Moats-Staats, B.M., Cool, C.D., Wynes, M.W., Stiles, A.D., and Riches, D.W., Human insulin-like growth factor-IA expression in transgenic mice promotes adenomatous hyperplasia but not pulmonary fibrosis, *Am J Physiol Lung Cell Mol Physiol,* 288, L805–L812, 2005.

66. Clinton, S.K., Lycopene: chemistry, biology, and implications for human health and disease, *Nutr Rev,* 56, 35–51, 1998.

67. Giovannucci, E., Tomatoes, tomato-based products, lycopene, and cancer: review of the epidemiologic literature, *J Natl Cancer Inst,* 91, 317–331, 1999.

68. Holick, C.N., Michaud, D.S., Stolzenberg-Solomon, R., Mayne, S.T., Pietinen, P., Taylor, P.R., Virtamo, J., and Albanes, D., Dietary carotenoids, serum {beta}-carotene, and retinol and risk of lung cancer in the alpha-tocopherol, beta-carotene cohort study, *Am J Epidemiol,* 156, 536–547, 2002.

69. Kim, D.J., Takasuka, N., Nishino, H., and Tsuda, H., Chemoprevention of lung cancer by lycopene, *Biofactors,* 13, 95–102, 2000.

70. Wang, X.D., Biological activity of lycopene against smoke-induced lung lesions: targeting the IGF-I/IGFBP-3 signal transduction pathway, in Packer, L., Kraemer, K., Obermuller-Jevicand, U., Sies, H., Eds., *Carotenoids and Retinoids: Molecular Aspects and Health Issues.* AOCS Press, Champaign, IL, pp. 168–181, 2005.

8 The Actions of the Vitamin D Receptor in Health and Malignancy; Polymorphic Associations and Gene Regulatory Actions

Moray J. Campbell and Kay W. Colston

CONTENTS

8.1   BACKGROUND

8.1.1   THE CANCER BURDEN

The clinical and societal impact of malignancy continues to be highly significant in the developed world and is becoming increasingly so in the developing world, despite significant progress in understanding disease etiology and generating novel therapies. The reasons for the sustained burden are numerous; they include the demographic transition occurring in many countries and the intrinsic complexity of the disease. The increased understanding of cancers has led to the development of a number of high-profile "targeted" therapies that are aimed at specific molecular lesions. Although many of these have generated significant clinical results, the development lead on these drugs also has significant associated financial costs that may prohibit their worldwide usage. This may change in the future as development lead times are reduced and targeting strategies improve. In the short-to-medium term, there is a need to understand the etiology of high-profile malignancies and develop preventative and therapeutic options that perhaps focus on shifting cancer from an acute to chronic disease.

8.1.2   COMMON AND COMPLEX ETIOLOGY OF BREAST, PROSTATE, AND COLON CANCER

The costs of these three cancers are very significant to the individual and to society. For example, there are approximately 1 million new cases of breast cancer diagnosed around the world every year; it comprises about 18% of all cancers in women. The impact is not restricted to the developed world, as some of the greatest increases of these cancer types are projected to occur in developing and emerging nations. Worryingly, though there is evidence of controlling the rate of increase in the developed world, there are significant consequences in terms of resource availability to treat these cancers in developing countries. Similar increases are also projected for prostate and colon cancer.

Significant improvements have been made in the management of these cancers since the 1970s with surgery, radiotherapy, chemotherapy, and in the case of prostate and breast cancer, endocrine therapies, providing significantly improved treatment modalities. Despite the improvements in disease-free survival, overall survival, and mortality with current recommended adjuvant therapy regimens, many issues remain unresolved, and the underlying causes for the development of these three high-profile cancers are still not clearly understood.

In the case of a minority of the cancer burden, known risks factors include a positive family history. Thus, familial breast cancers, linked to high-penetrant genetic mutations associated with the *BRCA1* and *BRCA2* gene loci, account for about 5% of all breast cancer cases, and drive an aggressive form of the cancer that is often typified by early-onset cases (< 30 yr).[1] Similarly, a number of gene targets have been implicated in the development of colon cancer. For example, the *APC* gene is a key regulator of the Wnt/β-catenin pathway and has been found to be mutated in kindreds with aggressive heritable forms of colon cancer.[2] Historically, this exclusive genetic causality has provided a paradigm for dissecting and understanding the etiology of cancer. Strikingly, despite the considerable resources that have been applied to hunting for further novel susceptibility loci in these cancers, they have not been identified. Thus, in breast cancer, a *BRCA3* gene has not emerged, and, equally, in prostate cancer, no strong penetrance genes have been identified.

An alternative contemporary view of the multifactorial etiology of these and other common cancers is that they include a contribution from an ill-defined combination of genetic factors with weak penetrance acting in response to a multitude of environmental factors.[3–7] Reflecting this complex etiology, the single greatest risk factor for all cancers is age, with the average age of onset of common cancers such as breast, prostate, and colon cancer in the sixth and seventh decades of life. These data fit more readily with models of cancer development that are multifactorial and require disruption of multiple mechanisms of cell restraint and tissue organization.[8] It is estimated that the development of most cancers require 4 to 7 disruptions to such pathways.[9,10]

The sporadic, temporal acquisition of a cancer phenotype is also compatible with models of disruption of the self-renewal of these epithelial tissues. It has become increasingly clear that these tissues, in common with other epithelial tissues and many other cell types in the adult human, are self-renewing and contain committed stem cell components.[11–16] These cells are slowly proliferating and are able to undergo asymmetric divisions to give rise to both other stem cells and transiently amplifying (TA) populations of progenitor cells that in turn give rise to the differentiated cell types, which typify the functions of these tissues and are subsequently lost through programmed cell death processes and replaced by newly differentiated TA cells. The mechanisms that control the intricate balance of these processes of division, differentiation, and programmed cell death are subjects of significant investigations. These studies have revealed common roles for Wnt and Hedgehog signaling and the actions of other signal transduction processes that govern cell cycle progression, with gene targets such as the cyclin-dependent kinase inhibitor p21[(waf1/cip1)] emerging as points of criticality upon which numerous signal pathways converge.

Stem cells of any tissue also have a high proliferative capacity and are the ideal candidates for tumorigenesis as they are programmed for self-renewal. It is likely to take fewer disruptions to maintain this activation than switching it on *de novo* in a more differentiated cell.[17] Furthermore, by self-renewing, stem cells are relatively long lived compared to other cells within tissues. Although it has become apparent that there are numerous mechanisms in place in stem cells to ensure genomic integrity, the longevity of these cells results in a greater likelihood of genetic, cytogenetic, or epigenetic disruptions accumulating or being passed on to daughter progenitors.[18]

8.1.3 Emerging Roles of Diet in Malignancy

It is becoming clear that environmental factors, through interacting with genetic components, play a significant role in determining the onset and severity of the overwhelming majority of cancers, which are sporadic in nature. It is unclear, however, what time point in an individual's life has to be modeled to capture the critical initiating or promoting events, which ultimately lead to overt cancer development in the sixth decade of life. The mechanistic understanding of the role that environmental risk factors play in cancer etiology is compounded by the necessity to attempt double-blind prospective studies of factors to establish clear links. Understandably, this is highly challenging. Perhaps the clearest risk factor for cancer development is the contribution of cigarette smoke to lung cancer. Considerable resources were required to elucidate what is now established as a clear causal relationship.[19]

Recently, the appreciation of the impact of diet on cancer has come significantly to the fore with a number of studies establishing unequivocal relationships between diet and cancer initiation and progression. Reflecting the accumulation of these data, the World Health Organization has now stated that diet forms the second-most preventable cause of cancer (after smoking). This impact will rise further due to demographic factors, and quite possibly due to changing dietary habits worldwide, this will contribute further to the projected increase in cancer incidence in preindustrialized nations.

High-profile malignancies such as breast, prostate, and colon cancer typify this scenario, in which the etiology of the disease reflects the cumulative impact of dietary factors over an individual's lifetime.[20–22] The relationship between diet and disease is already being exploited clinically, for example, in the SELECT trial to assess the chemoprevention potential of vitamin E and selenium in prostate cancer.[23–25] Reflecting the growing understanding of the significance of the relationships between diet, health, and disease, new scientific approaches are seeking to utilize genomic and postgenomic technologies to interrogate these mechanisms. The emerging field of nutrigenomics aims to dissect the impact of dietary factors on genomic regulation and, thereby, physiology and pathophysiology.[26–28]

Tissue self-renewal is controlled by intrinsic and extrinsic cues, including a range of niche signals and extrinsic hormonal and dietary cues, which appear to regulate many of the processes associated with differentiation and programmed cell death. The primary genomic sensor for many dietary and environmental (e.g., xenobiotic) factors is the nuclear receptor superfamily of ligand-activated transcription factors, which bind steroid hormones, vitamin micronutrients, and macronutrients such as fatty acids, lipids, and bile acids.[29–32] Thus, nuclear receptors integrate dietary extracellular signals into cell fate decisions such as cell cycle control, self-renewal, and xenobiotic clearance. These interrelationships are of particular pertinence to nuclear receptor biology because these receptors stand at an intersection of these various areas of research. Thus, nuclear receptors are central to the response to many dietary cues, play a role in governing cell proliferation and differentiation, and are disrupted in malignancy.

8.2 THE VITAMIN D RECEPTOR IS A MEMBER OF THE NUCLEAR RECEPTOR SUPERFAMILY

8.2.1 NUCLEAR RECEPTORS ALLOW A LOCAL RESPONSE TO LIPOPHILIC NUTRIENTS

The nuclear receptor superfamily of transcription factors (48 human members) binds with a range of affinities to lipid-derived hormonal and dietary factors and regulates gene targets (Table 8.1).[33] The family members can be classified broadly according to ligand affinities. The first group of receptors bind ligands with high affinity and is typified by the sex steroid hormone receptors (e.g., the estrogens receptor [ERα and β]), which sense estrogenic hormones and also a range of phytoestrogens and isoflavonoids. These receptors and the estrogen-related receptors (ERR) play a clear role in the development and regulation of the mammary gland, and constitute a central therapeutic axis in breast cancer.[34–40] Interestingly, their expression and corruption in the prostate and colon suggests a broader function.[41–46] A number of micronutrient ligands are also bound with high affinity by specific receptors. For example, the active metabolites of vitamin A and vitamin D are bound, respectively, by the retinoic acid and retinoid X receptors (RARs and RXRs)[47] and vitamin D receptor (VDR).[48] The second group of receptors, the adopted orphan receptors, bind more abundant macronutrients such as polyunsaturated fatty acids and bile acids with lower affinity, for example, the peroxisome proliferators-activated receptors (PPARs),[49–51] liver X receptors (LXRs),[52] and farnesoid X receptor (FXR).[53] Finally, a group of orphan receptors exists for which no ligands have been identified.[54]

The VDR was originally described for its central endocrine role in the maintenance of serum calcium levels. Similarly, the FXR and LXRs were described for their roles in regulating the metabolism of cholesterol, fatty and bile acids metabolism in the enterohepatic system. The expression of these receptors in nonclassical tissues, such as the prostate and breast, suggests a broader role in the local sensing of dietary lipid molecules (Table 8.1).[55,56] The response to fatty and bile acids is shared by other receptors such as RXRs[57] and the VDR, which can also respond to lithocholic acid (LCA), the secondary bile acid, to induce the cytochrome P450, CYP3A4.[58,59] Examination of the VDR, RARs, PPARs, FXR, and LXRs reveals that they have target genes[60] in common that regulate the cell cycle (e.g., p21[(waf1/cip1)61] and GADD45α[62,63]), differentiation (e.g., NKX3.1[64,65] and E-Cadherin[66,67]), and xenobiotic clearance via cytochrome P450s (e.g., CYP3A4[56,68–70]).

Collectively, the expression of a wider tissue expression of a compliment of nutrient-sensing receptors than hitherto suspected allows the local direct response to a wide range of dietary lipids. Thus, nuclear receptors provide a strong molecular

TABLE 8.1
Relative Expression of Dietary-Sensing Nuclear Receptors in Normal Breast, Prostate, and Colon Epithelium and Sample Dietary Ligands

Nuclear receptors	Relative abundance[1]			Dietary derived ligand
High affinity	Breast	Prostate	Colon	
ERα				Phytoestrogens, e.g. Genistein, and Flavonoids
ERβ				
ERRα				
ERRβ				
RARα				All *trans* retinoic acid
RARβ				
RARγ				
RXRα				9-cis retinoic acid, docosahexanoic acid
RXRβ				
RXRγ				
VDR				1α,25(OH)$_2$D$_3$ and Lithocholic acid
Broad affinity				
PPARα				Eicosapentaenoic acid
PPARδ				Linoleic acid
PPARγ				5,8,11,14-eicosatetraenoic acid
LXRα				24(S) hydroxycholesterol and cholesterol derivatives
LXRβ				Oxysterols
FXR				Chenodeoxycholic acid and other bile acids

[a] The relative abundance was determined *in silico* from publicly deposited SAGE data[33,] and the gradations of shading indicate the relative mRNA abundance. The darker shades indicate higher expression.

link between nutritional signals, gene regulation, and tissue maintenance. Supportively epidemiological and chemoprevention studies indicate that initiation or progression of cancer may relate to altered intake of micro- and macronutrients (e.g., the balance of omega 3 and omega 6 fatty acids) and cellular resistance to the receptors that sense these substances.[51,63,71] Collectively, these findings support the concept that the nuclear receptor superfamily acts as coordinated signaling conduits providing a functional link between hormonal, environmental, and dietary cues and tissue homeostasis.

8.2.2 LOCAL REMODELING OF CHROMATIN IS CENTRAL TO NUCLEAR RECEPTOR TRANSCRIPTIONAL FUNCTIONS

The nuclear receptors share a common architecture that includes defined regions for DNA recognition, ligand binding, and cofactor interactions. The DNA-binding domain recognizes specific nucleotide response elements (RE) in target gene enhancer/promoter regions. Most receptors preferentially form homo- or heterodimeric complexes; RXR is a central partner for VDR, PPARs, LXRs, and FXR. Therefore, simple REs are formed by two recognition motives, and their relative distance and orientation contributes to receptor binding specificity, and composite elements have been identified more recently.

In the absence of ligand, VDR-RXR dimer exists in an "*apo*" state, as part of large complexes (~2.0 MDa), associated with corepressors (e.g., NCoR2/SMRT) and bound to RE sequences. These complexes actively recruit a range of enzymes that posttranslationally modify histone tails, for example, histone deacetylases and methyltransferase, and thereby maintain a locally closed chromatin structure around RE sequences.[72] Ligand binding induces a so-called "*holo*" state, facilitating the association of the VDR-RXR dimer with coactivator complexes. A large number of interacting coactivator proteins have been described, which can be divided into multiple families including the p160 family, the non-p160 members, and members of the large "bridging" DRIP/TRAP/ARC complex, which links the receptor complex to the cointegrators CBP/p300 and basal transcriptional machinery.[30,31] These receptor coactivator complexes coordinate the activation of an antagonistic battery of enzymes such as histone acetyltransferases, and thereby induce the reorganization of local chromatin regions at the RE of the target gene promoter. The complex choreography of this event has recently emerged and involves cyclical rounds of promoter-specific complex assembly, gene transactivation, complex disassembly, and proteosome-mediated degradation[32,73,74] (Figure 8.1).

The expression, localization, and isoforms of corepressor complexes have emerged as critical to determine the spatiotemporal equilibrium between the antagonistic actions of the *apo* and *holo* NR megacomplexes, and thus determine target gene promoter responsiveness,[75–77] for example, in regulating NR function during neural cell differentiation, in determining cell-specific responses to steroid hormones, and in the inappropriate silencing of NR actions associated with neoplasia.[63,78,79]

It remains unclear to what extent the various histone modifications initiated by the apo and holo NR megacomplexes around gene promoter regions influence the subsequent transcriptional responsiveness of the promoter. It has been proposed that these modifications may form a stable and heritable "histone code," which determines the assembly of factors upon the chromatin template and controls individual promoter transcriptional responsiveness.[80–86] Functional studies of the SANT motif contained in the corepressor NCoR2/SMRT supports this latter idea.[87]

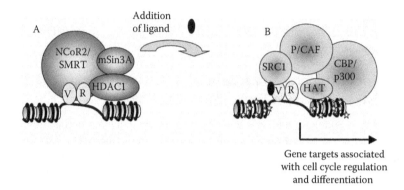

FIGURE 8.1 Ligand-activated switch of VDR and target genes. (A) In the absence of ligand ($1\alpha,25(OH)_2D_3$), the VDR-RXR heterodimer exists in the apo conformation associated with corepressors such as NCoR2/SMRT and actively represses gene transactivation through a range of posttranslational modifications of histone tails, thereby condensing local chromatin. (B) The addition of $1\alpha,25(OH)_2D_3$ induces conformational changes (holo conformation) in the ligand binding domain of the VDR and allows interactions with coactivator and cointegrator proteins that reverse the histone modifications and, thereby, facilitate transcription. A range of target genes associated with cell cycle regulation, apoptosis, adhesion, and others are consequently regulated.

8.2.3 OTHER FUNCTIONS OF VDR THAT CONTRIBUTE TO CELL REGULATORY ACTIONS

Other roles for the VDR have emerged, aside from the direct transcriptional effects. A number of workers have pursued the role for the VDR in nongenomic, rapid cellular effects. Recently, these studies have coincided with the elucidation of the actions of other nuclear receptors working at the cell membrane to bring about rapid effects mediated through the signal transduction process. These studies, for example, with the ERα, have demonstrated its expression and function in membrane processes.[88,89] Similarly, a role for VDR in these subcellular structures has emerged, which plays a role in modifying signal transduction processes, notably as an anti-apoptotic mechanism.[90,91] Another emergent area for the gene regulation by NRs, including the VDR, are a range of posttranscriptional effects that regulate mRNA stability, translation, and protein degradation,[92,93] although the mechanistic basis for these actions is less well understood.

8.3 THE VITAMIN D RECEPTOR

8.3.1 THE VDR: EXPRESSED IN A BROAD PANEL OF NONCALCEMIC TISSUES

Classically, the actions of vitamin D have been established as part of the endocrine systems that regulate serum calcium levels, in particular by regulating calcium absorption in the gut and regulating bone mineralization. Vitamin D status is dependent upon cutaneous synthesis initiated by solar radiation and also on dietary

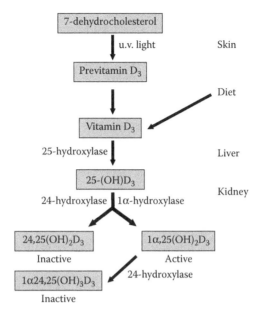

FIGURE 8.2 The metabolism of vitamin D_3. Renal synthesis is the major source of circulating $1\alpha,25(OH)_2D_3$. However, extrarenal generation of the active vitamin D metabolite may be of functional significance in other tissues such as breast, prostate, and colon. Most VDR-containing tissues also express 24-hydroxylase, the enzyme that catalyzes the initial step in the inactivation pathway for $25(OH)D_3$ and $1\alpha,25(OH)_2D_3$.

intake — a reduction of one or both sources leads to vitamin D insufficiency. Interestingly, the contribution from the UV-catalyzed cutaneous reaction is greater, contributing over 90% in a vitamin-D-sufficient individual. The correct and sufficient level of serum vitamin D is currently a matter of considerable debate.

Vitamin D is converted in the liver to 25-hydroxyvitamin D3 ($25[OH]D_3$), and circulating levels of this metabolite serve as a useful index of vitamin D status. A further hydroxylation occurs in the carbon 1 position by the recently cloned 25-hydroxyvitamin D-1α-hydroxylase (encoded by CYP27b1) to produce the bio-logically active metabolite. A second mitochondrial cytochrome P450 enzyme, the 24-hydroxylase (encoded by CYP24) enzyme, can utilize both $25(OH)D_3$ and $1\alpha,25(OH)_2D_3$ as substrates[11] and is the first step in the inactivation pathway for these metabolites (Figure 8.2).

8.3.2 AUTOCRINE VS. PARACRINE SIGNALING

Until recently, expression of the $25(OH)D_3$ activating enzyme, CYP27b, was thought to be restricted to the classical sites for endocrine synthesis of the biologically active form of the secosteroid hormone vitamin D, $1\alpha,25(OH)_2D_3$. However, the extra renal expression of CYP27b1 in nonclassical target tissues has raised the possibility of an autocrine/paracrine role for the local synthesis and signaling of $1\alpha,25(OH)_2D_3$.

Thus, 25(OH)D$_3$ may enter into an intracellular VDR signaling axis that coordinates the local synthesis, metabolism, and signal transduction of 1α,25(OH)$_2$D$_3$. The components of the axis have been shown to be dynamically regulated as CYP27b1 is repressed by 1α,25(OH)$_2$D$_3$ and, correspondingly, CYP24 is positively regulated by 1α,25(OH)$_2$D$_3$. Thus, elevated levels of 1α,25(OH)$_2$D$_3$ appear to block its synthesis and induce its own inactivation[94–96] and, therefore, represents a classical negative feedback loop. A number of workers have now found strong evidence for this local autocrine regulatory loop being expressed and operative in a wide range of noncalcemic tissues.[97–102] Thus, it has emerged that 1α,25(OH)$_2$D$_3$ is regulated in an endocrine manner, principally associated with its calcemic function and locally at an autocrine level, more likely associated with its role in regulation of cell proliferation and differentiation.

8.3.3 VDR Actions in Normal Tissues

The role for VDR actions in noncalcemic tissues has been the subject of intensive investigation, and a consistent theme that emerges is the regulation of target genes, which subsequently control cell growth, differentiation, and programmed cell death. *In vitro* 1α,25(OH)$_2$D$_3$ is able to regulate proliferation of a wide range of normal tissues including epithelial cells from the prostate, breast, and colon and myeloid CD 34 positive precursors.[103–107] Prostate and mammary glands and the lining of the gastrointestinal tract, all typify self-renewing tissues; for example, the lining of the colon is remodeled every 3 d. All these systems reveal various aspects of the interrelationships between diet, VDR, tissue maintenance, and cancer. In the case of the prostate and mammary gland, there is considerable postembryological development, primarily through adolescence. Thereafter in the adult, all three glands are maintained in a state of constant self-renewal, with committed stem cell components giving rise to multiple cell lineages.[108]

In mammals, the requirement for calcium increases during pregnancy and lactation to meet the increased needs of the fetal skeleton for mineralization and to provide calcium for milk. Thus, the mammary gland represents an intriguing area in which the endocrine, calcemic, and autocrine, cellular effects of the VDR appear to converge. During pregnancy and lactation, the circulating concentrations of 1α,25(OH)$_2$D$_3$ are elevated, leading to increased efficiency of intestinal calcium absorption. In addition to its importance in preservation of maternal calcium homeostasis during pregnancy and lactation, there is evidence that 1α,25(OH)$_2$D$_3$, acting through the VDR, plays a role in augmenting development, differentiation, and milk production in mammary glands. For example, early studies revealed that addition of 1α,25(OH)$_2$D$_3$ to the murine mammary gland increased the VDR expression and enhanced calcium uptake.[109]

The greatest insights have been gained more recently through the use of murine, transgenic, and knockout approaches. Four groups have independently generated *vdr*-deficient mice with a range of targeting strategies, for example, disrupting the zinc finger region of the DNA binding domain.[110–112] Disruption of the VDR results in a profound phenotype in these models, but is principally observed postweaning and is associated with the disruption of duodenal calcium absorption and bone mineralization, such as hypocalcemia, secondary hyperparathyroidism, osteomalacia, rickets, impaired bone formation, and elevated serum $1\alpha,25(OH)_2D_3$. In parallel, a range of more subtle effects are seen, and these are not shared by all the mice. These include uterine hypoplasia and impaired ovarian folliculogenesis, and male animals have reproductive dysfunction,[113] cardiac hypertrophy,[114] and enhanced thrombogenicity.[115] Importantly in the context of the current review, the more recent studies have revealed that female mice display altered mammary gland function, and the VDR ablated backgrounds have now been crossed into a range of tumorigenic models and support an antitumor chemoprevention role for VDR.

The mammary gland morphology in *vdr*-deficient mice supports a negative proliferative and prodifferentiative role for the VDR. Thus, the glands in the knockout animals display enhanced growth compared to their wild-type litter mates, and the glands become heavier with an elevated number of terminal end buds, greater ductal outgrowth, and enhanced secondary branch points.[104,116] This accelerated growth is exacerbated further during the pregnancy-associated proliferative burst, and, moreover, the widespread postlactation apoptosis associated with involution is delayed. Similarly, in cells derived from these animal and in *ex vivo* organ cultures, the response to exogenous estrogen and progesterone appears enhanced.[104]

The *vdr*-deficient mice have no overt prostate or colon phenotype; however, certainly in the case of the prostate, these glands differ in structure and function between humans and mice. However, studies in normal colonic crypts have identified the VDR in the upper portion, commensurate with a role in negatively regulating proliferation and promoting differentiation. Similarly, in the prostate, $1\alpha,25(OH)_2D_3$ cooperates with testosterone to induce differentiation in epithelial cells.

8.4 TRANSCRIPTIONAL AND CELLULAR EFFECTS OF THE VDR

In 1981, $1\alpha,25(OH)_2D_3$ was shown to inhibit human melanoma cells significantly *in vitro* at nanomolar concentrations[117] and, subsequently, $1\alpha,25(OH)_2D_3$ was found to cause differentiation in cultured mouse and human myeloid leukemic cells.[118,119] Following these studies, $1\alpha,25(OH)_2D_3$ has been demonstrated to have a range of antiproliferative effects in a wide panel of cancer cell lines, including those from prostate and breast.[48,66,105,120–130] Proliferation and differentiation of normal prostate epithelial cells is acutely regulated *in vitro* and *in vivo* by $1\alpha,25(OH)_2D_3$,[103,125] thereby justifying clinical trials in prostate cancer patients.[131–135] An overwhelming number of studies have used cancer cell lines to elucidate antiproliferative and prodifferentiative actions of the VDR, and, thus, the common models of VDR responses include MCF-7 breast cancer cells, LNCaP prostate cancer cells, and CaCo2 colon cancer cells.

A number of groups worldwide have undertaken comprehensive genomewide *in silico* and transcriptomic screens to elucidate the VDR transcriptome.[62,63,129,136–139] These studies have revealed broad consensus on certain targets, but have also highlighted variability. This may in part reflect experimental design, for example, undertaking these studies in cancer cell lines in which these processes are in part corrupted.[63]

The differences in part also reflect genuine tissue-specific differences of cofactor expression that alter the magnitude and extent of VDR transcriptional actions.

8.4.1 Cell Cycle Progression

The common antiproliferative function of the VDR in a range of cell models was shown by early studies to be associated with regulation of cell cycle progression, and subsequent *in vitro* studies focused on the characterization of gene targets that were modulated in association with these events. Subsequently, it emerged that a common feature of the antiproliferative actions of these vitamin D compounds is the arrest in G_0/G_1 of the cell cycle, associated with the upregulation of a number of cell cycle inhibitors including p21$^{(waf1/cip1)}$ [61,62,66,140] and p27$^{(kip1)}$.[92,141–144] A potential VDRE was discovered in the promoter of p21$^{(wafl/cip1)}$ gene, and mRNA was upregulated in p53-negative cell lines within 2 h exposure of $1\alpha,25(OH)_2D_3$ treatment, which suggests that this CDKI is a primary $1\alpha,25(OH)_2D_3$ responding gene.[61] Concomitant with these events is a downregulation of cyclin A and cyclin D1, decreases in kinase activities associated with, for example, Cdk2, and, ultimately, the dephosphorylation of the retinoblastoma protein and sequestration of E2F family members in a repressive complex.

How many of these events are directly mediated by VDR transcriptional activities and to what extent others are consequences of action is uncertain. For example, whereas the promoter/enhancer region of p21$^{(wafl/cip1)}$ contains several well-characterized VDRE, by contrast p27$^{(kip1)}$ appears to be regulated by a range of posttranscriptional mechanisms such as enhanced mRNA translation,[93] interacting with Sp1, which binds the p27$^{(kip1)}$ promoter,[92] and attenuating mechanisms that mediate its degradation.[145] Liganded VDR also decreases the level of cyclin E mRNA and thereby reduces the formation of cyclin E/CDK2 complexes.[145] Consequently, the reduced activity of these complexes prevents p27$^{(kip1)}$ phosphorylation and subsequent degradation. Thus, the $1\alpha,25(OH)_2D_3$ regulation of p27$^{(kip1)}$ appears complex and cell-type specific, as the elevation of p27$^{(kip1)}$ mRNA and protein are not consistently observed. This highlights the difficulty of establishing strict transcriptional targets and the range of posttranscriptional effects that appear in concert to regulate gene targets.

The upregulation of p21$^{(wafl/cip1)}$ and p27$^{(kip1)}$ principally mediates G_1 cell cycle arrest, but $1\alpha,25(OH)_2D_3$ has been shown to mediate a G_2/M cell cycle arrest in a number of cancer cell lines through the direct induction of GADD45α.[62,63,146] GADD45α inhibits the activation of mitosis-promoting cyclin B/CDK1 complexes.[147,148] Again, this regulation appears to combine direct gene transcription and a range of posttranscriptional mechanisms.

8.4.2 Programmed Cell Death

A common feature of certain cells, notably MCF-7 cells, is a profound induction of apoptosis, irrespective of p53 content. This may reflect the role that VDR plays in the involution of the postlactating mammary gland. The direct transcriptional targets that regulate these actions to an extent remain elusive although there is growing evidence of an involvement of the Bcl-2 family of proteins. Frequently, the induction of apoptosis is associated with an altered expression ratio between the antiapoptotic Bcl-2 family members and the proapoptotic BAX and BAK proteins, and the proapoptotic BAX protein being translocated from the cytosol to the mitochondria in MCF-7 cells.[121,149,150] Downregulation of Bcl-2 was also seen in $1\alpha,25(OH)_2D_3$-mediated apoptosis in colon and prostate cancer cell lines.[100,151] The importance of Bcl-2 became apparent when it was shown that overexpression of Bcl-2 can block $1\alpha,25(OH)_2D_3$-induced apoptosis in both MCF-7 (breast) and LNCaP (prostate) cancer cell lines.[151,152] Despite the apparent promotion of an active apatosome, the exact role of downstream caspases is unclear as broad spectrum inhibitors of their actions do not block apoptotic cell death. In such conditions, it is suggested that other proteases such as cathepsins mediate cell death.[152–154]

Programmed cell death following $1\alpha,25(OH)_2D_3$ treatment is also associated with a release of cytochrome C following loss of mitochondrial membrane integrity and an increase in the generation of reactive oxygen species (ROS).[155–158] $1\alpha,25(OH)_2D_3$ treatment involves the upregulation of the gene VDUP1 (vitamin-D-upregulated protein 1) that binds to the disulfide-reducing protein thioredoxin and inhibits its ability to neutralize ROS.[159,160] Thus, VDUP1 indirectly initiates oxidative-stress induced apoptosis. VDUP1 is also likely to relieve the direct inhibition of ASK1 (apoptosis signaling-regulated kinase 1), which is mediated by thioredoxin.[161]

Interestingly, the apoptotic responses in other cells, for example, LNCaP, appear to be delayed and not so pronounced, occurring up to 6 d posttreatment,[151] in which case, the apoptosis probably reflects less direct effects, but rather the integration of VDR signaling with other systems. Similarly, in other cell systems, including myeloid cells, $1\alpha,25(OH)_2D_3$ appears to mediate antiproliferative and prosurvival effects through the regulation of antiapoptotic target genes such as MCL-1.[162,163] In particular, myeloid cells undergo a profound monocytic differentiation in response to $1\alpha,25(OH)_2D_3$ treatment.[61,119,128,164] Taken together, these data would suggest that the extent and timing of apoptotic events arise through integration of $1\alpha,25(OH)_2D_3$ signaling with other cell signaling systems.

8.4.3 ADHESION AND MIGRATION

A number of investigators have highlighted the effect of $1\alpha,25(OH)_2D_3$ to regulate cellular homotypic adhesion and thereby suppress the invasive capacity of cells; many of these effects are associated with a more differentiated phenotype. A number of workers have demonstrated that in colon cancer cells, such as CaCo2 and HT29 cells, and primary cultures that $1\alpha,25(OH)_2D_3$ treatment elevates expression of a number of brush-border-associated enzymes such as alkaline phosphatase,[165–168] as well as intermediate filaments, vinculin, ZO-1, ZO-2, desmosomes, and E-cadherin.[67] E-cadherin is also regulated in other cell types such LNCaP and MCF-7 and may account for the suppression of the invasive phenotype displayed upon treatment with $1\alpha,25(OH)_2D_3$.[66,67,129,169] E-cadherin is a major component of the adherent junctions and essential for the maintenance of the epithelial phenotype through both maintaining homotypic cell adhesion and also sequestrating β-catenin and thereby attenuating the mitogenic effects of Frizelled/Wnt signaling. Reflecting this important dual role, E-cadherin is a frequent target of epigenetic silencing of promoter CpG island methylation in many cancer cell types.[170,171]

In an elegant series of studies, Munoz and coworkers have dissected the inter-relationships between the VDR, E-cadherin, and the Wnt signaling pathway in colon cancer cell lines and primary tumors. In these studies, the induction of E-cadherin was seen in subpopulations of SW480 colon cancer cells that express the VDR and respond to $1\alpha,25(OH)_2D_3$. Thus, in the presence of the $1\alpha,25(OH)_2D_3$, the VDR is able to limit the transcriptional effects of β-catenin by physically and directly binding it in the nucleus and secondly by upregulating E-cadherin to sequestrate β-catenin in the cytoplasm. In malignancy, these actions are corrupted through downregulation of VDR mRNA, which appears to be a direct consequence of binding by the transcriptional repressor SNAIL, itself a key regulator of the epithelial mesenchyme transition, which is overexpressed in colon cancer.[67,129,130,172]

8.4.4 GENOMIC INTEGRITY AND DNA REPAIR

An important and emergent area, both in terms of physiology and therapeutic exploitation, is the role the liganded VDR appears to play in maintaining genomic integrity and facilitating DNA repair. There appears to be close cooperation between VDR actions and those of p53. The p53 tumor suppressor pathway ensures genomic integrity in daughter cells by monitoring DNA damage and inducing cell cycle arrest and/or apoptosis in an attempt to repair or delete the fault.[173–175] Correlative data suggests that cells that respond to VDR actions generally have wild-type p53, suggesting that these signaling systems monitor and respond to dietary and environmental signals to negatively regulate mitosis.[31,176] At the molecular level, several target genes are shared by both signaling pathways, such as p21[(waf1/cip1)] and GADD45α.[63] Together, these findings suggest cooperativity.[177] Although this area has only recently emerged, there are a number of functional studies that support such cooperation, for example, $1\alpha,25(OH)_2D_3$ enhances ionizing radiation-induced apoptosis of LNCaP cells, which retain wild-type p53.[178]

The antiproliferative effect of $1\alpha,25(OH)_2D_3$ in MCF-7 and LNCaP cells has been associated with the induction of *BRCA1* mRNA and protein via transcriptional activation, again supporting a cooperative role in genomic surveillance.[179]

8.4.5 INTEGRATED SIGNALING

Collectively, these studies further demonstrate the integrated aspect of VDR signaling with other cell signaling systems and the importance of cell context to determine the phenotypic response. The cooperative actions with other nuclear receptors and with receptor tyrosine kinases will be examined to illustrate these concepts further.

Cross talk with other nuclear receptors. There is considerable evidence in the literature that the VDR cooperates and cross talks with other members of the NR1 subfamily of nuclear receptors. These range from direct physical interactions to regulation of the promoters of the other receptors. Greater complexity has emerged because the RE for the VDR have been found arranged in clusters or combined with the binding sites of other transcription factors to form more complex and integrated responsive regions, as found in the promoters of the cytochrome P450 enzymes CYP3A4, CYP24, and CYP27.[68–70,180–182] Also, there is evidence for more transient interactions through the exchange of cofactors such as the central dimeric RXR partner and the coordinated exchange of coactivators and corepressors. The cellular readout of these molecular interactions can be seen in a number of studies that demonstrate cooperativity between $1\alpha,25(OH)_2D_3$ and a range of other nuclear receptor ligands such as retinoids and those for the PPARs.[47,126,183–187]

More broadly, a range of cooperative actions have been identified between the VDR and the principal sex steroid hormone receptors in breast and prostate cells. For example, there appears to be reciprocal regulation of the VDR and ERα in breast cancer cells,[122] and phytoestrogens such as genistein induce the VDR.[188,189] Furthermore, $1\alpha,25(OH)_2D_3$ and genistein cooperate to increase the stability of the VDR protein and to upregulate p21[(wafl/cip1)] in breast cancer models *in vitro* and to cooperate *in vivo* to regulate gut epithelial turnover and differentiation.[190–192] These relationships are intricate as the VDR in turn is able to downregulate ERα.

Cross talk with receptor tyrosine kinases. Another concept to emerge is the integrated actions of the VDR with cell-membrane-located receptor tyrosine kinases. These studies have revealed a high degree of coregulation with members of the ERBB, TGF, and IGF families. These signals are highly contextual and include both downregulation of growth-promoting signals, such as IGF-I or ERBB1, as well as upregulation of negative growth regulation and increase in IGFBP-3.[193–195] Similarly, other pathways such as those mediated by the TGF family appear to be targeted with $1\alpha,25(OH)_2D_3$, for example, by upregulating the TGF-β2 receptor and a range of convergent effects.[196–202] Internally, the VDR enhances a number of signal transduction pathways, with proteins on the *p38* stress response pathway appearing to be both modulated and cooperatively acting with the VDR.[63,203–206] Again, the final phenotype response is divergent, depending upon cell type and, probably, transformation status. Future studies in normal cells, within tissue context, will address these issues.

8.5   *IN VIVO* ACTIONS OF THE VDR IN TUMOR MODELS

8.5.1   VDR KNOCKOUT TUMOR MODELS

The *vdr*-deficient animals have become extremely useful tools to elucidate the role for the VDR to act in a chemopreventive manner. A series of animals have been generated in which the VDR-ablated background has been crossed into one with a breast tumor disposition phenotype. Thus, crossing the *vdr*-deficient and heterozygote mice with mouse mammary tumor virus (MMTV)-*neu* transgenic mice has generated animals that show a degree of haplosufficiency with the tumor burden in the crossed mice being reduced with the presence of one wild-type *vdr* allele and further with wild-type *vdr*.[207] Alternatively, the knockout animals have been shown to demonstrate greater susceptibility to carcinogen challenge. For example, challenging these mice with DMBA induced more preneoplasic lesions in the mammary glands from *vdr* knockout than in wild-type mice.[208]

A parallel and larger series of studies have examined the ability of dietary or pharmacological addition of vitamin D compounds either to prevent tumor formation or inhibit the growth of exogenously added xenograft tumors. Many investigators have focused on establishing dietary regimes that recapitulate the epidemiological and laboratory findings. For example, multiple studies now suggest that a high-fat diet, with low levels of vitamin D, increases the risk of cancer development in a range of high-profile malignancies — notably, colon cancer (reviewed in Reference 209). A range of long-term studies have reported that wild-type mice fed with a Western-style diet (for example, high fat and phosphate and low vitamin D and calcium content) increased epithelial cell hyperproliferation. Equally acute exposure to these diets, for example, over 12 weeks, proved sufficient to induce colon-crypt hyperplasia — effects that could be ameliorated through the addition of calcium and vitamin D.[210–213]

A clear difficulty in recapitulating these effects is that mice are not humans; their spectrum of age-associated malignancies is different from humans, and other key metabolic differences exist. Recapitulating these lifetime effects are further compounded by the need to establish the window in which chemoprevention effects may play a role in either tumor initiation or progression.

8.5.2 OTHER TUMOR MODELS FOR VDR ACTIONS

Another important model in which to test chemoprevention and chemotherapy capacity is the Apc_{min} mouse. APC is a key negative regulator of β-catenin actions and has been found to be very commonly targeted for disruption through a variety of mechanisms in humans who develop colon cancer. Disruption in mice with a truncated *Apc* allele leads to a highly aggressive model of intestinal carcinogenesis in which the mutant mice develop neoplastic growth throughout the GI tract within weeks of birth. Therefore, the effects of Western-style diets, and in particular those in which vitamin D and calcium are deficient, have been tested in mutant Apc_{min} mice. The rate of polyp formation in this model was significantly increased when mice were fed a Western diet compared to animals on standard chow. The effects of $1\alpha,25(OH)_2D_3$ were modest to prevent polyp formation in this model and were associated with potent side effects (e.g., hypercalcemia) but were more pronounced and significant when a potent analog of $1\alpha,25(OH)_2D_3$ was used with reduced toxicity.[214]

An alternative to genetic backgrounds that drive carcinogenesis in murine and rat models is to expose test animals to cancer-initiating reagents and then to examine the effect of dietary components to again attenuate the previously established rates of tumor initiation and progression. The efficacy of $1\alpha,25(OH)_2D_3$ and its analogs have been extensively tested in these models, and a range of protective effects have been established against tumor initiation, progression, and invasion supporting chemoprevention and chemotherapy for $1\alpha,25(OH)_2D_3$ and its potent analogs. For example, immunodeficient mice injected with human breast cancer cell lines showed tumor suppression and reduced angiogenesis in response to $1\alpha,25(OH)_2D_3$,[215–217] and $1\alpha,25(OH)_2D_3$ reduced tumor size in chemically-induced tumors with *N*-methylnitrosourea and other carcinogens.[218–225]

A complementary approach to these studies has been to examine the capacity of $1\alpha,25(OH)_2D_3$ to interact with other dietary components that are known to be chemoprotective. One such strategy has focused on the ability to enhance local autocrine synthesis and signaling of $1\alpha,25(OH)_2D_3$. For example, phytoestrogens such as genistein are known to be protective, and *in vivo* soy or genistein feeding appears to increase the local expression of CYP27B1 and reduce CYP24 expression in the mouse colon, resulting in sustained elevated levels of $1\alpha,25(OH)_2D_3$.[188,192,226] These results would appear to support the concept that Asian diets, which are rich in phytoestrogens and vitamin D, may, in part, explain the traditionally low rates of breast, prostate, and colon cancer in this region.

Epidemiological evidence has shown that populations with a high incidence of colorectal cancer and consuming a high-fat and animal protein diet, excrete approximately twice the amount of secondary bile acids.[227–229] Unlike the primary bile acids, the secondary bile acids, such as LCA, are poorly reabsorbed into enterohepatic circulation and pass into the colon, and its concentration is higher than other secondary bile acids in patients with colorectal cancer[230,231] and can also promote colon cancer in animals. How LCA mediates these effects *in vivo* is unknown; however, *in vitro* studies have shown that LCA can induce DNA strand breaks, forms DNA adducts, and inhibits DNA repair enzymes.[232–235] Similarly, other secondary bile acids appear protumorigenic; for example, rats treated with the potent carcinogen azoxymethane (AOM) and fed a diet supplemented with the secondary bile acid deoxycholic acid develop more tumors than do animals treated with AOM alone.[236,237] By contrast, the tertiary bile acid ursodeoxycholic acid has been identified as a chemopreventive agent and is able to promote differentiation and inhibit proliferation of colon epithelial cells both *in vitro* and *in vivo*.[238,239]

Thus, the metabolism of cholesterol and synthesis of bile acids are critical. It has emerged that nuclear receptors play an integral role in determining bile acid levels by regulating synthesis and catabolism. Cholesterol is converted, primarily in the liver, by a feed-forward induction mediated by the LXRα and liver receptor homolog-1, which bind oxysterols and induce cholesterol 7-alpha-hydroxylase gene (CYP7A1), to generate bile acids.[240] Feedback repression is mediated by a complex containing the bile acid receptor (FXR), LRH-1, and the promoter-specific repressor, SHP,[241] which together repress transcription of CYP7A1 and, therefore, limit synthesis of bile acids.

The potentially toxic and tumorigenic effects of bile acids, such as LCA, are limited further by other nuclear receptors such as steroid and xenobiotic receptor (SXR)[240] constitutive androstane receptor, which induce a number of metabolizing and detoxifying enzymes such as CYP3A4 and glutathione S-transferase α and degrades bile acids such as LCA in the liver and intestine.[242] In parallel, the FXR has been shown to induce a range of target genes that may play other roles in controlling cell proliferation, such as the related NR, PPARα, hence providing molecular evidence for a local, paracrine, cross talk between the bile-acid-sensing receptor and cell proliferation.[243]

It has also been shown recently that the VDR can also bind and respond to LCA to induce metabolizing enzymes such as CYP3A4[58,59] and further reenforce the cross talk between bile acid milieu and colonic epithelial cell maintenance. Thus, the finding that oxysterols, bile acids, and some polyunsaturated fatty acids can bind and collectively activate LXRs, FXR, PPARs, SXR, CAR, RXR, and VDR, provides a strong molecular link between tissue homeostasis and the type and availability of nutrients, at least in the colon. The expression of the receptors in tissues outside the GI tract suggests a broader function too (Table 8.1).

Protection provided by SXR, FXR, and VDR activation may become compromised when the detoxification pathway is overwhelmed (e.g., by increased levels of LCA owing to sustained high-fat diets) or when other nuclear receptor ligands are deficient, for example, reduced signaling via the VDR in cases of vitamin D deficiency, and when diets have reduced levels of dietary-derived fatty acids that are known to be ligands for the PPARs.[57,244-246] Consistent with this model, there is an epidemiological relation between the incidence of colon cancer and Western-style, high-fat diets, and the highest death rates from colon cancer occur in areas with a high prevalence of rickets and underscores the integrated nature of dietary signaling.

8.6 MECHANISMS OF SUPPRESSION AND RESISTANCE TO THE ACTIONS OF THE VDR

8.6.1 REDUCED ENVIRONMENTAL AVAILABILITY OF $1\alpha,25(OH)_2D_3$

Epidemiological studies have demonstrated that the intensity of local sunlight is inversely correlated with risk of certain cancers including breast, prostatic, and colorectal carcinoma.[247-251] These findings suggest that the decreased availability of vitamin D, or its active metabolite, may negatively impact development of these cancer types. Dietary factors associated with risk reduction for breast cancer include a high ratio of vegetable-derived to total energy intake, a high fish intake,[252] as well as a high dietary vitamin D intake.[253] Another observed risk factor is latitude as it relates to UVB irradiation. Garland and associates[252,254,255] have reported that risk of fatal breast cancer in major urban areas of the U.S. appears to be inversely proportional to the intensity of sunlight and that synthesis of vitamin D from sunlight exposure may be associated with low risk for fatal breast cancer. These authors further suggest that differences in ultraviolet irradiation across the U.S. may account for the observed regional differences in breast cancer mortality.

Levels of $25(OH)D_3$, the major circulating metabolite of vitamin D, are directly related to dietary vitamin D intake and cutaneous synthesis in response to sunlight exposure. We have recently reported that $25(OH)D_3$ concentrations are significantly lower in breast cancer patients than in age-matched controls.[256] The activity of the renal 1α-hydroxylase enzyme is regulated such that circulating concentrations of $1\alpha,25(OH)_2D_3$ are maintained within a relatively narrow range in the face of substantial changes in serum $25(OH)D_3$ levels. However, in addition to uptake of $1\alpha,25(OH)_2D_3$ from the circulation, it is possible that breast cells locally generate $1\alpha,25(OH)_2D_3$ from $25(OH)D_3$ because breast cancer cells have been shown to express the $25(OH)D_3$ 1-hydroxylase. We have detected CYP27b1 mRNA and protein in breast cancer cell lines and primary tumors and, importantly, demonstrated enzyme activity,[102] suggesting that paracrine production of $1\alpha,25(OH)_2D_3$ could be important in maintenance of normal breast cell function. Thus, it could be postulated that low circulating concentrations of $25(OH)D_3$, arising either as a result of reduced exposure to sunlight or to dietary patterns, impair generation of $1\alpha,25(OH)_2D_3$ within breast tissue, increasing risk of tumor development.

Little is known about metabolism or half-life of $1\alpha,25(OH)_2D_3$ in normal breast or breast cancer cells. Catabolism of $1\alpha,25(OH)_2D_3$ is initiated via hydroxylation at the 24 position in the side chain, by the $25(OH)D_3$ 24-hydroxylase (CYP24). Comparative genome hybridization studies have found that CYP24 is amplified in human breast cancer.[257] Although the exact mechanism for this remains unclear, it is suggested that overexpression of the enzyme may abrogate growth control mediated by $1\alpha,25(OH)_2D_3$ via target cell inactivation of the hormone. We have demonstrated CYP24 elevation in primary breast tumors in relation to paired normal tissue, associated with altered patterns of $1\alpha,25(OH)_2D_3$ metabolism.[102]

Epidemiological studies have now linked the incidence of prostate cancer to vitamin D insufficiency as a result of either diet or environment. In 1990, Schwartz and colleagues suggested a role for vitamin D in decreasing the risk for prostate cancer based on the observation that mortality rates in the U.S. are inversely related to incident solar radiation.[251] Recently, a study of men in the San Francisco Bay area reported a reduced risk of advanced prostate cancer associated with high sun exposure.[258] In the U.K., a case-controlled study found a threefold increase in risk with low lifetime sun exposure.[259,260] As with breast, the proposed mechanism for the protective effects of sunlight on prostate cancer risk involves the generation of $1\alpha,25(OH)_2D_3$ from circulating $25(OH)D_3$ in prostate cells. It has been demonstrated that both normal and cancerous prostate cells express 1α-hydroxylase activity but that cancer cells have lower levels.[261–265] Prediagnostic serum levels of $25(OH)D_3$ have been assessed in several prospective studies with some,[266–268] but not others,[269] reporting increased risk among men with low circulating levels of the vitamin D metabolite, although there was some suggestion of an inverse relationship with advanced disease. Differences in the cutoff points for low $25(OH)D_3$ levels in these various studies could in part account for these findings and has recently been reviewed.[270]

As with breast and prostate cancer, some epidemiological studies have noted that colon cancer risk and mortality increase with increasing latitude. A study in the U.S. in Caucasian males demonstrated that age-adjusted colon and rectal cancer incidence showed an inverse relationship with solar radiation. Garland and Garland found that age-adjusted death rates from colon cancer in Caucasian males in the U.S. were nearly three times higher in northeastern states than in the more sunnier southern states.[252,255] A number of studies have attempted to examine the relationship between dietary vitamin D and colorectal cancer with equivocal results. To assess the combined effects of vitamin D from diet and cutaneous synthesis, Garland[271] studied the relationship between serum $25(OH)D_3$ levels and colon cancer. They found that $25(OH)D_3$ levels were significantly lower in cases than controls. A more recent study in women found an inverse association between $25(OH)D_3$ levels and risk of colorectal cancer. Benefit from higher $25(OH)D_3$ concentrations was observed for cancers at the distal colon and rectum but was not evident for those at the proximal colon.[272] No association with $1\alpha,25(OH)_2D_3$ levels was seen.

8.6.2 Cellular Resistance to the Actions of the VDR

A major limitation in the therapeutic exploitation of $1\alpha,25(OH)_2D_3$ in cancer therapies is the resistance of cells towards $1\alpha,25(OH)_2D_3$ because cancer and leukemic cell lines often display a spectrum of sensitivities including complete insensitivity to $1\alpha,25(OH)_2D_3$, irrespective of VDR expression.[66,67,128,273] A research focus has been to develop analogs of $1\alpha,25(OH)_2D_3$, and multiple studies have demonstrated that these compounds have some enhanced potency, but resistance remains an issue.

The molecular mechanisms for $1\alpha,25(OH)_2D_3$-insensitivity in cancer are emerging. We and others have demonstrated that the VDR is neither mutated nor is there a clear relationship between VDR expression and growth inhibition by $1\alpha,25(OH)_2D_3$.[274,275] Indeed, the PC-3 and DU 145 prostate cancer cell lines are not significantly inhibited by physiologically relevant doses of $1\alpha,25(OH)_2D_3$ and, consistent with this response, antiproliferative gene targets are not modulated.[66,179] The lack of an antiproliferative response is not reflected by an overall suppression of the capacity of these cells to perceive $1\alpha,25(OH)_2D_3$. VDR transactivation is sustained or even enhanced, as measured by induction of the highly $1\alpha,25(OH)_2D_3$-inducible CYP24 gene.[276]

Breast cancer cell lines also display a varied antiproliferative response to $1\alpha,25(OH)_2D_3$. For example, MCF-7 cells, which retain expression of ER α and β, displays antiproliferative sensitivity to $1\alpha,25(OH)_2D_3$ and readily undergoes apoptosis in response. By contrast, more aggressive cell lines with altered ER α and β expression profiles, for example, MDA-MB-231, are essentially insensitive to $1\alpha,25(OH)_2D_3$ antiproliferative effects[179,277–279] requiring high concentrations of $1\alpha,25(OH)_2D_3$ associated *in vivo* with dose-limiting hypercalcemic side effects. A number of established breast cancer cell lines that express transcriptionally active VDR fail to respond to the antiproliferative effects of $1\alpha,25(OH)_2D_3$, leading to the suggestion that a lack of functional VDR alone, again, cannot explain resistance.[280–282]

Several studies have assessed the relationship between VDR expression and clinical indices in patients with breast cancer. A high proportion (> 80%) of breast cancer biopsy specimens contain vitamin D receptors.[283] One report has suggested that VDR is upregulated at the protein level in breast carcinomas compared to normal breast tissue,[284,285] and there appears to be no significant correlation of VDR expression with expression of ER, lymph node status, tumor grade, or overall survival.[102,284,285] However, in a study of 136 patients with primary breast cancer, it was found that women with VDR-negative tumors relapsed significantly earlier than women with VDR-positive tumors. Also, patients with VDR-positive breast tumors have longer disease-free survival compared to those with VDR-negative tumors.[121]

8.6.3 Genetic Resistance

The gene that encodes the VDR protein is known to display polymorphic variation. Thus, polymorphisms in the 3′ and 5′ regions of the gene have been described and variously associated with risk of breast, prostatic, and colorectal carcinoma. However, it is not yet known in what way these differences in the gene may affect the translated protein. A start codon polymorphism has been reported in exon 2 at the

5′ end of the gene. This polymorphism is a $T{\to}C$ transition (ATC to ACG) three codons upstream from a second start codon that acts as the putative translation start site for alleles lacking the first start codon. The start codon polymorphism can be determined using the *fok* I restriction enzyme where "f" indicates the presence of the restriction site and the first ATC codon while F indicates its absence. Alleles with the ATG sequence at the first initiation site produce the full length, 427 amino acid VDR protein. In individuals with ACG sequence, initiation of translation occurs at the second ATG site, and the three NH2-terminal amino acids of the full-length VDR are missing. At the 3′ end of the gene, three polymorphisms have been identified that do not lead to any change in either the transcribed mRNA or the translated protein. The first two sequences generate *Bsm* I and *Apa* I restriction sites and are intronic, lying between exon 8 and exon 9.[121,286–288] The third polymorphism, which generates a *Taq* I restriction site, lies in exon 9 and leads to a silent codon change (from ATT to ATC) that both insert an isoleucine residue at position 352. These three polymorphisms are linked to a further gene variation, a variable-length adenosine sequence within the 3′ untranslated region (3′ UTR). The poly(A) sequence varies in length and can be segregated into two groups: long (L) sequences of 18 to 24 adenosines or short (S). Studies in the U.S. have indicated that these 3′ polymorphisms are in linkage disequilibrium in Caucasian populations such that 2 haplotypes are commonly observed: baTL (presence of *Bsm* I, *Apa* I restriction sites, absence of *Taq* I site, long poly(A) sequence) and BAtS (Figure 8.3).

Vitamin D and breast cancer. Recent studies have addressed the association between VDR genotype and breast cancer risk and progression. An Australian study

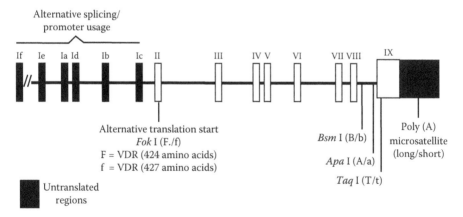

FIGURE 8.3 Polymorphisms in the human VDR gene. Exons shown as white rectangles contain the coding sequence. Black rectangles represent the 5′ and 3′ untranslated regions. There are six untranslated exons 5′ to exon 2, giving rise to alternative transcript sizes. Single-nucleotide polymorphisms have been identified in exon 2, intron 8, and exon 9. The polyadenosine (poly A) microsatellite in the 3′ UTR is present as long (A17–24) or short (A10–15) repeats. Only the *Fok* I polymorphism affects protein structure. The *Bsm* I, *Apa* I, *Taq* I, and poly A polymorphisms are in linkage disequilibrium in some populations.

determined *Apa* I and *Taq* I polymorphisms in patients with breast cancer and in 110 women with no history (family or personal) of breast cancer. Allele frequencies of the 3′ *Apa* I polymorphism showed a significant association with breast cancer risk whereas the *Taq* I polymorphism showed a similar trend but association was not significant.[289] Allele frequencies of the *Fok* I polymorphism were not found to be significantly different. A similar association was reported in a Japanese population in which the bb genotype conferred an almost fourfold increase in the risk of breast cancer.[290] A study of VDR polymorphisms and breast cancer risk in a London Caucasian population showed a significant association with *Bsm* I (odds ration *bb* vs. *BB* genotype 2.32).[288] The "L" poly(A) variant was also associated with a similar risk. These findings have recently been supported by a larger study in the same population in which controls were drawn from women attending breast screening and with a negative mammogram.[291] However, not all studies have shown such associations. Increased breast cancer risk among Latina women in the U.S. was associated with *SS/BB* genotypes.[292] Four reports showed no association between the *Taq* I polymorphism and breast cancer risk in Caucasians.[293–297] However, this last study reported an association between *TT* genotype and increased risk for lymph node metastases. Another study reported that the *bb* genotype conferred a fourfold higher risk of developing metastases compared to *BB*[298] and that the *AA* genotype is associated with metastases to bone.[299] Because there is strong genetic linkage between the 3 polymorphisms such that two haplotypes baTL and BAtS are almost always expressed in Caucasians, this latter study is not in agreement with the reports by Ruggiero et al. and Lundin. Because *Bsm* I, *Apa* I, and *Taq* I polymorphisms do not lead to changes in the VDR protein, it remains difficult to explain how these variations could modulate receptor function. To date, most studies have shown no correlation between these polymorphisms and abundance or stability of message or VDR protein expression. One report documented lower VDR mRNA levels in parathyroid tumors from baT homozygous individuals.[299] It is possible that in Caucasian subjects, the *Bsm/Apa* I/*Taq* I cluster does not influence VDR function but because of genetic linkage acts as a marker for the poly(A) sequence within the 3′ UTR. 3′ UTR sequences are known to be important in determining transcript stability.

When analyzed in isolation, the 5′ *Fok* I polymorphism was not associated with breast cancer risk in the studies of Bretherton-Watt et al. and Ingles et al. in Caucasian and Latina subjects, respectively. However, a small number of studies have carried out cross-genotyping analysis on the VDR polymorphisms and reported that this can reveal a positive association. A study by Ingles et al. of African-American women indicated that the *LS* and *LL* poly(A) variants had a 50% decreased risk of breast cancer compared to the *SS* but that this effect was limited to women who are homozygous for the absence of the *Fok* I restriction site (*FF*). The recent study by Guy et al.[291] reported that the *Fok* I variant modulated the increased risk associated with the *bb/LL* genotype such that possession of one or more F alleles together with the *bb/LL* genotype augmented breast cancer risk.

Some studies addressing functional activity have suggested that the shorter VDR protein encoded by the *F* allele is more transcriptionally active. Whitfield et al.[301]

found that there was no difference in transcriptional activity between the F and f VDR forms in human fibroblast cell lines. However, differences were seen when *Fok* I and poly(A) variants were assessed in isolation, such that maximal $1\alpha,25(OH)_2D_3$-induced transcriptional activity was seen in cells of the *FF/LL* genotype. It remains to be determined whether functional differences in the *Fok* I and poly(A) variants can be detected in cultured breast cancer cells.

Vitamin D and prostate cancer. Earlier studies suggested that polymorphisms in the VDR gene might also be associated with the risk factor of prostate cancer. Among these, a pilot study among non-Hispanic white subjects[302,303] showed an increased risk associated with the long form of the poly A microsatellite, and Ma et al.[304] observed an association with the bb genotype but only in men with decreased $25(OH)D_3$ concentrations. Ntais and coworkers performed a metaanalysis of 14 published studies with four common gene polymorphisms (*Taq* I, poly *A repeat, Bsm* I, and *Fok* I) in individuals of European, Asian, and African descent. They concluded from the study that these polymorphisms are unlikely to be major determinants of susceptibility to prostate cancer on a wide population basis.[305]

In the U.S., Cheteri et al.[306] studied Caucasian men for an association with risk of three polymorphisms (*Bsm* I, *Fok* I, and *poly A*). The frequency of genotypes was similar in cases and controls, although among men with localized disease, the bb genotype was associated with a modest increase in risk. Overall, these workers concluded that VDR gene polymorphisms are not predictors of prostate cancer risk.

Studies in a southern European population showed an association of VDR *T* allele with prostate cancer risk and, in particular, risk of cancer onset in men over the age of 66 yr. It was suggested that 50% of cases older than 66 yr could be attributed to the influence of this risk factor.[307] A study in the U.S. examined associations between prostate cancer risk and five polymorphisms in the VDR gene in young African Americans and Caucasians. Among Caucasians, there was no evidence for association between prostate cancer risk and alleles at any of the five polymorphic sites. However, among African Americans, prostate cancer risk was associated with homozygosity for the F allele at the *Fok* I site. Thus, it appears that the contribution of VDR genotypes to prostate cancer susceptibility might depend on the population studied.

Vitamin D and colorectal carcinoma. Experimental studies have shown that a Western-style diet with decreased levels of calcium and vitamin D increased the incidence of preneoplastic intestinal lesions in animal models of intestinal tumorigenesis, and dietary addition of calcium and vitamin D significantly reduced these changes. A number of studies have shown that calcium has a direct growth inhibitory and differentiation and apoptosis-inducing effect on normal and tumor cells, including those of the gastrointestinal tract. An antiproliferative effect of dietary action on intestinal cells could also result from binding to bile and fatty acids, which might reduce the proliferation-inducing effects of these compounds on the intestinal mucosa. *In vitro* studies have shown that the growth-inhibitory effects of vitamin D compounds on colon carcinoma cells are associated with cell cycle changes, modulation of growth factor signaling, and induction of apoptosis as has been shown for breast and prostate cancer.[209,211]

A further study has assessed the independent and joint effects of calcium supplementation and vitamin D status on colorectal adenoma recurrence. Results were also assessed in relation to VDR gene polymorphisms (*Taq* I and *Fok* I). In those subjects with serum 25(OH)D$_3$ levels above the median, calcium supplementation was associated with a reduced risk. VDR polymorphisms were not related to recurrence and did not modify the associations with vitamin D or calcium.[308] Ingles et al. reported no overall association between VDR gene polymorphisms and adenoma risk. However, patients with the *FF* genotype had increased risk of large adenomas compared to *Ff* and *ff* genotypes, and this relationship was of increased significance among low dietary calcium or vitamin D intake.[303,309] In contrast, a study confined to Singapore Chinese subjects reported that individuals with *ff* genotype had increased risk of colorectal cancer, and this effect was modified by both dietary calcium and fat. In individuals with either low calcium or fat intake, the risk associated with the ff genotype was increased.[310]

8.6.4 EPIGENETIC RESISTANCE

To date, no cytogenetic abnormalities of the VDR have been reported. Rather, a number of investigators have begun to explore epigenetic mechanisms that disrupt signaling. It has been proposed that apparent hormonal insensitivity is not determined solely by a linear relationship between the levels of $1\alpha,25(OH)_2D_3$ and the VDR, but rather that epigenetic events skew the responsiveness to selectively suppress responsiveness of target gene promoters.

Elevated corepressor expressions were frequently observed, most commonly involving NCoR2/SMRT, in malignant primary cultures and cell lines, with reduced $1\alpha,25(OH)_2D_3$ antiproliferative response, but not normal or BPH cultures, indicating that the ratio of VDR to corepressor is a more critical indicator of malignant status and $1\alpha,25(OH)_2D_3$ responsiveness. The significance of elevated corepressor levels in both cancer cell lines and primary cultures was observed, and it has been reasoned that this lesion could be targeted by cotreatment of ligand ($1\alpha,25(OH)_2D_3$) plus HDAC inhibitor (TSA) and supportively studies have demonstrated that the $1\alpha,25(OH)_2D_3$-response of the androgen-independent PC-3 cells was restored to levels indistinguishable from control normal prostate epithelial (PrEC) cells, by cotreatment with low doses of TSA. This reversal of $1\alpha,25(OH)_2D_3$ insensitivity provided the opportunity to examine patterns of global acetylation and expression of target genes. Microarray studies demonstrated that $1\alpha,25(OH)_2D_3$ plus TSA uniquely upregulated a group of "repressed" gene targets associated with the control of proliferation and induction of apoptosis, notably GADD45α and MAPK-APK2, a mediator of the p38 stress response pathway.[63,311]

Roles for both GADD45α and MAPK-APK2 have been demonstrated in cell lines that retain sensitivity to $1\alpha,25(OH)_2D_3$ signaling. For example, p38/MAPK-APK2 activation regulates $1\alpha,25(OH)_2D_3$-induced HL-60 myeloid differentiation,[312] and upregulation of GADD45α is a functional part of the antiproliferative action of EB1089 (an analog of $1\alpha,25(OH)_2D_3$) in SCC25 squamous carcinoma cells[62] and $1\alpha,25(OH)_2D_3$ in ovarian cancer cell lines.[146] These studies highlight these targets as key to mediating the antiproliferative action of $1\alpha,25(OH)_2D_3$. A siRNA approach demonstrated the significant role that NCoR2/SMRT plays in regulating this response, with its repression resulting in profound enhancement of the induction of GADD45α in response to $1\alpha,25(OH)_2D_3$.[63,311] These data support a central role for elevated NCoR2/SMRT levels in suppressing the induction of key target genes, resulting in loss of sensitivity to the antiproliferative action of $1\alpha,25(OH)_2D_3$.

Parallel studies demonstrated that the spectrum of reduced $1\alpha,25(OH)_2D_3$ responsiveness between nonmalignant breast epithelial cells and cancer cell lines was again not determined solely by a linear relationship between the levels of $1\alpha,25(OH)_2D_3$ and the VDR. Rather, elevated corepressor levels, notably NCoR1, in breast cancer cell lines and primary tumors were common and determined the sensitivity towards $1\alpha,25(OH)_2D_3$. In turn, these antiproliferative responses were either attenuated by overexpression of NCoR1 or increased by targeting the NCoR1 complex with HDAC inhibitors. Furthermore, gene regulation data support the concept that elevated corepressors such as NCoR1 are reducing the capacity of the VDR to act as a transcription factor for antiproliferative target genes. Namely, to suppress the mRNA accumulation of the antiproliferative gene targets (p21[(wafl/cip1)], GADD45α, and VDUP-1) in MDA-MB-231 cells treated with $1\alpha,25(OH)_2D_3$ compared to MCF-12A cells. These genes become more inducible in the TSA-based cotreatments with vitamin D_3 compounds in MDA-MB-231 cells.[313,314]

Interestingly, the pronounced and frequent increase in NCoR1 corepressor levels in the primary tumor material positively associated with increased, rather than decreased, VDR mRNA levels. These data suggest that the VDR is retained in tumors and may actually provide a benefit. These findings, together with studies by Miller et al.[274] and Friedrich et al.,[284] suggest that the VDR is not overtly disrupted by genetic or cytogenetic mechanisms in cancer, but rather that epigenetic mechanisms attenuate the transcriptional responsiveness. A number of reasons may explain these phenomena. Firstly, the elevation of both VDR and NCoR1 may drive *apo* receptor complexes to assemble on the promoter/enhancer region of target genes and, therefore, form a template for subsequent, more stable, epigenetic silencing of these regions. Secondly, it may allow cytoplasmic VDR actions to suppress apoptosis via nontranscriptional interactions.[91]

Hence, it has been proposed that deregulated tissue-specific corepressors inappropriately sustain histone deacetylation around the VDRE or target gene promoter regions, and shift the dynamic equilibrium between *apo* and *holo* receptor conformations to favor transcriptional repression (e.g., GADD45α, , VDUP-1). As a result, VDR gene targets are less responsive in $1\alpha,25(OH)_2D_3$-insensitive cancer cells compared to nonmalignant counterparts. Furthermore, targeting cotreatment of vitamin D_3 compounds plus TSA generates a temporal window where the equilibrium point between *apo* and *holo* complexes is shifted to favor a more transcriptionally permissive environment and allow the gene target to be modulated in a unique and significantly greater manner than either agent alone; notably, p21[(wafl/cip1)] and GADD45α.

Taken together, these studies suggest that increased expression of different corepressors disrupts the actions of the VDR, and is a relatively common event in solid tumors and adds to a growing body of data that places the expression of CoA/CoR milieu as being critical to determine nuclear receptor actions.[315–327]

8.7 FUTURE PERSPECTIVES

Historically, researchers have studied the abilities of single-nuclear receptors to regulate a discrete group of gene targets and influence cell function. This has led to substantial knowledge concerning many of these receptors individually. Cell and organism function, however, depends on the dynamic interaction of a collection of receptors through the networks that link them. The current lack of an integral view of how these interactions bring about function and dysfunction of the aging human individual can be attributed to the relatively recent limitation of available techniques and tools to undertake such studies. The implementation of the new postgenomic techniques together with bioinformatics and systems-biology methodology to generate an integral view of the processes by which cells, tissues, and organisms interact with diet. Therefore, the transition from a reductionist to an integrative, systems-biology approach will be required.[328] This transition will allow VDR processes to be described in the dynamic interaction with other nuclear receptors, and between cellular components to identify critical nodes of control.

A common goal of many researchers around the world is to understand how dietary intervention based on knowledge of nutritional requirement, nutritional status, and genotype (i.e., "intelligent nutrition") can be used to prevent, ameliorate, or cure chronic disease. Just as pharmacogenomics has led to the concept of "personalized medicine" and "designer drugs," so will nutrigenomics open the way for "personalized nutrition." In other words, by understanding our nutritional needs, our nutritional status, and our genotype, nutrigenomics will enable better individual management of health and well-being by precisely matching diet to unique physiological genetic makeup. A critical step to promoting this understanding is to construct mathematical models using systems biology approaches to define how these interactions can work. Ultimately, this will deliver a predicative, preventative, and personalized understanding of individual dietary interactions.

REFERENCES

1. Lacroix, M. and Leclercq, G. The portrait of hereditary breast cancer. *Breast Cancer Res. Treat.*, 89: 297–304, 2005.
2. Jo, W.S. and Chung, D.C. Genetics of hereditary colorectal cancer. *Semin. Oncol.*, 32: 11–23, 2005.
3. Balmain, A., Gray, J., and Ponder, B. The genetics and genomics of cancer. *Nat. Genet.*, 33 (Suppl.): 238–244, 2003.
4. Cook, J.D., Davis, B.J., Cai, S.L., Barrett, J.C., Conti, C.J., and Walker, C.L. Interaction between genetic susceptibility and early-life environmental exposure determines tumor-suppressor-gene penetrance. *Proc. Natl. Acad. Sci. U.S.A.*, 102: 8644–8649, 2005.
5. Kotnis, A., Sarin, R., and Mulherkar, R. Genotype, phenotype and cancer: role of low penetrance genes and environment in tumor susceptibility. *J. Biosci.*, 30: 93–102, 2005.

6. Caceres, D.D., Iturrieta, J., Acevedo, C., Huidobro, C., Varela, N., and Quinones, L. Relationship among metabolizing genes, smoking and alcohol used as modifier factors on prostate cancer risk: exploring some gene–gene and gene–environment interactions. *Eur. J. Epidemiol.*, 20: 79–88, 2005.

7. Heavey, P.M., McKenna, D., and Rowland, I.R. Colorectal cancer and the relationship between genes and the environment. *Nutr. Cancer*, 48: 124–141, 2004.

8. Hanahan, D. and Weinberg, R.A. The hallmarks of cancer. *Cell*, 100: 57–70, 2000.

9. Bellacosa, A. Genetic hits and mutation rate in colorectal tumorigenesis: versatility of Knudson's theory and implications for cancer prevention. *Genes Chromosomes Cancer*, 38: 382–388, 2003.

10. Futreal, P.A., Kasprzyk, A., Birney, E., Mullikin, J.C., Wooster, R., and Stratton, M.R. Cancer and genomics. *Nature*, 409: 850–852, 2001.

11. Reya, T. and Clevers, H. Wnt signalling in stem cells and cancer. *Nature*, 434: 843–850, 2005.

12. Al Hajj, M. and Clarke, M.F. Self-renewal and solid tumor stem cells. *Oncogene*, 23: 7274–7282, 2004.

13. Al Hajj, M., Becker, M.W., Wicha, M., Weissman, I., and Clarke, M.F. Therapeutic implications of cancer stem cells. *Curr. Opin. Genet. Dev.*, 14: 43–47, 2004.

14. Dontu, G., Al Hajj, M., Abdallah, W.M., Clarke, M.F., and Wicha, M.S. Stem cells in normal breast development and breast cancer. *Cell Prolif.*, 36 (Suppl. 1): 59–72, 2003.

15. De Marzo, A.M., Nelson, W.G., Meeker, A.K., and Coffey, D.S. Stem cell features of benign and malignant prostate epithelial cells. *J. Urol.*, 160: 2381–2392, 1998.

16. Huss, W.J., Gray, D.R., Werdin, E.S., Funkhouser, W.K., Jr., and Smith, G.J. Evidence of pluripotent human prostate stem cells in a human prostate primary xenograft model. *Prostate*, 60: 77–90, 2004.

17. Reya, T., Morrison, S.J., Clarke, M.F., and Weissman, I.L. Stem cells, cancer, and cancer stem cells. *Nature*, 414: 105–111, 2001.

18. Beachy, P.A., Karhadkar, S.S., and Berman, D.M. Tissue repair and stem cell renewal in carcinogenesis. *Nature*, 432: 324–331, 2004.

19. Hecht, S.S. Tobacco smoke carcinogens and lung cancer. *J. Natl. Cancer Inst.*, 91: 1194–1210, 1999.

20. Astorg, P. Dietary n-6 and n-3 polyunsaturated fatty acids and prostate cancer risk: a review of epidemiological and experimental evidence. *Cancer Causes Control*, 15: 367–386, 2004.

21. Boyle, P., Severi, G., and Giles, G.G. The epidemiology of prostate cancer. *Urol. Clin. N. Am.*, 30: 209–217, 2003.

22. Messina, M.J. Emerging evidence on the role of soy in reducing prostate cancer risk. *Nutr. Rev.*, 61: 117–131, 2003.

23. Djavan, B., Zlotta, A., Schulman, C., Teillac, P., Iversen, P., Boccon, G.L., Bartsch, G., and Marberger, M. Chemotherapeutic prevention studies of prostate cancer. *J. Urol.*, 171: S10–S13, 2004.

24. Pathak, S.K., Sharma, R.A., and Mellon, J.K. Chemoprevention of prostate cancer by diet-derived antioxidant agents and hormonal manipulation (review). *Int. J. Oncol.*, 22: 5–13, 2003.

25. Surh, Y.J. Cancer chemoprevention with dietary phytochemicals. *Nat. Rev. Cancer*, 3: 768–780, 2003.

26. Agoulnik, I.U., Krause, W.C., Bingman, W.E., III, Rahman, H.T., Amrikachi, M., Ayala, G.E., and Weigel, N.L. Repressors of androgen and progesterone receptor action. *J. Biol. Chem.*, 278: 31136–31148, 2003.

27. Cohen, R.N., Brzostek, S., Kim, B., Chorev, M., Wondisford, F.E., and Hollenberg, A.N. The specificity of interactions between nuclear hormone receptors and core-pressors is mediated by distinct amino acid sequences within the interacting domains. *Mol. Endocrinol.*, 15: 1049–1061, 2001.

28. Hu, X., Li, Y., and Lazar, M.A. Determinants of CoRNR-dependent repression complex assembly on nuclear hormone receptors. *Mol. Cell Biol.*, 21: 1747–1758, 2001.

29. Belandia, B. and Parker, M.G. Nuclear receptors: a rendezvous for chromatin remodeling factors. *Cell*, 114: 277–280, 2003.

30. Hermanson, O., Glass, C.K., and Rosenfeld, M.G. Nuclear receptor coregulators: multiple modes of modification. *Trends Endocrinol. Metab.*, 13: 55–60, 2002.

31. Nagy, L. and Schwabe, J.W. Mechanism of the nuclear receptor molecular switch. *Trends Biochem. Sci.*, 29: 317–324, 2004.

32. Reid, G., Hubner, M.R., Metivier, R., Brand, H., Denger, S., Manu, D., Beaudouin, J., Ellenberg, J., and Gannon, F. Cyclic, proteasome-mediated turnover of unliganded and liganded ER alpha on responsive promoters is an integral feature of estrogen signaling. *Mol. Cell*, 11: 695–707, 2003.

33. Lal, A., Lash, A.E., Altschul, S.F., Velculescu, V., Zhang, L., McLendon, R.E., Marra, M.A., Prange, C., Morin, P.J., Polyak, K., Papadopoulos, N., Vogelstein, B., Kinzler, K.W., Strausberg, R.L., and Riggins, G.J. A public database for gene expression in human cancers. *Cancer Res.*, 59: 5403–5407, 1999.

34. Barkhem, T., Nilsson, S., and Gustafsson, J.A. Molecular mechanisms, physiological consequences and pharmacological implications of estrogen receptor action. *Am. J. Pharmacogenomics*, 4: 19–28, 2004.

35. Bentrem, D., Fox, J.E., Pearce, S.T., Liu, H., Pappas, S., Kupfer, D., Zapf, J.W., and Jordan, V.C. Distinct molecular conformations of the estrogen receptor alpha complex exploited by environmental estrogens. *Cancer Res.*, 63: 7490–7496, 2003.

36. Brosens, J.J., Tullet, J., Varshochi, R., and Lam, E.W. Steroid receptor action. *Best. Pract. Res. Clin. Obstet. Gynaecol.*, 18: 265–283, 2004.

37. Brown, P.H. and Lippman, S.M. Chemoprevention of breast cancer. *Breast Cancer Res. Treat.*, 62: 1–17, 2000.

38. Cheng, G., Weihua, Z., Warner, M., and Gustafsson, J.A. Estrogen receptors ER alpha and ER beta in proliferation in the rodent mammary gland. *Proc. Natl. Acad. Sci. U.S.A.*, 101: 3739–3746, 2004.

39. Giguere, V. To ERR in the estrogen pathway. *Trends Endocrinol. Metab.*, 13: 220–225, 2002.

40. Jacobs, M.N. and Lewis, D.F. Steroid hormone receptors and dietary ligands: a selected review. *Proc. Nutr. Soc.*, 61: 105–122, 2002.

41. Adams, J.Y., Leav, I., Lau, K.M., Ho, S.M., and Pflueger, S.M. Expression of estrogen receptor beta in the fetal, neonatal, and prepubertal human prostate. *Prostate*, 52: 69–81, 2002.

42. Jarred, R.A., McPherson, S.J., Bianco, J.J., Couse, J.F., Korach, K.S., and Risbridger, G.P. Prostate phenotypes in estrogen-modulated transgenic mice. *Trends Endocrinol. Metab.*, 13: 163–168, 2002.

43. Lau, K. M., LaSpina, M., Long, J., and Ho, S. M. Expression of estrogen receptor (ER)-alpha and ER-beta in normal and malignant prostatic epithelial cells: regulation by methylation and involvement in growth regulation. *Cancer Res.*, 60: 3175–3182, 2000.

44. Gustafsson, J.A. What pharmacologists can learn from recent advances in estrogen signalling. *Trends Pharmacol. Sci.*, 24: 479–485, 2003.

45. Krishnan, K., Campbell, S., Abdel-Rahman, F., Whaley, S., and Stone, W.L. Cancer chemoprevention drug targets. *Curr. Drug Targets*, 4: 45–54, 2003.

46. Di Leo, A., Messa, C., Cavallini, A., and Linsalata, M. Estrogens and colorectal cancer. *Curr. Drug Targets Immune Endocr. Metab. Disord.*, 1: 1–12, 2001.

47. Campbell, M.J., Park, S., Uskokovic, M.R., Dawson, M.I., and Koeffler, H.P. Expression of retinoic acid receptor-beta sensitizes prostate cancer cells to growth inhibition mediated by combinations of retinoids and a 19-nor hexafluoride vitamin D3 analog. *Endocrinology*, 139: 1972–1980, 1998.

48. Skowronski, R.J., Peehl, D.M., and Feldman, D. Vitamin D and prostate cancer: 1,25 dihydroxyvitamin D3 receptors and actions in human prostate cancer cell lines. *Endocrinology*, 132: 1952–1960, 1993.

49. Collett, G.P., Betts, A.M., Johnson, M.I., Pulimood, A.B., Cook, S., Neal, D.E., and Robson, C.N. Peroxisome proliferator-activated receptor alpha is an androgen-responsive gene in human prostate and is highly expressed in prostatic adenocarcinoma. *Clin. Cancer Res.*, 6: 3241–3248, 2000.

50. Mueller, E., Smith, M., Sarraf, P., Kroll, T., Aiyer, A., Kaufman, D.S., Oh, W., Demetri, G., Figg, W.D., Zhou, X.P., Eng, C., Spiegelman, B.M., and Kantoff, P.W. Effects of ligand activation of peroxisome proliferator-activated receptor gamma in human prostate cancer. *Proc. Natl. Acad. Sci. U.S.A.,* 97: 10990–10995, 2000.

51. Stephen, R.L., Gustafsson, M.C., Jarvis, M., Tatoud, R., Marshall, B.R., Knight, D., Ehrenborg, E., Harris, A.L., Wolf, C.R., and Palmer, C.N. Activation of peroxisome proliferator-activated receptor delta stimulates the proliferation of human breast and prostate cancer cell lines. *Cancer Res.*, 64: 3162–3170, 2004.

52. Fukuchi, J., Kokontis, J.M., Hiipakka, R.A., Chuu, C.P., and Liao, S. Antiproliferative effect of liver X receptor agonists on LNCaP human prostate cancer cells. *Cancer Res.*, 64: 7686–7689, 2004.

53. Mohan, R. and Heyman, R.A. Orphan nuclear receptor modulators. *Curr. Top. Med. Chem.*, 3: 1637–1647, 2003.

54. Zhang, X.K. Vitamin A and apoptosis in prostate cancer. *Endocr. Relat. Cancer*, 9: 87–102, 2002.

55. Bjorkhem, I., Meaney, S., and Diczfalusy, U. Oxysterols in human circulation: which role do they have? *Curr. Opin. Lipidol.*, 13: 247–253, 2002.

56. Francis, G.A., Fayard, E., Picard, F., and Auwerx, J. Nuclear receptors and the control of metabolism. *Annu. Rev. Physiol.*, 65: 261–311, 2003.

57. Goldstein, J.T., Dobrzyn, A., Clagett-Dame, M., Pike, J.W., and DeLuca, H.F. Isolation and characterization of unsaturated fatty acids as natural ligands for the retinoid-X receptor. *Arch. Biochem. Biophys.*, 420: 185–193, 2003.

58. Adachi, R., Shulman, A.I., Yamamoto, K., Shimomura, I., Yamada, S., Mangelsdorf, D.J., and Makishima, M. Structural determinants for vitamin D receptor response to endocrine and xenobiotic signals. *Mol. Endocrinol.*, 18: 43–52, 2004.

59. Makishima, M., Lu, T.T., Xie, W., Whitfield, G.K., Domoto, H., Evans, R.M., Haussler, M.R., and Mangelsdorf, D.J. Vitamin D receptor as an intestinal bile acid sensor. *Science*, 296: 1313–1316, 2002.

60. Anderson, S.P., Dunn, C., Laughter, A., Yoon, L., Swanson, C., Stulnig, T.M., Steffensen, K.R., Chandraratna, R.A., Gustafsson, J.A., and Corton, J.C. Overlapping transcriptional programs regulated by the nuclear receptors peroxisome proliferator-activated receptor {alpha}, retinoid X receptor and liver X receptor in mouse liver. *Mol. Pharmacol.*, 2004.

61. Liu, M., Lee, M.H., Cohen, M., Bommakanti, M., and Freedman, L.P. Transcriptional activation of the Cdk inhibitor p21 by vitamin D3 leads to the induced differentiation of the myelomonocytic cell line U937. *Genes Dev.*, 10: 142–153, 1996.

62. Akutsu, N., Lin, R., Bastien, Y., Bestawros, A., Enepekides, D.J., Black, M.J., and White, J.H. Regulation of gene Expression by 1alpha,25-dihydroxyvitamin D3 and its analog EB1089 under growth-inhibitory conditions in squamous carcinoma cells. *Mol. Endocrinol.*, 15: 1127–1139, 2001.

63. Khanim, F.L., Gommersall, L.M., Wood, V.H., Smith, K.L., Montalvo, L., O'Neill, L.P., Xu, Y., Peehl, D.M., Stewart, P.M., Turner, B.M., and Campbell, M.J. Altered SMRT levels disrupt vitamin D(3) receptor signalling in prostate cancer cells. *Oncogene*, 23: 6712–6725, 2004.

64. Bieberich, C.J., Fujita, K., He, W.W., and Jay, G. Prostate-specific and androgen-dependent expression of a novel homeobox gene. *J. Biol. Chem.*, 271: 31779–31782, 1996.

65. Gregory, C.W., Hamil, K.G., Kim, D., Hall, S.H., Pretlow, T.G., Mohler, J.L., and French, F.S. Androgen receptor expression in androgen-independent prostate cancer is associated with increased expression of androgen-regulated genes. *Cancer Res.*, 58: 5718–5724, 1998.

66. Campbell, M.J., Elstner, E., Holden, S., Uskokovic, M., and Koeffler, H.P. Inhibition of proliferation of prostate cancer cells by a 19-nor-hexafluoride vitamin D3 analogue involves the induction of p21waf1, p27kip1 and E-cadherin. *J. Mol. Endocrinol.*, 19: 15–27, 1997.

67. Palmer, H.G., Gonzalez-Sancho, J.M., Espada, J., Berciano, M.T., Puig, I., Baulida, J., Quintanilla, M., Cano, A., de Herreros, A.G., Lafarga, M., and Munoz, A. Vitamin D(3) promotes the differentiation of colon carcinoma cells by the induction of E-cadherin and the inhibition of beta-catenin signaling. *J. Cell Biol.*, 154: 369–387, 2001.

68. Gnerre, C., Blattler, S., Kaufmann, M.R., Looser, R., and Meyer, U.A. Regulation of CYP3A4 by the bile acid receptor FXR: evidence for functional binding sites in the CYP3A4 gene. *Pharmacogenetics*, 14: 635–645, 2004.

69. Hukkanen, J., Vaisanen, T., Lassila, A., Piipari, R., Anttila, S., Pelkonen, O., Raunio, H., and Hakkola, J. Regulation of CYP3A5 by glucocorticoids and cigarette smoke in human lung-derived cells. *J. Pharmacol. Exp. Ther.*, 304: 745–752, 2003.

70. Jurutka, P.W., Thompson, P.D., Whitfield, G.K., Eichhorst, K.R., Hall, N., Dominguez, C.E., Hsieh, J.C., Haussler, C. A., and Haussler, M.R. Molecular and functional comparison of 1,25-dihydroxyvitamin D(3) and the novel vitamin D receptor ligand, lithocholic acid, in activating transcription of cytochrome P450 3A4. *J. Cell Biochem.*, 2004.

71. Sporn, M.B. New agents for chemoprevention of prostate cancer. *Eur. Urol.*, 35: 420–423, 1999.

72. Fischle, W., Dequiedt, F., Hendzel, M. J., Guenther, M.G., Lazar, M.A., Voelter, W., and Verdin, E. Enzymatic activity associated with class II HDACs is dependent on a multiprotein complex containing HDAC3 and SMRT/N-CoR. *Mol. Cell*, 9: 45–57, 2002.

73. Vaisanen, S., Dunlop, T.W., Frank, C., and Carlberg, C. Using chromatin immuno-precipitation to monitor 1alpha,25-dihydroxyvitamin D(3)-dependent chromatin activity on the human CYP24 promoter. *J. Steroid Biochem. Mol. Biol.*, 89–90: 277–279, 2004.

74. Metivier, R., Penot, G., Hubner, M.R., Reid, G., Brand, H., Kos, M., and Gannon, F. Estrogen receptor-alpha directs ordered, cyclical, and combinatorial recruitment of cofactors on a natural target promoter. *Cell*, 115: 751–763, 2003.

75. Goodson, M.L., Jonas, B.A., and Privalsky, M.L. Alternative mRNA splicing of SMRT creates functional diversity by generating corepressor isoforms with different affinities for different nuclear receptors. *J. Biol. Chem.*, 280, 7493–7503, 2005.

76. Germain, P., Iyer, J., Zechel, C., and Gronemeyer, H. Co-regulator recruitment and the mechanism of retinoic acid receptor synergy. *Nature*, 415: 187–192, 2002.

77. Jepsen, K. and Rosenfeld, M.G. Biological roles and mechanistic actions of co-repressor complexes. *J. Cell Sci.*, 115: 689–698, 2002.

78. Hermanson, O., Jepsen, K., and Rosenfeld, M.G. N-CoR controls differentiation of neural stem cells into astrocytes. *Nature*, 419: 934–939, 2002.

79. Shang, Y. and Brown, M. Molecular determinants for the tissue specificity of SERMs. *Science*, 295: 2465–2468, 2002.

80. Jenuwein, T. and Allis, C.D. Translating the histone code. *Science*, 293: 1074–1080, 2001.

81. Turner, B.M. Cellular memory and the histone code. *Cell*, 111: 285–291, 2002.

82. Yoon, H.G., Choi, Y., Cole, P.A., and Wong, J. Reading and function of a histone code involved in targeting corepressor complexes for repression. *Mol. Cell Biol.*, 25: 324–335, 2005.

83. Turner, B.M. Histone acetylation and an epigenetic code. *Bioessays*, 22: 836–845, 2000.

84. Turner, B.M. Histone acetylation as an epigenetic determinant of long-term transcriptional competence. *Cell Mol. Life Sci.*, 54: 21–31, 1998.

85. Turner, B.M. Decoding the nucleosome. *Cell*, 75: 5–8, 1993.

86. Turner, B.M. Histone acetylation and control of gene expression. *J. Cell Sci.*, 99 (Pt. 1): 13–20, 1991.

87. Yu, J., Li, Y., Ishizuka, T., Guenther, M.G., and Lazar, M.A. A SANT motif in the SMRT corepressor interprets the histone code and promotes histone deacetylation. *EMBO J.*, 22: 3403–3410, 2003.

88. Walters, M.R. and Nemere, I. Receptors for steroid hormones: membrane-associated and nuclear forms. *Cell Mol. Life Sci.*, 61: 2309–2321, 2004.

89. Revankar, C.M., Cimino, D.F., Sklar, L.A., Arterburn, J.B., and Prossnitz, E.R. A transmembrane intracellular estrogen receptor mediates rapid cell signaling. *Science*, 307: 1625–1630, 2005.

90. Norman, A.W., Mizwicki, M.T., and Norman, D.P. Steroid-hormone rapid actions, membrane receptors and a conformational ensemble model. *Nat. Rev. Drug Discov.*, 3: 27–41, 2004.

91. Vertino, A.M., Bula, C.M., Chen, J.R., Almeida, M., Han, L., Bellido, T., Kousteni, S., Norman, A.W., and Manolagas, S.C. Nongenotropic, anti-apoptotic signaling of 1alpha, 25(OH)2-vitamin D3 and analogs through the ligand binding domain (LBD) of the vitamin D receptor (VDR) in osteoblasts and osteocytes: mediation by Src, PI3, and JNK kinases. *J. Biol. Chem.*, 280, 14130–14137, 2005.

92. Huang, Y.C., Chen, J.Y., and Hung, W.C. Vitamin D3 receptor/Sp1 complex is required for the induction of p27Kip1 expression by vitamin D3. *Oncogene*, 23: 4856–4861, 2004.

93. Hengst, L. and Reed, S.I. Translational control of p27Kip1 accumulation during the cell cycle. *Science*, 271: 1861–1864, 1996.

94. Takeyama, K., Kitanaka, S., Sato, T., Kobori, M., Yanagisawa, J., and Kato, S. 25-Hydroxyvitamin D3 1alpha-hydroxylase and vitamin D synthesis. *Science*, 277: 1827–1830, 1997.

Jones, G., Ramshaw, H., Zhang, A., Cook, R., Byford, V., White, J., and Petkovich, M. Expression and activity of vitamin D-metabolizing cytochrome P450s (CYP1alpha and CYP24) in human nonsmall cell lung carcinomas. *Endocrinology*, 140: 3303–3310, 1999.

96. Jones, G., Strugnell, S.A., and Deluca, H.F. Current understanding of the molecular actions of vitamin D. *Physiol Rev.*, 78: 1193–1231, 1998.

97. Zehnder, D., Bland, R., Williams, M.C., McNinch, R.W., Howie, A.J., Stewart, P.M., and Hewison, M. Extrarenal expression of 25-hydroxyvitamin d(3)-1 alpha-hydroxylase. *J. Clin. Endocrinol. Metab.*, 86: 888–894, 2001.

98. Schwartz, G.G., Whitlatch, L.W., Chen, T.C., Lokeshwar, B.L., and Holick, M.F. Human prostate cells synthesize 1,25-dihydroxyvitamin D3 from 25-hydroxyvitamin D3. *Cancer Epidemiol. Biomarkers Prev.*, 7: 391–395, 1998.

99. Schwartz, G.G., Eads, D., Rao, A., Cramer, S.D., Willingham, M.C., Chen, T.C., Jamieson, D.P., Wang, L., Burnstein, K.L., Holick, M.F., and Koumenis, C. Pancreatic cancer cells express 25-hydroxyvitamin D-1 alpha-hydroxylase and their proliferation is inhibited by the prohormone 25-hydroxyvitamin D3. *Carcinogenesis*, 25: 1015–1026, 2004.

100. Diaz, L., Sanchez, I., Avila, E., Halhali, A., Vilchis, F., and Larrea, F. Identification of a 25-hydroxyvitamin D3 1alpha-hydroxylase gene transcription product in cultures of human syncytiotrophoblast cells. *J. Clin. Endocrinol. Metab.*, 85: 2543–2549, 2000.

101. Friedrich, M., Villena-Heinsen, C., Axt-Fliedner, R., Meyberg, R., Tilgen, W., Schmidt, W., and Reichrath, J. Analysis of 25-hydroxyvitamin D3-1alpha-hydroxylase in cervical tissue. *Anticancer Res.*, 22: 183–186, 2002.

102. Townsend, K., Banwell, C.M., Guy, M., Colston, K.W., Mansi, J.L., Stewart, P.M., Campbell, M.J., and Hewison, M. Autocrine metabolism of vitamin D in normal and malignant breast tissue. *Clin. Cancer Res.*, 11: 3579–3586, 2005.

103. Konety, B.R., Schwartz, G.G., Acierno, J.S., Jr., Becich, M.J., and Getzenberg, R.H. The role of vitamin D in normal prostate growth and differentiation. *Cell Growth Differ.*, 7: 1563–1570, 1996.

104. Zinser, G., Packman, K., and Welsh, J. Vitamin D(3) receptor ablation alters mammary gland morphogenesis. *Development*, 129: 3067–3076, 2002.

105. Tong, W.M., Bises, G., Sheinin, Y., Ellinger, A., Genser, D., Potzi, R., Wrba, F., Wenzl, E., Roka, R., Neuhold, N., Peterlik, M., and Cross, H.S. Establishment of primary cultures from human colonic tissue during tumor progression: vitamin-D responses and vitamin-D-receptor expression. *Int. J. Cancer*, 75: 467–472, 1998.

106. Ratnam, A.V., Bikle, D.D., Su, M.J., and Pillai, S. Squamous carcinoma cell lines fail to respond to 1,25-Dihydroxyvitamin D despite normal levels of the vitamin D receptor. *J. Invest. Dermatol.*, 106: 522–525, 1996.

107. Rashid, S.F., Mountford, J.C., Gombart, A.F., and Campbell, M.J. 1alpha,25-dihydroxyvitamin D(3) displays divergent growth effects in both normal and malignant cells. *Steroids*, 66: 433–440, 2001.

108. Richardson, G.D., Robson, C.N., Lang, S.H., Neal, D.E., Maitland, N.J., and Collins, A.T. CD133, a novel marker for human prostatic epithelial stem cells. *J. Cell Sci.*, 117: 3539–3545, 2004.

109. Mezzetti, G., Monti, M.G., Casolo, L.P., Piccinini, G., and Moruzzi, M.S. 1,25-Dihydroxycholecalciferol-dependent calcium uptake by mouse mammary gland in culture. *Endocrinology*, 122: 389–394, 1988.

110. Li, Y.C., Pirro, A.E., Amling, M., Delling, G., Baron, R., Bronson, R., and Demay, M.B. Targeted ablation of the vitamin D receptor: an animal model of vitamin D-dependent rickets type II with alopecia. *Proc. Natl. Acad. Sci. U.S.A.*, 94: 9831–9835, 1997.

111. Yoshizawa, T., Handa, Y., Uematsu, Y., Takeda, S., Sekine, K., Yoshihara, Y., Kawakami, T., Arioka, K., Sato, H., Uchiyama, Y., Masushige, S., Fukamizu, A., Matsumoto, T., and Kato, S. Mice lacking the vitamin D receptor exhibit impaired bone formation, uterine hypoplasia and growth retardation after weaning. *Nat. Genet.*, 16: 391–396, 1997.

112. Erben, R.G., Soegiarto, D.W., Weber, K., Zeitz, U., Lieberherr, M., Gniadecki, R., Moller, G., Adamski, J., and Balling, R. Deletion of deoxyribonucleic acid binding domain of the vitamin D receptor abrogates genomic and nongenomic functions of vitamin D. *Mol. Endocrinol.*, 16: 1524–1537, 2002.

113. Yoshizawa, T., Handa, Y., Uematsu, Y., Takeda, S., Sekine, K., Yoshihara, Y., Kawakami, T., Arioka, K., Sato, H., Uchiyama, Y., Masushige, S., Fukamizu, A., Matsumoto, T., and Kato, S. Mice lacking the vitamin D receptor exhibit impaired bone formation, uterine hypoplasia and growth retardation after weaning. *Nat. Genet.*, 16: 391–396, 1997.

114. Xiang, W., Kong, J., Chen, S., Cao, L.P., Qiao, G., Zheng, W., Liu, W., Li, X., Gardner, D.G., and Li, Y.C. Cardiac hypertrophy in vitamin D receptor knockout mice: role of the systemic and cardiac renin-angiotensin systems. *Am. J. Physiol. Endocrinol. Metab.*, 288: E125–E132, 2005.

115. Aihara, K., Azuma, H., Akaike, M., Ikeda, Y., Yamashita, M., Sudo, T., Hayashi, H., Yamada, Y., Endoh, F., Fujimura, M., Yoshida, T., Yamaguchi, H., Hashizume, S., Kato, M., Yoshimura, K., Yamamoto, Y., Kato, S., and Matsumoto, T. Disruption of nuclear vitamin D receptor gene causes enhanced thrombogenicity in mice. *J. Biol. Chem.*, 279: 35798–35802, 2004.

116. Zinser, G.M. and Welsh, J. Accelerated mammary gland development during pregnancy and delayed postlactational involution in vitamin D3 receptor null mice. *Mol. Endocrinol.*, 18: 2208–2223, 2004.

117. Colston, K., Colston, M. J., and Feldman, D. 1,25-dihydroxyvitamin D3 and malignant melanoma: the presence of receptors and inhibition of cell growth in culture. *Endocrinology*, 108: 1083–1086, 1981.

118. Miyaura, C., Abe, E., Kuribayashi, T., Tanaka, H., Konno, K., Nishii, Y., and Suda, T. 1 alpha,25-Dihydroxyvitamin D3 induces differentiation of human myeloid leukemia cells. *Biochem. Biophys. Res. Commun.*, 102: 937–943, 1981.

119. Abe, E., Miyaura, C., Sakagami, H., Takeda, M., Konno, K., Yamazaki, T., Yoshiki, S., and Suda, T. Differentiation of mouse myeloid leukemia cells induced by 1 alpha,25-dihydroxyvitamin D3. *Proc. Natl. Acad. Sci. U.S.A.*, 78: 4990–4994, 1981.

120. Colston, K., Colston, M.J., Fieldsteel, A.H., and Feldman, D. 1,25-dihydroxyvitamin D3 receptors in human epithelial cancer cell lines. *Cancer Res.*, 42: 856–859, 1982.

121. Colston, K.W., Berger, U., and Coombes, R.C. Possible role for vitamin D in controlling breast cancer cell proliferation. *Lancet,* 1: 188–191, 1989.

122. Love-Schimenti, C.D., Gibson, D.F., Ratnam, A.V., and Bikle, D.D. Antiestrogen potentiation of antiproliferative effects of vitamin D3 analogues in breast cancer cells. *Cancer Res.*, 56: 2789–2794, 1996.

123. Mehta, R.G., Hussain, E.A., Mehta, R.R., and Das Gupta, T.K. Chemoprevention of mammary carcinogenesis by 1alpha-hydroxyvitamin D5, a synthetic analog of vitamin D. *Mutat. Res.*, 523–524: 253–264, 2003.

124. Welsh, J., Wietzke, J.A., Zinser, G.M., Smyczek, S., Romu, S., Tribble, E., Welsh, J.C., Byrne, B., and Narvaez, C.J. Impact of the Vitamin D3 receptor on growth-regulatory pathways in mammary gland and breast cancer. *J. Steroid Biochem. Mol. Biol.*, 83: 85–92, 2002.

125. Peehl, D.M., Skowronski, R.J., Leung, G.K., Wong, S.T., Stamey, T.A., and Feldman, D. Antiproliferative effects of 1,25-dihydroxyvitamin D3 on primary cultures of human prostatic cells. *Cancer Res.*, 54: 805–810, 1994.

126. Elstner, E., Campbell, M.J., Munker, R., Shintaku, P., Binderup, L., Heber, D., Said, J., and Koeffler, H.P. Novel 20-epi-vitamin D3 analog combined with 9-cis-retinoic acid markedly inhibits colony growth of prostate cancer cells. *Prostate*, 40: 141–149, 1999.

127. Koike, M., Elstner, E., Campbell, M.J., Asou, H., Uskokovic, M., Tsuruoka, N., and Koeffler, H.P. 19-nor-hexafluoride analogue of vitamin D3: a novel class of potent inhibitors of proliferation of human breast cell lines. *Cancer Res.*, 57: 4545–4550, 1997.

128. Munker, R., Norman, A., and Koeffler, H.P. Vitamin D compounds: effect on clonal proliferation and differentiation of human myeloid cells. *J. Clin. Invest*, 78: 424–430, 1986.

129. Palmer, H.G., Sanchez-Carbayo, M., Ordonez-Moran, P., Larriba, M.J., Cordon-Cardo, C., and Munoz, A. Genetic signatures of differentiation induced by 1alpha,25-dihydroxyvitamin D3 in human colon cancer cells. *Cancer Res.*, 63: 7799–7806, 2003.

130. Palmer, H.G., Larriba, M.J., Garcia, J.M., Ordonez-Moran, P., Pena, C., Peiro, S., Puig, I., Rodriguez, R., De La, F.R., Bernad, A., Pollan, M., Bonilla, F., Gamallo, C., de Herreros, A.G., and Munoz, A. The transcription factor SNAIL represses vitamin D receptor expression and responsiveness in human colon cancer. *Nat. Med.*, 2004.

131. Beer, T.M., Eilers, K.M., Garzotto, M., Egorin, M.J., Lowe, B.A., and Henner, W.D. Weekly high-dose calcitriol and docetaxel in metastatic androgen-independent prostate cancer. *J. Clin. Oncol.*, 21: 123–128, 2003.

132. Beer, T.M., Myrthue, A., and Eilers, K.M. Rationale for the development and current status of calcitriol in androgen-independent prostate cancer. *World J. Urol.*, 23: 28–32, 2005.

133. Beer, T.M., Myrthue, A., Garzotto, M., O'Hara, M.F., Chin, R., Lowe, B.A., Montalto, M.A., Corless, C.L., and Henner, W.D. Randomized study of high-dose pulse calcitriol or placebo prior to radical prostatectomy. *Cancer Epidemiol. Biomarkers Prev.*, 13: 2225–2232, 2004.

134. Beer, T.M., Garzotto, M., and Katovic, N.M. High-dose calcitriol and carboplatin in metastatic androgen-independent prostate cancer. *Am. J. Clin. Oncol.*, 27: 535–541, 2004.

135. Trump, D.L., Hershberger, P.A., Bernardi, R.J., Ahmed, S., Muindi, J., Fakih, M., Yu, W.D., and Johnson, C.S. Anti-tumor activity of calcitriol: pre-clinical and clinical studies. *J. Steroid Biochem. Mol. Biol.*, 89–90: 519–526, 2004.

136. Eelen, G., Verlinden, L., Van Camp, M., Mathieu, C., Carmeliet, G., Bouillon, R., and Verstuyf, A. Microarray analysis of 1alpha,25-dihydroxyvitamin D3-treated MC3T3-E1 cells. *J. Steroid Biochem. Mol. Biol.*, 89–90: 405–407, 2004.

137. Eelen, G., Verlinden, L., Van Camp, M., van Hummelen, P., Marchal, K., de Moor, B., Mathieu, C., Carmeliet, G., Bouillon, R., and Verstuyf, A. The effects of 1alpha,25-dihydroxyvitamin D3 on the expression of DNA replication genes. *J. Bone Miner. Res.*, 19: 133–146, 2004.

138. Guzey, M., Luo, J., and Getzenberg, R.H. Vitamin D3 modulated gene expression patterns in human primary normal and cancer prostate cells. *J. Cell Biochem.*, 93: 271–285, 2004.

139. Lin, R., Nagai, Y., Sladek, R., Bastien, Y., Ho, J., Petrecca, K., Sotiropoulou, G., Diamandis, E.P., Hudson, T.J., and White, J.H. Expression profiling in squamous carcinoma cells reveals pleiotropic effects of vitamin D3 analog EB1089 signaling on cell proliferation, differentiation, and immune system regulation. *Mol. Endocrinol.*, 16: 1243–1256, 2002.

140. Zhuang, S.H. and Burnstein, K.L. Antiproliferative effect of 1alpha,25-dihydroxyvitamin D3 in human prostate cancer cell line LNCaP involves reduction of cyclin-dependent kinase 2 activity and persistent G1 accumulation. *Endocrinology*, 139: 1197–1207, 1998.

141. Yang, E.S. and Burnstein, K.L. Vitamin D inhibits G1 to S progression in LNCaP prostate cancer cells through p27Kip1 stabilization and Cdk2 mislocalization to the cytoplasm. *J. Biol. Chem.*, 278: 46862–46868, 2003.

142. Ryhanen, S., Jaaskelainen, T., Mahonen, A., and Maenpaa, P.H. Inhibition of MG-63 cell cycle progression by synthetic vitamin D3 analogs mediated by p27, Cdk2, cyclin E, and the retinoblastoma protein. *Biochem. Pharmacol.*, 66: 495–504, 2003.

143. Lin, R., Wang, T.T., Miller, W.H., Jr., and White, J.H. Inhibition of F-Box protein p45(SKP2) expression and stabilization of cyclin-dependent kinase inhibitor p27(KIP1) in vitamin D analog-treated cancer cells. *Endocrinology*, 144: 749–753, 2003.

144. Liu, W., Asa, S.L., and Ezzat, S. Vitamin D and its analog EB1089 induce p27 accumulation and diminish association of p27 with Skp2 independent of PTEN in pituitary corticotroph cells. *Brain Pathol.*, 12: 412–419, 2002.

145. Li, P., Li, C., Zhao, X., Zhang, X., Nicosia, S.V., and Bai, W. p27(Kip1) stabilization and G(1) arrest by 1,25-dihydroxyvitamin D(3) in ovarian cancer cells mediated through down-regulation of cyclin E/cyclin-dependent kinase 2 and Skp1-Cullin-F-box protein/Skp2 ubiquitin ligase. *J. Biol. Chem.*, 279: 25260–25267, 2004.

146. Jiang, F., Li, P., Fornace, A. J., Jr., Nicosia, S.V., and Bai, W. G2/M arrest by 1,25-dihydroxyvitamin D3 in ovarian cancer cells mediated through the induction of GADD45 via an exonic enhancer. *J. Biol. Chem.*, 278: 48030–48040, 2003.

147. Jin, S., Mazzacurati, L., Zhu, X., Tong, T., Song, Y., Shujuan, S., Petrik, K.L., Rajasekaran, B., Wu, M., and Zhan, Q. Gadd45a contributes to p53 stabilization in response to DNA damage. *Oncogene*, 22: 8536–8540, 2003.

148. Jin, S., Fan, F., Fan, W., Zhao, H., Tong, T., Blanck, P., Alomo, I., Rajasekaran, B., and Zhan, Q. Transcription factors Oct-1 and NF-YA regulate the p53-independent induction of the GADD45 following DNA damage. *Oncogene*, 20: 2683–2690, 2001.

149. Danielsson, C., Mathiasen, I.S., James, S.Y., Nayeri, S., Bretting, C., Hansen, C.M., Colston, K.W., and Carlberg, C. Sensitive induction of apoptosis in breast cancer cells by a novel 1,25-dihydroxyvitamin D3 analogue shows relation to promoter selectivity. *J. Cell Biochem.*, 66: 552–562, 1997.

150. Welsh, J. Vitamin D and breast cancer: insights from animal models. *Am. J. Clin. Nutr.*, 80: 1721S–1724S, 2004.

151. Blutt, S.E., McDonnell, T.J., Polek, T.C., and Weigel, N.L. Calcitriol-induced apoptosis in LNCaP cells is blocked by overexpression of Bcl-2. *Endocrinology*, 141: 10–17, 2000.

152. Mathiasen, I.S., Lademann, U., and Jaattela, M. Apoptosis induced by vitamin D compounds in breast cancer cells is inhibited by Bcl-2 but does not involve known caspases or p53. *Cancer Res.*, 59: 4848–4856, 1999.

153. Weitsman, G.E., Ravid, A., Liberman, U.A., and Koren, R. Vitamin D enhances caspase-dependent and independent TNF-induced breast cancer cell death: the role of reactive oxygen species. *Ann. N.Y. Acad. Sci.*, 1010: 437–440, 2003.

154. Pirianov, G. and Colston, K.W. Interaction of vitamin D analogs with signaling pathways leading to active cell death in breast cancer cells. *Steroids*, 66: 309–318, 2001.

155. Weitsman, G.E., Koren, R., Zuck, E., Rotem, C., Liberman, U.A., and Ravid, A. Vitamin D sensitizes breast cancer cells to the action of H(2)O(2): mitochondria as a convergence point in the death pathway. *Free Radic. Biol. Med.*, 39: 266–278, 2005.

156. Ravid, A. and Koren, R. The role of reactive oxygen species in the anticancer activity of vitamin D. *Recent Results Cancer Res.*, 164: 357–367, 2003.

157. Weitsman, G.E., Ravid, A., Liberman, U.A., and Koren, R. Vitamin D enhances caspase-dependent and -independent TNFalpha-induced breast cancer cell death: the role of reactive oxygen species and mitochondria. *Int. J. Cancer*, 106: 178–186, 2003.

158. Narvaez, C.J., Byrne, B.M., Romu, S., Valrance, M., and Welsh, J. Induction of apoptosis by 1,25-dihydroxyvitamin D3 in MCF-7 Vitamin D3-resistant variant can be sensitized by TPA. *J. Steroid Biochem. Mol. Biol.*, 84: 199–209, 2003.

159. Jeon, J.H., Lee, K.N., Hwang, C.Y., Kwon, K.S., You, K.H., and Choi, I. Tumor suppressor VDUP1 increases p27kip1 stability by inhibiting JAB1. *Cancer Res.*, 65: 4485–4489, 2005.

160. Yang, X., Young, L.H., and Voigt, J.M. Expression of a vitamin D-regulated gene (VDUP-1) in untreated- and MNU-treated rat mammary tissue. *Breast Cancer Res. Treat.*, 48: 33–44, 1998.

161. Saitoh, M., Nishitoh, H., Fujii, M., Takeda, K., Tobiume, K., Sawada, Y., Kawabata, M., Miyazono, K., and Ichijo, H. Mammalian thioredoxin is a direct inhibitor of apoptosis signal-regulating kinase (ASK) 1. *EMBO J.*, 17: 2596–2606, 1998.

162. Wang, X. and Studzinski, G.P. Antiapoptotic action of 1,25-dihydroxyvitamin D3 is associated with increased mitochondrial MCL-1 and RAF-1 proteins and reduced release of cytochrome c. *Exp. Cell Res.*, 235: 210–217, 1997.

163. Sauer, B., Ruwisch, L., and Kleuser, B. Antiapoptotic action of 1alpha,25-dihydroxyvitamin D3 in primary human melanocytes. *Melanoma Res.*, 13: 339–347, 2003.

164. Bunce, C.M., Mountford, J.C., French, P.J., Mole, D.J., Durham, J., Michell, R.H., and Brown, G. Potentiation of myeloid differentiation by anti-inflammatory agents, by steroids and by retinoic acid involves a single intracellular target, probably an enzyme of the aldoketoreductase family. *Biochim. Biophys. Acta*, 1311: 189–198, 1996.

165. Bischof, M.G., Redlich, K., Schiller, C., Chirayath, M.V., Uskokovic, M., Peterlik, M., and Cross, H.S. Growth inhibitory effects on human colon adenocarcinoma-derived Caco-2 cells and calcemic potential of 1 alpha,25-dihydroxyvitamin D3 analogs: structure-function relationships. *J. Pharmacol. Exp. Ther.*, 275: 1254–1260, 1995.

166. Shabahang, M., Buras, R.R., Davoodi, F., Schumaker, L.M., Nauta, R.J., Uskokovic, M.R., Brenner, R.V., and Evans, S.R. Growth inhibition of HT-29 human colon cancer cells by analogues of 1,25-dihydroxyvitamin D3. *Cancer Res.*, 54: 4057–4064, 1994.

167. Cross, H.S., Farsoudi, K.H., and Peterlik, M. Growth inhibition of human colon adenocarcinoma-derived Caco-2 cells by 1,25-dihydroxyvitamin D3 and two synthetic analogs: relation to in vitro hypercalcemic potential. *Naunyn Schmiedebergs Arch. Pharmacol.*, 347: 105–110, 1993.

168. Giuliano, A.R., Franceschi, R.T., and Wood, R.J. Characterization of the vitamin D receptor from the Caco-2 human colon carcinoma cell line: effect of cellular differentiation. *Arch. Biochem. Biophys.*, 285: 261–269, 1991.

169. Krill, D., Stoner, J., Konety, B.R., Becich, M.J., and Getzenberg, R.H. Differential effects of vitamin D on normal human prostate epithelial and stromal cells in primary culture. *Urology*, 54: 171–177, 1999.

170. Debruyne, P., Vermeulen, S., and Mareel, M. The role of the E-cadherin/catenin complex in gastrointestinal cancer. *Acta Gastroenterol. Belg.*, 62: 393–402, 1999.

171. Morin, P.J. beta-catenin signaling and cancer. *Bioessays*, 21: 1021–1030, 1999.

172. Larriba, M.J. and Munoz, A. SNAIL vs. vitamin D receptor expression in colon cancer: therapeutics implications. *Br. J. Cancer*, 2005.

173. Hofseth, L.J., Hussain, S.P., and Harris, C.C. p53: 25 years after its discovery. *Trends Pharmacol. Sci.*, 25: 177–181, 2004.

174. Fridman, J.S. and Lowe, S.W. Control of apoptosis by p53. *Oncogene*, 22: 9030–9040, 2003.

175. Haupt, S., Berger, M., Goldberg, Z., and Haupt, Y. Apoptosis — the p53 network. *J. Cell Sci.*, 116: 4077–4085, 2003.

176. Altucci, L. and Gronemeyer, H. Nuclear receptors in cell life and death. *Trends Endocrinol. Metab*, 12: 460–468, 2001.

177. Sengupta, S. and Wasylyk, B. Physiological and pathological consequences of the interactions of the p53 tumor suppressor with the glucocorticoid, androgen, and estrogen receptors. *Ann. N.Y. Acad. Sci.*, 1024: 54–71, 2004.

178. Dunlap, N., Schwartz, G.G., Eads, D., Cramer, S.D., Sherk, A.B., John, V., and Koumenis, C. 1alpha,25-dihydroxyvitamin D(3) (calcitriol) and its analogue, 19-nor-1alpha,25(OH)(2)D(2), potentiate the effects of ionising radiation on human prostate cancer cells. *Br. J. Cancer*, 89: 746–753, 2003.

179. Campbell, M.J., Gombart, A.F., Kwok, S.H., Park, S., and Koeffler, H.P. The anti-proliferative effects of 1alpha,25(OH)2D3 on breast and prostate cancer cells are associated with induction of BRCA1 gene expression. *Oncogene*, 19: 5091–5097, 2000.

180. Szanto, A., Benko, S., Szatmari, I., Balint, B.L., Furtos, I., Ruhl, R., Molnar, S., Csiba, L., Garuti, R., Calandra, S., Larsson, H., Diczfalusy, U., and Nagy, L. Transcriptional Regulation of Human CYP27 Integrates Retinoid, Peroxisome Proliferator-Activated Receptor, and Liver X Receptor Signaling in Macrophages. *Mol. Cell Biol.*, 24: 8154–8166, 2004.

181. Lehmann, J.M., McKee, D.D., Watson, M.A., Willson, T. M., Moore, J.T., and Kliewer, S.A. The human orphan nuclear receptor PXR is activated by compounds that regulate CYP3A4 gene expression and cause drug interactions. *J. Clin. Invest.*, 102: 1016–1023, 1998.

182. Dwivedi, P.P., Omdahl, J.L., Kola, I., Hume, D.A., and May, B.K. Regulation of rat cytochrome P450C24 (CYP24) gene expression: evidence for functional cooperation of Ras-activated Ets transcription factors with the vitamin D receptor in 1,25-dihydroxyvitamin D(3)-mediated induction. *J. Biol. Chem.*, 275: 47–55, 2000.

183. Schrader, M., Bendik, I., Becker-Andre, M., and Carlberg, C. Interaction between retinoic acid and vitamin D signaling pathways. *J. Biol. Chem.*, 268: 17830–17836, 1993.

184. Blutt, S.E., Allegretto, E.A., Pike, J.W., and Weigel, N.L. 1,25-dihydroxyvitamin D3 and 9-cis-retinoic acid act synergistically to inhibit the growth of LNCaP prostate cells and cause accumulation of cells in G1. *Endocrinology*, 138: 1491–1497, 1997.

185. Peehl, D.M., Krishnan, A.V., and Feldman, D. Pathways mediating the growth-inhibitory actions of vitamin D in prostate cancer. *J. Nutr.*, 133: 2461S–2469S, 2003.

186. Dunlop, T.W., Vaisanen, S., Frank, C., Molnar, F., Sinkkonen, L., and Carlberg, C. The human peroxisome proliferator-activated receptor delta gene is a primary target of 1alpha,25-dihydroxyvitamin D3 and its nuclear receptor. *J. Mol. Biol.*, 349: 248–260, 2005.

187. James, S.Y., Mackay, A.G., and Colston, K.W. Vitamin D derivatives in combination with 9-cis retinoic acid promote active cell death in breast cancer cells. *J. Mol. Endocrinol.*, 14: 391–394, 1995.

188. Cross, H.S., Kallay, E., Lechner, D., Gerdenitsch, W., Adlercreutz, H., and Armbrecht, H.J. Phytoestrogens and vitamin D metabolism: a new concept for the prevention and therapy of colorectal, prostate, and mammary carcinomas. *J. Nutr.*, 134: 1207S–1212S, 2004.

189. Kallay, E., Adlercreutz, H., Farhan, H., Lechner, D., Bajna, E., Gerdenitsch, W., Campbell, M., and Cross, H.S. Phytoestrogens regulate vitamin D metabolism in the mouse colon: relevance for colon tumor prevention and therapy. *J. Nutr.*, 132: 3490S–3493S, 2002.

190. Swami, S., Krishnan, A.V., Peehl, D.M., and Feldman, D. Genistein potentiates the growth inhibitory effects of 1,25-dihydroxyvitamin D(3) in DU145 human prostate cancer cells: role of the direct inhibition of CYP24 enzyme activity. *Mol. Cell Endocrinol.*, 2005.

191. Rao, A., Coan, A., Welsh, J.E., Barclay, W.W., Koumenis, C., and Cramer, S.D. Vitamin D receptor and p21/WAF1 are targets of genistein and 1,25-dihydroxyvitamin D3 in human prostate cancer cells. *Cancer Res.*, 64: 2143–2147, 2004.

192. Lechner, D. and Cross, H.S. Phytoestrogens and 17beta-estradiol influence vitamin D metabolism and receptor expression-relevance for colon cancer prevention. *Recent Results Cancer Res.*, 164: 379–391, 2003.

193. Rozen, F. and Pollak, M. Inhibition of insulin-like growth factor I receptor signaling by the vitamin D analogue EB1089 in MCF-7 breast cancer cells: a role for insulin-like growth factor binding proteins. *Int. J. Oncol.*, 15: 589–594, 1999.

194. Huynh, H., Pollak, M., and Zhang, J.C. Regulation of insulin-like growth factor (IGF) II and IGF binding protein 3 autocrine loop in human PC-3 prostate cancer cells by vitamin D metabolite 1,25(OH)2D3 and its analog EB1089. *Int. J. Oncol.*, 13: 137–143, 1998.

195. Rozen, F., Yang, X.F., Huynh, H., and Pollak, M. Antiproliferative action of vitamin D-related compounds and insulin-like growth factor-binding protein 5 accumulation. *J. Natl. Cancer Inst.*, 89: 652–656, 1997.

196. Weikkolainen, K., Keski-Oja, J., and Koli, K. Expression of latent TGF-beta binding protein LTBP-1 is hormonally regulated in normal and transformed human lung fibroblasts. *Growth Factors*, 21: 51–60, 2003.

197. Han, S.H., Jeon, J.H., Ju, H.R., Jung, U., Kim, K.Y., Yoo, H.S., Lee, Y.H., Song, K.S., Hwang, H.M., Na, Y.S., Yang, Y., Lee, K.N., and Choi, I. VDUP1 upregulated by TGF-beta1 and 1,25-dihydorxyvitamin D3 inhibits tumor cell growth by blocking cell-cycle progression. *Oncogene*, 22: 4035–4046, 2003.

198. Bizzarri, M., Cucina, A., Valente, M.G., Tagliaferri, F., Borrelli, V., Stipa, F., and Cavallaro, A. Melatonin and vitamin D3 increase TGF-beta1 release and induce growth inhibition in breast cancer cell cultures. *J. Surg. Res.*, 110: 332–337, 2003.

199. Cao, Z., Flanders, K.C., Bertolette, D., Lyakh, L.A., Wurthner, J.U., Parks, W.T., Letterio, J.J., Ruscetti, F.W., and Roberts, A.B. Levels of phospho-Smad2/3 are sensors of the interplay between effects of TGF-beta and retinoic acid on monocytic and granulocytic differentiation of HL-60 cells. *Blood*, 101: 498–507, 2003.

200. Koli, K., Saharinen, J., Hyytiainen, M., Penttinen, C., and Keski-Oja, J. Latency, activation, and binding proteins of TGF-beta. *Microsc. Res. Tech.*, 52: 354–362, 2001.

201. Jung, C.W., Kim, E.S., Seol, J.G., Park, W.H., Lee, S.J., Kim, B.K., and Lee, Y.Y. Antiproliferative effect of a vitamin D3 analog, EB1089, on HL-60 cells by the induction of TGF-beta receptor. *Leuk. Res.*, 23: 1105–1112, 1999.

202. Lian, J.B. and Stein, G.S. The developmental stages of osteoblast growth and differentiation exhibit selective responses of genes to growth factors (TGF beta 1) and hormones (vitamin D and glucocorticoids). *J. Oral Implantol.*, 19: 95–105, 1993.

203. Qi, X., Tang, J., Pramanik, R., Schultz, R.M., Shirasawa, S., Sasazuki, T., Han, J., and Chen, G. p38 MAPK activation selectively induces cell death in K-ras-mutated human colon cancer cells through regulation of vitamin D receptor. *J. Biol. Chem.*, 279: 22138–22144, 2004.

204. Ji, Y., Kutner, A., Verstuyf, A., Verlinden, L., and Studzinski, G.P. Derivatives of vitamins D2 and D3 activate three MAPK pathways and upregulate pRb expression in differentiating HL60 cells. *Cell Cycle*, 1: 410–415, 2002.

205. Pepper, C., Thomas, A., Hoy, T., Milligan, D., Bentley, P., and Fegan, C. The vitamin D3 analog EB1089 induces apoptosis via a p53-independent mechanism involving p38 MAP kinase activation and suppression of ERK activity in B-cell chronic lymphocytic leukemia cells in vitro. *Blood*, 101: 2454–2460, 2003.

206. Qi, X., Pramanik, R., Wang, J., Schultz, R.M., Maitra, R.K., Han, J., DeLuca, H.F., and Chen, G. The p38 and JNK pathways cooperate to trans-activate vitamin D receptor via c-Jun/AP-1 and sensitize human breast cancer cells to vitamin D(3)-induced growth inhibition. *J. Biol. Chem.*, 277: 25884–25892, 2002.

207. Zinser, G.M. and Welsh, J. Vitamin D receptor status alters mammary gland morphology and tumorigenesis in MMTV-neu mice. *Carcinogenesis*, 25, 2361–2372, 2004.

208. Zinser, G.M., Sundberg, J.P., and Welsh, J. Vitamin D(3) receptor ablation sensitizes skin to chemically induced tumorigenesis. *Carcinogenesis*, 23: 2103–2109, 2002.

209. Lamprecht, S.A. and Lipkin, M. Chemoprevention of colon cancer by calcium, vitamin D and folate: molecular mechanisms. *Nat. Rev. Cancer*, 3: 601–614, 2003.

210. Lipkin, M. and Newmark, H.L. Vitamin D, calcium and prevention of breast cancer: a review. *J. Am. Coll. Nutr.*, 18: 392S–397S, 1999.

211. Lipkin, M., Reddy, B., Newmark, H., and Lamprecht, S. A. Dietary factors in human colorectal cancer. *Annu. Rev. Nutr.*, 19: 545–586, 1999.

212. Xue, L., Lipkin, M., Newmark, H., and Wang, J. Influence of dietary calcium and vitamin D on diet-induced epithelial cell hyperproliferation in mice. *J. Natl. Cancer Inst.*, 91: 176–181, 1999.

213. Yang, K., Edelmann, W., Fan, K., Lau, K., Leung, D., Newmark, H., Kucherlapati, R., and Lipkin, M. Dietary modulation of carcinoma development in a mouse model for human familial adenomatous polyposis. *Cancer Res.*, 58: 5713–5717, 1998.

214. Huerta, S., Irwin, R.W., Heber, D., Go, V.L., Koeffler, H.P., Uskokovic, M.R., and Harris, D.M. 1alpha,25-(OH)(2)-D(3) and its synthetic analogue decrease tumor load in the Apc(min) mouse. *Cancer Res.*, 62: 741–746, 2002.

215. Nakagawa, K., Sasaki, Y., Kato, S., Kubodera, N., and Okano, T. 22-Oxa-1alpha,25-dihydroxyvitamin D3 inhibits metastasis and angiogenesis in lung cancer. *Carcinogenesis*, 26: 1044–1054, 2005.

216. Yildiz, F., Kars, A., Cengiz, M., Yildiz, O., Akyurek, S., Selek, U., Ozyigit, G., and Atahan, I.L. 1,25-Dihydroxy vitamin D3: can it be an effective therapeutic option for aggressive fibromatosis. *Med. Hypotheses*, 64: 333–336, 2005.

217. Bernardi, R.J., Johnson, C.S., Modzelewski, R.A., and Trump, D.L. Antiproliferative effects of 1alpha,25-dihydroxyvitamin D(3) and vitamin D analogs on tumor-derived endothelial cells. *Endocrinology*, 143: 2508–2514, 2002.

218. Lucia, M.S., Anzano, M.A., Slayter, M.V., Anver, M.R., Green, D.M., Shrader, M.W., Logsdon, D.L., Driver, C.L., Brown, C.C., and Peer, C.W., Chemopreventive activity of tamoxifen, N-(4-hydroxyphenyl)retinamide, and the vitamin D analogue Ro24-5531 for androgen-promoted carcinomas of the rat seminal vesicle and prostate. *Cancer Res.*, 55: 5621–5627, 1995.

219. Anzano, M.A., Smith, J.M., Uskokovic, M.R., Peer, C.W., Mullen, L.T., Letterio, J.J., Welsh, M.C., Shrader, M.W., Logsdon, D.L., Driver, C.L., and . 1 alpha,25-Dihydroxy-16-ene-23-yne-26,27-hexafluorocholecalciferol (Ro24-5531), a new deltanoid (vitamin D analogue) for prevention of breast cancer in the rat. *Cancer Res.*, 54: 1653–1656, 1994.

220. Mehta, R.G. Stage-specific inhibition of mammary carcinogenesis by 1alpha-hydroxyvitamin D5. *Eur. J. Cancer*, 40: 2331–2337, 2004.

221. Cope, M.B., Steele, V.E., Eto, I., Juliana, M.M., Hill, D.L., and Grubbs, C.J. Prevention of methylnitrosourea-induced mammary cancers by 9-cis-retinoic acid and/or vitamin D3. *Oncol. Rep.*, 9: 533–537, 2002.

222. He, R.K. and Gascon-Barre, M. Influence of the vitamin D status on the early hepatic response to carcinogen exposure in rats. *J. Pharmacol. Exp. Ther.*, 281: 464–469, 1997.

223. Otoshi, T., Iwata, H., Kitano, M., Nishizawa, Y., Morii, H., Yano, Y., Otani, S., and Fukushima, S. Inhibition of intestinal tumor development in rat multi-organ carcinogenesis and aberrant crypt foci in rat colon carcinogenesis by 22-oxa-calcitriol, a synthetic analogue of 1 alpha, 25-dihydroxyvitamin D3. *Carcinogenesis*, 16: 2091–2097, 1995.

224. Belleli, A., Shany, S., Levy, J., Guberman, R., and Lamprecht, S.A. A protective role of 1,25-dihydroxyvitamin D3 in chemically induced rat colon carcinogenesis. *Carcinogenesis*, 13: 2293–2298, 1992.

225. Colston, K.W., Pirianov, G., Bramm, E., Hamberg, K.J., and Binderup, L. Effects of Seocalcitol (EB1089) on nitrosomethyl urea-induced rat mammary tumors. *Breast Cancer Res. Treat.*, 80: 303–311, 2003.

226. Cross, H.S., Kallay, E., Khorchide, M., and Lechner, D. Regulation of extrarenal synthesis of 1,25-dihydroxyvitamin D3 — relevance for colonic cancer prevention and therapy. *Mol. Aspects Med.*, 24: 459–465, 2003.

227. Mohamed, T., Sato, H., Kurosawa, T., and Oikawa, S. Bile acid extraction rate in the liver of cows fed high-fat diet and lipid profiles in the portal and hepatic veins. *J. Vet. Med. A Physiol. Pathol. Clin. Med.*, 49: 151–156, 2002.

228. Roy, C.C., Fournier, L.A., Chartrand, L., Lepage, G., and Yousef, I. Effect of diversion of pancreatic secretions on biliary lipids and bile salt kinetics in the rat. *J. Pediatr. Gastroenterol. Nutr.*, 2: 152–158, 1983.

229. Cummings, J.H., Wiggins, H.S., Jenkins, D.J., Houston, H., Jivraj, T., Drasar, B.S., and Hill, M.J. Influence of diets high and low in animal fat on bowel habit, gastrointestinal transit time, fecal microflora, bile acid, and fat excretion. *J. Clin. Invest.*, 61: 953–963, 1978.

230. Debruyne, P.R., Bruyneel, E.A., Karaguni, I.M., Li, X., Flatau, G., Muller, O., Zimber, A., Gespach, C., and Mareel, M.M. Bile acids stimulate invasion and haptotaxis in human colorectal cancer cells through activation of multiple oncogenic signaling pathways. *Oncogene*, 21: 6740–6750, 2002.

231. Kishida, T., Taguchi, F., Feng, L., Tatsuguchi, A., Sato, J., Fujimori, S., Tachikawa, H., Tamagawa, Y., Yoshida, Y., and Kobayashi, M. Analysis of bile acids in colon residual liquid or fecal material in patients with colorectal neoplasia and control subjects. *J. Gastroenterol.*, 32: 306–311, 1997.

232. Pool-Zobel, B.L. and Leucht, U. Induction of DNA damage by risk factors of colon cancer in human colon cells derived from biopsies. *Mutat. Res.*, 375: 105–115, 1997.

233. Nair, P. and Turjman, N. Role of bile acids and neutral sterols in familial cancer syndromes of the colon. *Dis. Colon Rectum*, 26: 629–632, 1983.

234. Narisawa, T., Reddy, B.S., and Weisburger, J.H. Effect of bile acids and dietary fat on large bowel carcinogenesis in animal models. *Gastroenterol. Jpn.*, 13: 206–212, 1978.

235. Reddy, B.S. Role of bile metabolites in colon carcinogenesis: animal models. *Cancer*, 36: 2401–2406, 1975.

236. Baijal, P.K., Fitzpatrick, D.W., and Bird, R.P. Comparative effects of secondary bile acids, deoxycholic and lithocholic acids, on aberrant crypt foci growth in the post-initiation phases of colon carcinogenesis. *Nutr. Cancer*, 31: 81–89, 1998.

237. Hori, T., Matsumoto, K., Sakaitani, Y., Sato, M., and Morotomi, M. Effect of dietary deoxycholic acid and cholesterol on fecal steroid concentration and its impact on the colonic crypt cell proliferation in azoxymethane-treated rats. *Cancer Lett.*, 124: 79–84, 1998.

238. Wali, R.K., Stoiber, D., Nguyen, L., Hart, J., Sitrin, M.D., Brasitus, T., and Bisson-nette, M. Ursodeoxycholic acid inhibits the initiation and postinitiation phases of azoxymethane-induced colonic tumor development. *Cancer Epidemiol. Biomarkers Prev.*, 11: 1316–1321, 2002.

239. Momen, M.A., Monden, Y., Houchi, H., and Umemoto, A. Effect of ursodeoxycholic acid on azoxymethane-induced aberrant crypt foci formation in rat colon: in vitro potential role of intracellular Ca2+. *J. Med. Invest.*, 49: 67–73, 2002.

240. Xie, W., Radominska-Pandya, A., Shi, Y., Simon, C.M., Nelson, M.C., Ong, E.S., Wax-man, D.J., and Evans, R.M. An essential role for nuclear receptors SXR/PXR in detox-ification of cholestatic bile acids. *Proc. Natl. Acad. Sci. U.S.A.*, 98: 3375–3380, 2001.

241. Lu, T.T., Makishima, M., Repa, J.J., Schoonjans, K., Kerr, T.A., Auwerx, J., and Mangelsdorf, D.J. Molecular basis for feedback regulation of bile acid synthesis by nuclear receptors. *Mol. Cell*, 6: 507–515, 2000.

242. Goodwin, B., Glass, C.K., and Umetani, M.G. Identification of modification. *Trends Endocrinol. Metab.*, 13: 55–60, 2002.

243. Pineda, T.I., Claudel, T., Duval, C., Kosykh, V., Fruchart, J.C., and Staels, B. Bile acids induce the expression of the human peroxisome proliferator-activated receptor alpha gene via activation of the farnesoid X receptor. *Mol. Endocrinol.*, 17: 259–272, 2003.

244. Kitareewan, S., Burka, L.T., Tomer, K.B., Parker, C.E., Deterding, L.J., Stevens, R.D., Forman, B.M., Mais, D.E., Heyman, R.A., McMorris, T., and Weinberger, C. Phytol metabolites are circulating dietary factors that activate the nuclear receptor RXR. *Mol. Biol. Cell*, 7: 1153–1166, 1996.

245. LeMotte, P.K., Keidel, S., and Apfel, C. M. Phytanic acid is a retinoid X receptor ligand. *Eur. J. Biochem.*, 236: 328–333, 1996.

246. Radominska-Pandya, A. and Chen, G. Photoaffinity labeling of human retinoid X receptor beta (RXRbeta) with 9-cis-retinoic acid: identification of phytanic acid, docosahexaenoic acid, and lithocholic acid as ligands for RXRbeta. *Biochemistry*, 41: 4883–4890, 2002.

247. Grant, W.B. and Garland, C.F. A critical review of studies on vitamin D in relation to colorectal cancer. *Nutr. Cancer*, 48: 115–123, 2004.

248. Grant, W.B. A multicountry ecologic study of risk and risk reduction factors for prostate cancer mortality. *Eur. Urol.*, 45: 271–279, 2004.

249. Grant, W.B. An estimate of premature cancer mortality in the U.S. due to inadequate doses of solar ultraviolet-B radiation. *Cancer*, 94: 1867–1875, 2002.

250. Grant, W.B. An ecologic study of dietary and solar ultraviolet-B links to breast carcinoma mortality rates. *Cancer*, 94: 272–281, 2002.

251. Schwartz, G.G. and Hulka, B.S. Is vitamin D deficiency a risk factor for prostate cancer? (Hypothesis). *Anticancer Res.*, 10: 1307–1311, 1990.

252. Garland, F.C., Garland, C.F., Gorham, E.D., and Young, J.F. Geographic variation in breast cancer mortality in the United States: a hypothesis involving exposure to solar radiation. *Prev. Med.*, 19: 614–622, 1990.

253. John, E.M., Schwartz, G.G., Dreon, D.M., and Koo, J. Vitamin D and breast cancer risk: the NHANES I epidemiologic follow-up study, 1971–1975 to 1992. National Health and Nutrition Examination Study. *Cancer Epidemiol. Biomarkers Prev.*, 8: 399–406, 1999.

254. Gorham, E.D., Garland, F.C., and Garland, C.F. Sunlight and breast cancer incidence in the USSR. *Int. J. Epidemiol.*, 19: 820–824, 1990.

255. Garland, C.F. and Garland, F.C. Do sunlight and vitamin D reduce the likelihood of colon cancer? *Int. J. Epidemiol.*, 9: 227–231, 1980.

256. Lowe, L.C., Guy, M., Mansi, J.L., Peckitt, C., Bliss, J., Wilson, R.G., and Colston, K.W. Plasma 25-hydroxy vitamin D concentrations, vitamin D receptor genotype and breast cancer risk in a U.K. Caucasian population. *Eur. J. Cancer*, 41: 1164–1169, 2005.

257. Albertson, D.G., Ylstra, B., Segraves, R., Collins, C., Dairkee, S.H., Kowbel, D., Kuo, W.L., Gray, J.W., and Pinkel, D. Quantitative mapping of amplicon structure by array CGH identifies CYP24 as a candidate oncogene. *Nat. Genet.*, 25: 144–146, 2000.

258. John, E.M., Schwartz, G.G., Koo, J., Van Den, B.D., and Ingles, S.A. Sun exposure, vitamin D receptor gene polymorphisms, and risk of advanced prostate cancer. *Cancer Res.*, 65: 5470–5479, 2005.

259. Luscombe, C.J., Fryer, A.A., French, M.E., Liu, S., Saxby, M.F., Jones, P.W., and Strange, R.C. Exposure to ultraviolet radiation: association with susceptibility and age at presentation with prostate cancer. *Lancet*, 358: 641–642, 2001.

260. Luscombe, C.J., French, M.E., Liu, S., Saxby, M.F., Jones, P.W., Fryer, A.A., and Strange, R.C. Prostate cancer risk: associations with ultraviolet radiation, tyrosinase and melanocortin-1 receptor genotypes. *Br. J. Cancer*, 85: 1504–1509, 2001.

261. Jacobs, E.T., Giuliano, A.R., Martinez, M.E., Hollis, B.W., Reid, M.E., and Marshall, J.R. Plasma levels of 25-hydroxyvitamin D, 1,25-dihydroxyvitamin D and the risk of prostate cancer. *J. Steroid Biochem. Mol. Biol.*, 89–90: 533–537, 2004.

262. Ma, J.F., Nonn, L., Campbell, M.J., Hewison, M., Feldman, D., and Peehl, D.M. Mechanisms of decreased Vitamin D 1alpha-hydroxylase activity in prostate cancer cells. *Mol. Cell Endocrinol.*, 221: 67–74, 2004.

263. Wang, L., Whitlatch, L.W., Flanagan, J.N., Holick, M.F., and Chen, T.C. Vitamin D autocrine system and prostate cancer. *Recent Results Cancer Res.*, 164: 223–237, 2003.

264. Chen, T.C., Wang, L., Whitlatch, L.W., Flanagan, J.N., and Holick, M.F. Prostatic 25-hydroxyvitamin D-1alpha-hydroxylase and its implication in prostate cancer. *J. Cell Biochem.*, 88: 315–322, 2003.

265. Hsu, J.Y., Feldman, D., McNeal, J.E., and Peehl, D.M. Reduced 1alpha-hydroxylase activity in human prostate cancer cells correlates with decreased susceptibility to 25-hydroxyvitamin D3-induced growth inhibition. *Cancer Res.*, 61: 2852–2856, 2001.

266. Tuohimaa, P., Lyakhovich, A., Aksenov, N., Pennanen, P., Syvala, H., Lou, Y.R., Ahonen, M., Hasan, T., Pasanen, P., Blauer, M., Manninen, T., Miettinen, S., Vilja, P., and Ylikomi, T. Vitamin D and prostate cancer. *J. Steroid Biochem. Mol. Biol.*, 76: 125–134, 2001.

267. Ahonen, M.H., Tenkanen, L., Teppo, L., Hakama, M., and Tuohimaa, P. Prostate cancer risk and prediagnostic serum 25-hydroxyvitamin D levels (Finland). *Cancer Causes Control*, 11: 847–852, 2000.

268. Tuohimaa, P., Tenkanen, L., Ahonen, M., Lumme, S., Jellum, E., Hallmans, G., Stattin, P., Harvei, S., Hakulinen, T., Luostarinen, T., Dillner, J., Lehtinen, M., and Hakama, M. Both high and low levels of blood vitamin D are associated with a higher prostate cancer risk: a longitudinal, nested case-control study in the Nordic countries. *Int. J. Cancer*, 108: 104–108, 2004.

269. Gann, P.H., Ma, J., Hennekens, C.H., Hollis, B.W., Haddad, J.G., and Stampfer, M.J. Circulating vitamin D metabolites in relation to subsequent development of prostate cancer. *Cancer Epidemiol. Biomarkers Prev.*, 5: 121–126, 1996.

270. Giovannucci, E. The epidemiology of vitamin D and cancer incidence and mortality: a review (U.S.). *Cancer Causes Control*, 16: 83–95, 2005.

271. Garland, C., Shekelle, R.B., Barrett-Connor, E., Criqui, M.H., Rossof, A.H., and Paul, O. Dietary vitamin D and calcium and risk of colorectal cancer: a 19-year prospective study in men. *Lancet*, 1: 307–309, 1985.

272. Feskanich, D., Ma, J., Fuchs, C.S., Kirkner, G.J., Hankinson, S.E., Hollis, B.W., and Giovannucci, E.L. Plasma vitamin D metabolites and risk of colorectal cancer in women. *Cancer Epidemiol. Biomarkers Prev.*, 13: 1502–1508, 2004.

273. Kubota, T., Koshizuka, K., Koike, M., Uskokovic, M., Miyoshi, I., and Koeffler, H.P. 19-nor-26,27-bishomo-vitamin D3 analogs: a unique class of potent inhibitors of proliferation of prostate, breast, and hematopoietic cancer cells. *Cancer Res.*, 58: 3370–3375, 1998.

274. Miller, C.W., Morosetti, R., Campbell, M.J., Mendoza, S., and Koeffler, H.P. Integrity of the 1,25-dihydroxyvitamin D3 receptor in bone, lung, and other cancers. *Mol. Carcinog.*, 19: 254–257, 1997.

275. Zhuang, S.H., Schwartz, G.G., Cameron, D., and Burnstein, K.L. Vitamin D receptor content and transcriptional activity do not fully predict antiproliferative effects of vitamin D in human prostate cancer cell lines. *Mol. Cell Endocrinol.*, 126: 83–90, 1997.

276. Miller, G.J., Stapleton, G.E., Hedlund, T.E., and Moffat, K.A. Vitamin D receptor expression, 24-hydroxylase activity, and inhibition of growth by 1alpha,25-dihydroxyvitamin D3 in seven human prostatic carcinoma cell lines. *Clin. Cancer Res.*, 1: 997–1003, 1995.

277. Banwell, C.M., Colston, K.W., O'Neill, L.P., Stewart, P.M., Turner, B.M., and Campbell, M.J. Elevated expression of the nuclear receptor co-repressor (NCoR1) attenuates vitamin D receptor signalling in breast cancer cells. Submitted. 2005.

278. Banwell, C.M., O'Neill, L.P., Uskokovic, M.R., and Campbell, M.J. Targeting 1alpha,25-dihydroxyvitamin D3 antiproliferative insensitivity in breast cancer cells by co-treatment with histone deacetylation inhibitors. *J. Steroid Biochem. Mol. Biol.*, 89–90: 245–249, 2004.

279. Elstner, E., Linker-Israeli, M., Said, J., Umiel, T., de Vos, S., Shintaku, I. P., Heber, D., Binderup, L., Uskokovic, M., and Koeffler, H.P. 20-epi-vitamin D3 analogues: a novel class of potent inhibitors of proliferation and inducers of differentiation of human breast cancer cell lines. *Cancer Res.*, 55: 2822–2830, 1995.

280. Narvaez, C.J., Zinser, G., and Welsh, J. Functions of 1alpha,25-dihydroxyvitamin D(3) in mammary gland: from normal development to breast cancer. *Steroids*, 66: 301–308, 2001.

281. Narvaez, C.J. and Welsh, J. Differential effects of 1,25-dihydroxyvitamin D3 and tetradecanoylphorbol acetate on cell cycle and apoptosis of MCF-7 cells and a vitamin D3-resistant variant. *Endocrinology*, 138: 4690–4698, 1997.

282. Mork, H.C., Danielsson, C., and Carlberg, C. The potent anti-proliferative effect of 20-epi analogues of 1,25 dihydroxyvitamin D3 in human breast-cancer MCF-7 cells is related to promoter selectivity. *Int. J. Cancer*, 67: 739–742, 1996.

283. Eisman, J.A., Suva, L.J., Sher, E., Pearce, P.J., Funder, J.W., and Martin, T.J. Frequency of 1,25-dihydroxyvitamin D3 receptor in human breast cancer. *Cancer Res.*, 41: 5121–5124, 1981.

284. Friedrich, M., Axt-Fliedner, R., Villena-Heinsen, C., Tilgen, W., Schmidt, W., and Reichrath, J. Analysis of vitamin D-receptor (VDR) and retinoid X-receptor alpha in breast cancer. *Histochem. J.*, 34: 35–40, 2002.

285. Friedrich, M., Meyberg, R., Axt-Fliedner, R., Villena-Heinsen, C., Tilgen, W., Schmidt, W., and Reichrath, J. Vitamin D receptor (VDR) expression is not a prognostic factor in cervical cancer. *Anticancer Res.*, 22: 299–304, 2002.

286. Guy, M., Lowe, L.C., Bretherton-Watt, D., Mansi, J.L., Peckitt, C., Bliss, J., Wilson, R.G., Thomas, V., and Colston, K.W. Vitamin D receptor gene polymorphisms and breast cancer risk. *Clin. Cancer Res.*, 10: 5472–5481, 2004.

287. Guy, M., Lowe, L.C., Bretherton-Watt, D., Mansi, J. L., and Colston, K.W. Approaches to evaluating the association of vitamin D receptor gene polymorphisms with breast cancer risk. *Recent Results Cancer Res.*, 164: 43–54, 2003.

288. Bretherton-Watt, D., Given-Wilson, R., Mansi, J.L., Thomas, V., Carter, N., and Colston, K.W. Vitamin D receptor gene polymorphisms are associated with breast cancer risk in a U.K. Caucasian population. *Br. J. Cancer*, 85: 171–175, 2001.

289. Curran, J.E., Vaughan, T., Lea, R.A., Weinstein, S.R., Morrison, N.A., and Griffiths, L.R. Association of a vitamin D receptor polymorphism with sporadic breast cancer development. *Int. J. Cancer*, 83: 723–726, 1999.

290. Yamagata, M., Nakajima, S., Tokita, A., Sakai, N., Yanagihara, I., Yabuta, K., and Ozono, K. Analysis of the stable levels of messenger RNA derived from different polymorphic alleles in the vitamin D receptor gene. *J. Bone Miner. Metab.*, 17: 164–170, 1999.

291. Guy, M., Lowe, L.C., Bretherton-Watt, D., Mansi, J.L., Peckitt, C., Bliss, J., Wilson, R.G., Thomas, V., and Colston, K.W. Vitamin D receptor gene polymorphisms and breast cancer risk. *Clin. Cancer Res.*, 10: 5472–5481, 2004.

292. Ingles, S.A., Garcia, D.G., Wang, W., Nieters, A., Henderson, B.E., Kolonel, L.N., Haile, R.W., and Coetzee, G.A. Vitamin D receptor genotype and breast cancer in Latinas (United States). *Cancer Causes Control*, 11: 25–30, 2000.

293. Dunning, A.M., Healey, C.S., Pharoah, P.D., Teare, M.D., Ponder, B.A., and Easton, D.F. A systematic review of genetic polymorphisms and breast cancer risk. *Cancer Epidemiol. Biomarkers Prev.*, 8: 843–854, 1999.

294. Dunning, A.M., McBride, S., Gregory, J., Durocher, F., Foster, N.A., Healey, C.S., Smith, N., Pharoah, P.D., Luben, R.N., Easton, D.F., and Ponder, B.A. No association between androgen or vitamin D receptor gene polymorphisms and risk of breast cancer. *Carcinogenesis*, 20: 2131–2135, 1999.

295. Goode, E.L., Dunning, A.M., Kuschel, B., Healey, C.S., Day, N.E., Ponder, B.A., Easton, D.F., and Pharoah, P.P. Effect of germ-line genetic variation on breast cancer survival in a population-based study. *Cancer Res.*, 62: 3052–3057, 2002.

296. Newcomb, P.A., Kim, H., Trentham-Dietz, A., Farin, F., Hunter, D., and Egan, K.M. Vitamin D receptor polymorphism and breast cancer risk. *Cancer Epidemiol. Biomarkers Prev.*, 11: 1503–1504, 2002.

297. Lundin, A.C., Soderkvist, P., Eriksson, B., Bergman-Jungestrom, M., and Wingren, S. Association of breast cancer progression with a vitamin D receptor gene polymorphism: south-east Sweden Breast Cancer Group. *Cancer Res.*, 59: 2332–2334, 1999.

298. Ruggiero, M., Pacini, S., Aterini, S., Fallai, C., Ruggiero, C., and Pacini, P. Vitamin D receptor gene polymorphism is associated with metastatic breast cancer. *Oncol. Res.*, 10: 43–46, 1998.

299. Schondorf, T., Eisberg, C., Wassmer, G., Warm, M., Becker, M., Rein, D.T., and Gohring, U.J. Association of the vitamin D receptor genotype with bone metastases in breast cancer patients. *Oncology*, 64: 154–159, 2003.

300. Carling, T., Rastad, J., Akerstrom, G., and Westin, G. Vitamin D receptor (VDR) and parathyroid hormone messenger ribonucleic acid levels correspond to polymorphic VDR alleles in human parathyroid tumors. *J. Clin. Endocrinol. Metab.*, 83: 2255–2259, 1998.

301. Whitfield, G.K., Remus, L.S., Jurutka, P.W., Zitzer, H., Oza, A.K., Dang, H.T., Haussler, C.A., Galligan, M.A., Thatcher, M.L., Encinas, D.C., and Haussler, M.R. Functionally relevant polymorphisms in the human nuclear vitamin D receptor gene. *Mol. Cell Endocrinol.*, 177: 145–159, 2001.

302. Ingles, S.A., Ross, R.K., Yu, M.C., Irvine, R.A., La Pera, G., Haile, R.W., and Coetzee, G.A. Association of prostate cancer risk with genetic polymorphisms in vitamin D receptor and androgen receptor. *J. Natl. Cancer Inst.*, 89: 166–170, 1997.

303. Ingles, S.A., Coetzee, G.A., Ross, R.K., Henderson, B.E., Kolonel, L.N., Crocitto, L., Wang, W., and Haile, R.W. Association of prostate cancer with vitamin D receptor haplotypes in African-Americans. *Cancer Res.*, 58: 1620–1623, 1998.

304. Ma, J., Stampfer, M.J., Gann, P.H., Hough, H.L., Giovannucci, E., Kelsey, K.T., Hennekens, C.H., and Hunter, D.J. Vitamin D receptor polymorphisms, circulating vitamin D metabolites, and risk of prostate cancer in United States physicians. *Cancer Epidemiol. Biomarkers Prev.*, 7: 385–390, 1998.

305. Ntais, C., Polycarpou, A., and Ioannidis, J.P. Vitamin D receptor gene polymorphisms and risk of prostate cancer: a meta-analysis. *Cancer Epidemiol. Biomarkers Prev.*, 12: 1395–1402, 2003.

306. Cheteri, M.B., Stanford, J.L., Friedrichsen, D.M., Peters, M.A., Iwasaki, L., Langlois, M.C., Feng, Z., and Ostrander, E.A. Vitamin D receptor gene polymorphisms and prostate cancer risk. *Prostate*, 59: 409–418, 2004.

307. Medeiros, R., Morais, A., Vasconcelos, A., Costa, S., Pinto, D., Oliveira, J., and Lopes, C. The role of vitamin D receptor gene polymorphisms in the susceptibility to prostate cancer of a southern European population. *J. Hum. Genet.*, 47: 413–418, 2002.

308. Grau, M.V., Baron, J.A., Sandler, R.S., Haile, R.W., Beach, M.L., Church, T.R., and Heber, D. Vitamin D, calcium supplementation, and colorectal adenomas: results of a randomized trial. *J. Natl. Cancer Inst.*, 95: 1765–1771, 2003.

309. Ingles, S.A., Wang, J., Coetzee, G.A., Lee, E.R., Frankl, H.D., and Haile, R.W. Vitamin D receptor polymorphisms and risk of colorectal adenomas (U.S.). *Cancer Causes Control*, 12: 607–614, 2001.

310. Wong, H.L., Seow, A., Arakawa, K., Lee, H.P., Yu, M.C., and Ingles, S.A. Vitamin D receptor start codon polymorphism and colorectal cancer risk: effect modification by dietary calcium and fat in Singapore Chinese. *Carcinogenesis*, 24: 1091–1095, 2003.

311. Rashid, S.F., Moore, J.S., Walker, E., Driver, P.M., Engel, J., Edwards, C.E., Brown, G., Uskokovic, M.R., and Campbell, M.J. Synergistic growth inhibition of prostate cancer cells by 1 alpha,25 Dihydroxyvitamin D(3) and its 19-nor-hexafluoride analogs in combination with either sodium butyrate or trichostatin A. *Oncogene*, 20: 1860–1872, 2001.

312. Wang, X., Rao, J., and Studzinski, G.P. Inhibition of p38 MAP kinase activity up-regulates multiple MAP kinase pathways and potentiates 1,25-dihydroxyvitamin D(3)-induced differentiation of human leukemia HL60 cells. *Exp. Cell Res.*, 258: 425–437, 2000.

313. Banwell, C.M., Singh, R., Stewart, P.M., Uskokovic, M.R., and Campbell, M.J. Antiproliferative signalling by 1,25(OH)$_2$D$_3$ in prostate and breast cancer is suppressed by a mechanism involving histone deacetylation. *Recent Results Cancer Res.*, 164, 83–98, 2003.

314. Banwell, C.M., O'Neill, L.P., Uskokovic, M.R., and Campbell, M.J. Targeting 1alpha,25-dihydroxyvitamin D3 antiproliferative insensitivity in breast cancer cells by co-treatment with histone deacetylation inhibitors, *J. Steroid Biochem. Mol. Biol.*, 89–90, 245–249, 2004.

315. Ishii, S., Yamada, M., Satoh, T., Monden, T., Hashimoto, K., Shibusawa, N., Onigata, K., Morikawa, A., and Mori, M. Aberrant dynamics of histone deacetylation at the thyrotropin-releasing hormone gene in resistance to thyroid hormone. *Mol. Endocrinol.*, 2004.

316. Krogsdam, A.M., Nielsen, C.A., Neve, S., Holst, D., Helledie, T., Thomsen, B., Bendixen, C., Mandrup, S., and Kristiansen, K. Nuclear receptor corepressor-dependent repression of peroxisome-proliferator-activated receptor delta-mediated transactivation. *Biochem. J.*, 363: 157–165, 2002.

317. Weston, A.D., Blumberg, B., and Underhill, T.M. Active repression by unliganded retinoid receptors in development: less is sometimes more. *J. Cell Biol.*, 161: 223–228, 2003.

318. Picard, F., Kurtev, M., Chung, N., Topark-Ngarm, A., Senawong, T., Oliveira, R.M., Leid, M., McBurney, M.W., and Guarente, L. Sirt1 promotes fat mobilization in white adipocytes by repressing PPAR-gamma. *Nature*, 429: 771–776, 2004.

319. Gnanapragasam, V.J., Leung, H.Y., Pulimood, A.S., Neal, D.E., and Robson, C.N. Expression of RAC 3, a steroid hormone receptor co-activator in prostate cancer. *Br. J. Cancer*, 85: 1928–1936, 2001.

320. Feldman, B.J. and Feldman, D. The development of androgen-independent prostate cancer. *Nat. Rev. Cancer*, 1: 34–45, 2001.

321. Planas-Silva, M.D., Shang, Y., Donaher, J.L., Brown, M., and Weinberg, R.A. AIB1 enhances estrogen-dependent induction of cyclin D1 expression. *Cancer Res.*, 61: 3858–3862, 2001.

322. Kawashima, H., Takano, H., Sugita, S., Takahara, Y., Sugimura, K., and Nakatani, T. A novel steroid receptor co-activator protein (SRAP) as an alternative form of steroid receptor RNA-activator gene: expression in prostate cancer cells and enhancement of androgen receptor activity. *Biochem. J.*, 369: 163–171, 2003.

323. Jiang, W.G., Douglas-Jones, A., and Mansel, R.E. Expression of peroxisome-proliferator activated receptor-gamma (PPARgamma) and the PPARgamma co-activator, PGC-1, in human breast cancer correlates with clinical outcomes. *Int. J. Cancer*, 106: 752–757, 2003.

324. Hudelist, G., Czerwenka, K., Kubista, E., Marton, E., Pischinger, K., and Singer, C.F. Expression of sex steroid receptors and their co-factors in normal and malignant breast tissue: AIB1 is a carcinoma-specific co-activator. *Breast Cancer Res. Treat.*, 78: 193–204, 2003.

325. Kollara, A., Kahn, H. J., Marks, A., and Brown, T. J. Loss of androgen receptor associated protein 70 (ARA70) expression in a subset of HER2-positive breast cancers. *Breast Cancer Res. Treat.*, 67: 245–253, 2001.

326. Grignani, F., De Matteis, S., Nervi, C., Tomassoni, L., Gelmetti, V., Cioce, M., Fanelli, M., Ruthardt, M., Ferrara, F.F., Zamir, I., Seiser, C., Grignani, F., Lazar, M.A., Minucci, S., and Pelicci, P.G. Fusion proteins of the retinoic acid receptor-alpha recruit histone deacetylase in promyelocytic leukaemia. *Nature*, 391: 815–818, 1998.
327. Lin, R.J., Nagy, L., Inoue, S., Shao, W., Miller, W.H., Jr., and Evans, R.M. Role of the histone deacetylase complex in acute promyelocytic leukaemia. *Nature*, 391: 811–814, 1998.
328. Westerhoff, H.V. and Palsson, B.O. The evolution of molecular biology into systems biology. *Nat. Biotechnol.*, 22: 1249–1252, 2004.

9 The Role of Alcohol Dehydrogenase Polymorphism in Alcohol-Associated Carcinogenesis

Helmut K. Seitz and Felix Stickel

CONTENTS

9.1 INTRODUCTION

Alcoholism is a commonly occurring disease, and in some societies up to 3% of the adult population shows alcohol dependency [1]. However, even in heavy drinkers the occurrence of certain alcohol-associated organ injuries is rather low. Only 10 to 15% of heavy drinkers develop, for example, cirrhosis of the liver [2], and only a small percentage develops cancer. Chronic alcohol consumption is indeed a risk factor for cancer of the upper aerodigestive tract (UADT) including the oral cavity, oropharynx, hypopharynx, and esophagus, of the liver in the presence of cirrhosis, of the large intestine, and of the breast [3]. The amount of alcohol is obviously not the only determinant for organ injury; genetic and environmental factors may modulate and determine organ damage and/or carcinogenesis. It has been convincingly shown that acetaldehyde (AA), rather than alcohol itself, is carcinogenic [4]. Thus, the amount of AA to which cells or tissues are exposed following alcohol ingestion may

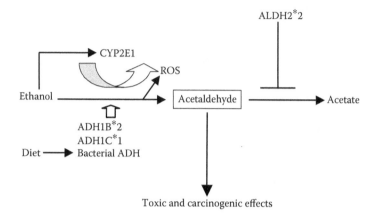

FIGURE 9.1 Ethanol metabolism and its influence by various alcohol dehydrogenase (*ADH*) alleles and acetaldehyde dehydrogenase (*ALDH*). *ADH1B* and *ADH1C* show polymorphism with the alleles *ADH1B*2* and *ADH1C*1*, which code for rapid metabolizing enzymes leading to increased acetaldehyde (AA) concentrations. *ALDH2*2* codes for an enzyme with low activity, resulting in a decreased metabolism of AA leading to elevated AA concentrations. Gastrointestinal bacteria may also contain ADH and contribute to luminal ethanol metabolism, which is influenced by diets. Finally, chronic ethanol consumption results in the induction of cytochrome P4502E1 (CYP2E1), which metabolizes ethanol to AA and, in addition, produces reactive oxygen species (ROS).

be of great importance and may, among other factors, influence carcinogenesis. The AA concentration in tissues depends on its production and degradation (Figure 9.1). In the present overview, the role of AA in carcinogenesis and the genetic factors modulating AA levels will be discussed in detail. For discussions on other factors involved in alcohol-associated carcinogenesis, recent review articles [3–5] may be referred.

9.2 ACETALDEHYDE — A CARCINOGEN

There is increasing evidence that AA, rather than alcohol itself, is responsible for the cocarcinogenic effect of alcohol [6]. AA is highly toxic, mutagenic, and carcinogenic. AA interferes at many sites with DNA synthesis and repair and can, consequently, result in tumor development [7]. Numerous *in vitro* and *in vivo* experiments in prokaryotic and eukaryotic cell cultures as well as in animal models have shown that AA has direct mutagenic and carcinogenic effects. It causes point mutations in the hypoxanthine-guanine phosphoribosyl transferase locus in human lymphocytes and induces sister chromatid exchanges and gross chromosomal aberrations [8–10]. It induces inflammation and metaplasia of tracheal epithelium, delays cell cycle progression, and enhances cell injury associated with hyperregeneration [6,11]. Thus, when AA was administered in drinking water to rodents [12], the mucosa lesions of the UADT resembled those following chronic alcohol ingestion [13]. It has also been shown that AA interferes with the DNA repair machinery. AA directly inhibits O6-methyl-guanyltransferase, an enzyme important for the repair of adducts caused by alkylating agents [14]. Moreover, when inhaled, AA causes nasopharyngeal and laryngeal carcinoma [15]. AA also binds rapidly to cellular proteins and DNA, resulting in morphological and functional impairment of the cell and in an immunological cascade reaction. The binding to DNA and the formation of stable adducts represent one mechanism by which AA could trigger the occurrence of replication errors and/or mutations in oncogenes or tumor suppressor genes [16]. The occurrence of stable DNA adducts has been shown in various organs of alcohol-fed rodents and in the leukocytes of alcoholics [17]. In addition, it has been shown that the major stable DNA adduct N^2-ethyl-2-deoxyguanosine (N^2-Et-dG) can indeed be used efficiently by eukaryotic DNA polymerase [18]. Although N^2-Et-dG has been shown to form in DNA samples from white blood cells of human alcoholics and in the liver of rats that were administered ethanol in the drinking water, there is relatively little evidence that this lesion is mutagenic, and the biological significance of the lesion is unclear. However, this lesion can be detected in human urine samples, suggesting that it may be useful as a biomarker of AA-related DNA damage [19]. More recent data has shown that in the presence of basic amino acids or histones, AA reacts with deoxyguanosine in DNA to form a different DNA adduct, 1, N^2-propano-dG (PdG) [19]. In contrast to N^2-Et-dG, PdG has been shown to be a mutagenic DNA lesion *in vivo* in mammalian cells. These AA-associated effects occurred at AA concentrations from 40 to 1000 μM, which are similar to concentrations observed in human saliva following alcohol ingestion [20]. It has been recently shown that the polyamines, spermine and spermidine, can also facilitate the formation of PdG from AA and dG at AA concentrations as low as 80 μM. According to the International Agency for Research on Cancer (IARC), there is sufficient evidence to identify AA as a carcinogen in experimental animals [7].

AA is produced from ethanol by alcohol dehydrogenase (ADH) or cytochrome P4502E1 (CYP2E1). Seven isoenzymes exist for ADH, and almost every tissue contains ADH activity. ADH2 is only present in the liver and ADH4, only in the upper gastrointestinal mucosa (for a review, see Reference 21). *ADH1B* and *ADH1C* are polymorphic, and thus, depending on the presence of either one of the diverse polymorphic sites, they code for enzymes capable of producing different amounts of AA [22]. The amount of AA produced by CYP2E1 is relatively small. However, in chronic alcoholics, CYP2E1 is induced, and this pathway contributes to up to 30% of the overall ethanol metabolism [23]. This CYP2E1-dependent microsomal ethanol-oxidizing system (MEOS) also produces reactive oxygen species (ROS), which may be of importance in alcohol-associated carcinogenesis [24,25]. ROS results in lipid peroxidation (LPO). LPO-derived reactive hydroxyalkenals can form promutagenic exocyclic etheno-DNA adducts *in vivo*. A recent study in rodents showed that both acute and short-term ethanol exposures increased approximately twofold the hepatic concentrations of 1,N^6-ethenodeoxyadenosine (εdA) and 3,N^4-ethenodeoxycytidine (εdC) in DNA [26], which was similar to the increase induced by carcinogens such as urethane [27]. ε-DNA adducts probably play a causal role in the initiation and progression of liver carcinogenesis as they produce base pair substitution mutations in various organisms and mammalian cells. εdA can lead to $AT \to GC$ transitions and to $AT \to TA$ and $AT \to CG$ transversions [28,29]. εdC can cause $CG \to AT$ transversions and $CG \to TA$ transitions [30,31], and N^2, 3-etheno-deoxyguanosine, which is also formed *in vivo* from LPO products, can lead to $GC \to AT$ transitions [31]. In addition, CYP2E1 activates various procarcinogens present in diet and tobacco smoke to their ultimate carcinogens [32]. For more details, one may refer to a recent review article [33]. It is, however, noteworthy that an induction of CYP2E1 with all its negative side effects occurs at an alcohol dose of 40 g/d within one week of regular alcohol ingestion and varies significantly interindividually [34].

Increased AA concentrations may also occur when its detoxification is inadequate. AA is metabolized by acetaldehyde dehydrogenases (ALDHs) (for a review, see Reference 35). The most important ALDH is acetaldehyde dehydrogenase 2 (ALDH2), with a high affinity to AA, which eliminates even trace amounts of AA. Mutations of ALDH2, as seen in more than 40% of Asians, result in elevated serum AA concentrations and cancer [6].

9.3 *ALDH2* MUTATION AND ITS ROLE IN ALCOHOL-ASSOCIATED CARCINOGENESIS

Recent and striking evidence for the causal role of AA in ethanol-associated UADT carcinogenesis derives from genetic linkage studies in alcoholics. Individuals who accumulate AA because of polymorphism and/or mutation in the gene coding for enzymes responsible for AA generation and detoxification have been shown to have an increased cancer risk. In Japan as well as in other Asian countries, a high percentage of individuals carry a mutation of the *ALDH2* gene. In humans, there are at least four to five classes of ALDH isoenzymes [21]. Mitochondrial class 2 ALDH (ALDH2) is primarily responsible for AA oxidation. Human ALDH2 enzyme is polymorphic, with two distinct alleles: *ALDH2*1* and *ALDH2*2*. *ALDH2*2* results from a single-point mutation in chromosome 6. Individuals homozygous for the mutated *ALDH2*2* allele are completely devoid of ALDH2 activity, whereas heterozygous individuals showing the *ALDH2*1*, 2 genotype reveal only 30 to 50% of the normal ALDH activity. Blood AA levels of *ALDH2*2* homozygous individuals are 6 to 20 times higher compared to *ALDH2*1* individuals, in whom AA is hardly detectable after alcohol consumption. The elevated AA concentrations cause unpleasant side effects (flush syndrome) that protect these individuals from alcoholism. However, heterozygous individuals may become heavy drinkers or even alcoholics [6].

Yokoyama et al. [36] were the first to report that the heterozygous mutation of the *ALDH2* gene (*ALDH2*1,2*) is a strong risk factor for esophageal cancer in everyday drinkers and alcoholics [36,37]. A comprehensive study of the *ALDH2* genotype and cancer prevalence in Japanese alcoholics showed that the frequency of inactive ALDH2 increased remarkably among alcoholics with cancer of the oral cavity, oropharynx, hypopharynx, larynx, esophagus, and colorectum [38]. It is important to note that these individuals also have high AA levels in their saliva, and thus AA is delivered directly to the surface mucosa of the UADT in such individuals [39].

9.4 POLYMORPHISM OF ALCOHOL DEHYDROGENASE AND ITS POSSIBLE ROLE IN ALCOHOL-ASSOCIATED CARCINOGENESIS

9.4.1 GASTROINTESTINAL CANCER

In addition to the mutation of the *ALDH2* gene, polymorphisms of alcohol dehydrogenase 1B (*ADH1B*) and alcohol dehydrogenase 1C (*ADH1C*) may also modulate AA levels. Whereas the *ADH1B*2* allele encodes for an enzyme that is approximately 40 times more active than the enzyme encoded by the *ADH1B*1* allele, *ADH1C*1* transcription leads to an ADH isoenzyme 2.5 times more active than that from *ADH1C*2*. However, the *ADH1B*2* allele frequency is high in Asians but low in Caucasians. It protects from alcoholism because of the high amount of AA produced and its toxic side effects [6,40]. Because of the low *ADH1B*2* allele frequency and the lack of *ALDH2* mutations in Caucasians, *ADH1C* polymorphism and its role in alcohol-associated carcinogenesis can ideally be investigated in Caucasian populations.

Studies on *ADH1C* polymorphism in Caucasians and UADT cancer have shown contradictory results. Whereas an increased risk of oropharyngeal and laryngeal cancer in individuals with the *ADH1C*1* allele has been reported [41,42], others could not confirm such an association in case–control studies [43–47]. One reason for this discrepancy is the fact that in all these studies, the percentage of cancer patients with high alcohol intake was rather low, sometimes extremely low. In the study by Sturgis et al. [44] the amount of alcohol ingested was not even reported. Thus, it is not surprising that a pooled analysis of all the studies published so far led to the conclusion that the *ALDH1C* allele is not a risk factor for alcohol-associated carcinogenesis [48]. Visapää et al. studied 107 alcoholic patients with high alcohol ingestion and oropharyngeal, laryngeal, hypopharyngeal, and esophageal cancer to compare their *ADH1C* genotype with 103 age-matched alcoholics with a similar alcohol consumption but without cancer, and they observed a significantly increased cancer risk in individuals with the *ADH1C*1* allele [49]. This was found to be associated with significantly elevated AA levels in the saliva of individuals homozygous for *ADH1C*1* [49]. Increased salivary AA levels in these individuals as in individuals with ineffective ALDH activity may explain their increased cancer risk because AA comes into direct contact with the mucosa. In this context, it is interesting to note that AA-fed rats showed a severe hyperregeneration of the upper gastrointestinal mucosa [12]; this is very similar to the morphological changes observed after chronic alcohol consumption [13]. These changes were only observed when the animals had functionally intact salivary glands. After sialoadenectomy, this proliferation disappeared, which supports the hypothesis that salivary AA is involved in carcinogenesis. In this context, it has to be pointed out that chronic alcohol consumption alters salivary morphology and function [50].

Morphometric analyses in rats that were fed alcohol for over 6 months showed an enlargement of the nuclei of the basal cells in the oral mucosa associated with an increased percentage of cells in the S phase and a reduction of the epithelial thickness, indicating mucosal atrophy and hyperproliferation [51]. A similar finding of hyperproliferation was reported for the esophageal mucosa in rats chronically fed ethanol [13].

In a more recent extended study, Stickel et al. were also able to demonstrate that *ADH1C*1* allele is a significant risk factor for hepatocellular cancer in heavy drinkers with cirrhosis of the liver [52]. These data are in contrast to the results reported by Yokoyama and coworkers [38], who could not find any effect of *ALDH2* genotype on hepatocellular cancer development in alcoholics. One explanation could be that in the Japanese population a high prevalence of hepatitis B and C is present, and this may have influenced the negative results.

AA can also be produced by oral bacteria. Significant amounts of AA can be detected in the saliva of healthy volunteers after ingestion of a moderate dose of alcohol, which is 10 to 20 times higher compared to systemic blood AA levels even at a higher alcohol intake [20]. Salivary AA concentrations following ethanol ingestion can be significantly reduced by using the antiseptic chlorhexidine prior to alcohol intake, emphasizing the important role of oral bacteria in AA production [20]. It has been shown that alcoholics with oropharyngeal cancer have very high salivary AA concentrations [53]. This may be due to the fact that smoking [54] and poor oral hygiene [55], both frequently observed in alcoholics, result in high salivary AA concentrations due to bacterial AA production. Very recently it has been shown that smoking rapidly changes the oral bacterial flora from Gram-negative to Gram-positive bacteria, which leads to AA concentrations 50 to 60% higher compared to those observed without smoking [56]. Indeed, Gram-positive bacteria are capable of producing higher amounts of AA than Gram-negative bacteria. In addition, *Candida albicans*, frequently found in the microbial environment of smokers, converts alcohol to AA. The data imply that smokers exposed to moderate amounts of alcohol produce higher AA concentrations compared to nonsmokers. Apart from that, poor oral hygiene is associated with bacterial overgrowth, parodontitis, and caries and also increases salivary AA concentrations. In this context, it seems worthwhile to mention that nonpathogenic *Neisseria* species isolated from oral cavity produce significant amounts of AA [56].

AA can also be produced by fecal bacteria. It has been shown that the amount of AA per gram of tissue is highest for the colonic mucosa compared to all other tissues in the body. This is primarily due to the production of AA from fecal bacteria, as animal studies with germ-free rats have shown [57]. AA has toxic effects on the colon mucosa, resulting in a decreased number of cells in the functional compartment of the colonic crypt. This AA-mediated toxicity is answered by a secondary compensatory hyperregeneration that increases crypt cell production rates and an extension of the proliferative compartment towards the lumen of the crypt [11,58,59]. Such a change in crypt cell dynamics represents a condition associated with increased risk for colorectal cancer [60–62]. The alcohol-associated hyperregeneration of the colonic mucosa is especially pronounced with increasing age [11]. This may have practical implications as age alone is a risk factor for colorectal cancer. The hyperproliferative colorectal mucosa observed in animals was recently confirmed in alcoholics [63]. Here again, the significant extension of the proliferative compartment of the rectal crypt has been documented. Although AA production from fecal bacteria obviously dominates in the colon, it has been recently observed that individuals carrying in homozygosity the *ADH1C*1* allele also exhibit an increased risk for colorectal cancer because they produce more AA, as already discussed earlier [Seitz, personal communication]. A similar observation was made by Tiemersma et al. [64], who found an increased risk of colorectal cancer in subjects with higher alcohol consumption and the *ADH1C*1.1* homozygous genotype.

9.4.2 BREAST CANCER

Numerous studies have demonstrated chronic alcohol consumption to be, even at moderate doses, a significant risk factor for the development of breast cancer [3,65–68]. The possible mechanisms of alcohol-associated breast cancer still remain unclear. Coutelle et al., found that even moderate alcohol consumers with one *ADH1C*1* allele have an increased risk of developing alcohol-associated breast cancer [69].

Patients with breast cancer exhibited an *ADH1C*1* allele frequency of 62%, which differed significantly from that of age-matched controls with high alcohol intake but without cancer [69]. The *ADH1C* genotypes in women with breast cancer were to the same irrespective of whether they consumed more or less than 20 g of alcohol per day. This may emphasize the effect observed in many epidemiological studies that even intake of small doses of alcohol is a risk factor for breast cancer. It is, however, noteworthy that it was not possible to compare women with breast cancer and alcohol consumption with women who completely abstained from alcohol. Only seven women stated that they had zero alcohol intake. Because of this small number, a statistical analysis was not meaningful. Our findings are in accordance with the results of a case–control study reported by Freudenheim et al. [70], which was performed in the U.S. with 500 patients with breast cancer and age-matched controls. This study gave evidence of an increased risk among pre- (OR 2.3, 95% CI 1.2–4.3) but not postmenopausal women (OR 1.1, 95% CI 0.7–1.7) those associated with *ADH1C*1.1* genotype compared to those associated with *ADH1C*1.2* and *ADH1C*2.2* genotypes. At particular risk were premenopausal women homozygous for the *ADH1C*1* allele with an alcohol intake above the median (OR 3.6, 95% CI 1.5–8.8), in contrast to lighter drinkers with the *ADH1C*2.2* or *ADH1C1*1.2* genotypes.

ADH1C is also involved in steroid hormone metabolism [71,72], and there is some evidence that ethanol enhances the expression of estrogen receptors of the breast [73–76]. Finally, it should be pointed out that alcohol may lead to decreased retinoic acid concentrations in some tissues [77]. Low retinoid acid levels lead to the activation of the *AP1* gene with hyperregeneration, a condition favoring carcinogenesis [78]. However, retinoic acid levels in breast tissue under alcohol conditions are still not known.

It is well known that alcohol ingestion leads to increased estradiol levels in all phases of the menstrual cycle, predominately in the midphase, where estrogen levels are already relatively high. Most studies showed a positive correlation between alcohol intake and serum estrogen levels when alcohol was administered in high doses [79–82]. Because breast cancer risk increases in relation to the time exposure of estrogens over a lifetime, it seems possible that chronic alcohol intake, even at lower doses, increases this exposure dramatically.

9.5 SUMMARY AND CONCLUSION

Chronic alcohol consumption and heavy smoking are the major risk factors for UADT, including the oropharynx, hypopharynx, larynx, and esophagus cancers. Alcoholic liver cirrhosis is also a precancerous condition. Furthermore, chronic alcohol ingestion even at a moderate dosage enhances carcinogenesis in the colorectum and breast, especially in individuals with increased susceptibility to cancer. Evidence has accumulated that acetaldehyde is predominantly responsible for the alcohol-associated carcinogenesis because acetaldehyde is carcinogenic, mutagenic, binds to DNA and protein, destructs folate, and results in secondary hyperregeneration. Acetaldehyde is produced by various alcohol dehydrogenases in the liver and in the gastrointestinal tract by gastrointestinal bacteria. Acetaldehyde is degraded by acetaldehyde dehydrogenases to acetate. Both generation and degradation of acetaldehyde are modulated by polymorphisms or mutations of the genes responsible for the enzymes involved. Thus, a genetic susceptibility towards alcohol-associated cancer exists. In addition, cigarette smoke and some alcoholic beverages also contain acetaldehyde.

Other mechanisms by which alcohol stimulates carcinogenesis include the induction of cytochrome P4502E1 associated with (1) an enhanced production of free radicals and enhanced activation of various procarcinogens present in alcoholic beverages and in diets, in association with tobacco smoke, (2) a change in the metabolism and distribution of carcinogens, (3) alterations in cell cycle behavior such as cell cycle duration leading to hyperproliferation, (4) nutritional deficiencies, such as methyl, vitamin E, folate, pyridoxalphosphate, zinc, and selenium deficiencies, and (5) alterations of the immune system, eventually resulting in an increased susceptibility to certain virus infections such as hepatits B virus and hepatitis C virus. In addition, local mechanisms within specific tissues may be of particular importance. Such mechanisms lead to tissue injury such as cirrhosis of the liver, a major prerequisite for hepatocellular carcinoma. Also, an alcohol-mediated increase in estradiols may be, at least in part, responsible for breast cancer risk. Thus, all these mechanisms functioning in concert actively modulate carcinogenesis and lead to its stimulation.

REFERENCES

1. Jahrbuch Sucht 2003, Gensthacht: Neuland Verlagsgesellschaft.
2. Bellantini, S. et al., Drinking habits as co-factors of risk for alcohol-induced liver damage, *Gut,* 41, 845–850, 1997.
3. Pöschl, G. and Seitz, H.K., Alcohol and cancer, *Alcohol Alcohol*, 39, 155–156, 2004.
4. Seitz, H.K., Stickel, F., and Homann, N., Pathogenetic mechanisms of upper aerodigestive tract cancer in alcoholics, *Int J Cancer*, 108, 483–487, 2004.

5. Pöschl, G. et al., Alcohol and cancer: genetic and nutritional aspects, *Proc Nutr Soc,* 63, 65–71, 2004.
6. Seitz, H.K. et al., Alcohol and cancer, *Alcohol Clin Exp Res,* 25; 137–143, 2001.
7. Anonymous, Acetaldehyde, *IARC Monogr Eval Carcinog Risk Chem Hum*, 36, 1985.
8. Dellarco, V.L., A mutagenicity assessment of acetaldehyde, *Mutat Res*, 195, 1–20, 1988.
9. Helander, A. and Lindahl-Kiessling, K., Increased frequency of acetaldehyde-induced sister-chromatide exchanges in human lymphocytes treated with an aldehyde dehydrogenase inhibitor, *Mutat Res*, 264, 103–107, 1991.
10. Obe, G., Jonas, R., and Schmidt, S., Metabolism of ethanol *in vitro* produces a compound which induces sister-chromatid exchanges in human peripheral lymphocytes *in vitro*: acetaldehyde not ethanol is mutagenetic, *Mutat Res,* 174, 47–51, 1986.
11. Simanowski, U.A. et al., Enhancement of ethanol induced rectal mucosal hyper-regeneration with age in F244 rats, *Gut,* 35, 1102–1106, 1994.
12. Homann, N. et al., Effects of acetaldehyde on cell regeneration and differentiation of the upper gastrointestinal tract mucosa, *J Natl Cancer Inst*, 89, 1692–1697, 1997.
13. Simanowski, U.A. et al., Esophageal epithelial hyperregeneration following chronic ethanol ingestion: effect of age and salivary gland function, *J Natl Cancer Inst*, 85, 2030–2033, 1993.
14. Espina, N. et al., In vitro and in vivo inhibitory effect of ehtanol and acetaldehyde on O6-methylguanine transferase, *Carcionogenesis,* 9, 761–766, 1988.
15. Woutersen, R.A. et al., Inhalation toxicity of acetaldehyde in rats: III, Carcinogenicity study, *Toxicology,* 41, 213–231, 1986.
16. Fang, J.L. and Vaca, C.E., Development of a 32P-postlabeling method for the analysis of adducts arising through the reaction of acetaldehyde with 2-deoxyguanosine-3′-monophosphate and DNA, *Carcinogenesis,* 16, 2177–2185, 1995.
17. Fang, J.L. and Vaca, C.E., Detection of DNA adducts of acetaldehyde in peripheral white blood cells of alcohol abusers, *Carcinogenesis*, 18, 627–632, 1997.
18. Matsuda, T. et al., Effective utilization of N2-ethyl-2-deoxyguanosine triphosphate during DNA synthesis catalyzed by mammalian replicative DNA polymerases, *Biochemistry,* 38, 929–935, 1999.
19. Brooks, P.J. and Theruvathu, J.A., Mechanisms of acetaldehyde induced DNA damage, *Alcohol*, 35, 187–193, 2005.
20. Homann, N. et al., High acetaldehyde levels in saliva after ethanol consumption: methodological aspects and pathogenetic implications, *Carinogenesis*, 18, 1739–1743, 1997.
21. Seitz, H.K. and Oneta, C.M., Gastrointestinal alcohol dehydrogenases, *Nutr Rev*, 56, 52–60, 1998.
22. Bosron, W.F. and Li, T.K., Genetic polymorphism of human liver alcohol and aldehyde dehydrogenase, and their relationship to alcohol metabolism and alcoholism, *Hepatology,* 6, 502–510, 1986.
23. Lieber, C.S., Alcohol and the liver 1994 update, *Gastroenterology* 106, 1085, 1994.
24. Stickel, F. et al., Cocarcinogenic effects of alcohol in hepatocarcinogenesis, *Gut,* 51, 132–139, 2002.
25. Frank, A. et al., Immunohistochemical detection of 1, N⁶-ethenodeoxyadenosine in nuclei of human liver affected by diseases predisposing to hepato carcinogenesis, *Carcinogenesis*, 25, 1027–1031, 2004.
26. Navasumrit, P. et al., Ethanol enhances the formation of endogenously and exogenously derived adducts in rat hepatic DNA, *Mutat Res*, 479, 81–94, 2001.

27. Bartsch, H. and Nair, J., New DNA-based biomarkers for oxidative stress and cancer chemoprevention studies, *Eur J Cancer*, 36, 1229–1234, 2000.

28. Basu, A.K. et al., Mutagenic and genotoxic effects of three vinyl chloride-induced DNA lesions: 1, N[6]-ethenoadenine, 3, N[4]-ethenocytosine, and 4-amino-5-(imidazol-2-yl) imidazole, *Biochemistry*, 32, 12793–12801, 1993.

29. Pandya, G.A. and Moriya, M., 1, N[6]-ethenoadenosine, a DNA adduct highly mutagenic in mammalian cells, *Biochemistry*, 35, 11487–11492, 1996.

30. Palejwala, V.A. et al., Quantitative multiplex sequence analysis of mutational hot spots, frequency and specificity of mutations induced by a site-specific ethenocytosine in M13 viral DNA, *Biochemistry*, 32, 4105–4111, 1993.

31. Moriya, M. et al., Mutagenic potency of exocyclic DNA adducts: marked differences between *Escherichia coli* and simian kidney cells, *Proc Natl Acad Sci USA,* 91, 11899–11903, 1994.

32. Seitz, H.K. and Oswald, B., Effect of ethanol on procarcinogen activation, in *Alcohol and Cancer*, Watson, R.R., Ed., CRC Press, Boca Raton, Ann Arbor, London, Tokyo, 1992, 55–72.

33. Seitz, H.K., Pöschl, G., and Simanowski, U.A., Alcohol and cancer, in *Recent Developments in Alcoholism*, Vol. 14, The Consequences of Alcoholism, Galanther, M., Ed., Plenum Press, London, 1998, pp. 68–96.

34. Oneta, C.M. et al., Dynamics of Cytochrome P4502E1 activity in man: induction by ethanol and disappearance during withdrawal phase, *J Hepatol*, 36, 47–52, 2002.

35. Pares, X. and Farres, J., Alcohol and aldehyde dehydrogenases in the gastrointestinal tract, in *Alcohol and the Gastrointestinal Tract*, Preedy, V.R. and Watson Ronald, R., Eds., CRC Press, Boca Raton, New York, London, Tokyo, 1996.

36. Yokoyama, A. et al., Multiple primary esophageal and concurrent aerodigestive tract cancer and the aldehyde dehydrogenase-2 genotype of Japanese alcoholics, *Cancer,* 77, 1986–1990, 1996.

37. Yokoyama, A. et al., Alcohol and aldehyde gene polymorphisms influence susceptibility to esophageal cancer in Japanese alcoholics, *Alcohol Clin Exp Res*, 23, 1705–1710, 1999.

38. Yokoyama, A. et al., Alcohol-related cancers and aldehydrogenase-2 in Japanese alcoholics, *Carcinogenesis,* 19, 1383–1387, 1998.

39. Väkeväinen, S. et al., High salivary acetaldehyde after a moderate dose of alcohol in ALDH2-deficient subjects: strong evidence for the local carcinogenic action of acetaldehyde, *Alcohol Clin Exp Res*, 24, 873–877, 2000.

40. Borras, E. et al., Genetic polymorphism of alcohol dehydrogenase in Europeans: the ADH2*2 allele decreases the risk for alcoholism and is associated with ADH3*1, *Hepatology,* 31, 984–989, 2000.

41. Harty, L.C. et al., Alcohol dehydrogenase 3 genotype and risk of oral cavity and pharyngeal cancers, *J Natl Cancer Inst,* 89, 1698–1705, 1997.

42. Coutelle, C. et al., Laryngeal and oropharyngeal cancer, and alcohol dehydrogenase 3 and glutathine S-transferase M1 polymorphism, *Hum Genet,* 99, 319–325, 1997.

43. Olshan, A.F. et al., Risk of head and neck cancer and the alcohol dehydrogenase 3 genotype, *Carcinogenesis*, 22, 57–61, 2001.

44. Sturgis, E.M. et al., Alcohol dehydrogenase 3 genotype is not associated with risk of squamous cell carcinoma of the oral cavity and pharynx, *Cancer Epidemiol Biomarkers Prev*, 10, 273–275, 2001.

45. Schwartz, S.M. et al., Oral squamous cell cancer risk in relation to alcohol consumption and alcohol dehydrogenase 3 genotypes, *Cancer Epidemiol Biomarkers Prev*, 10, 1137–1144, 2001.

46. Zavras, A.I. et al., Interaction between a single nucleotide polymorphism in the alcohol dehydrogenase 3 gene, alcohol consumption and oral cancer risk, *Int J Cancer*, 97, 526–530, 2002.

47. Risch, A. et al., Laryngeal cancer risk in Caucasians is associated with alcohol and tobacco consumption but not modified by genetic polymorphisms in class 1 alcohol dehydrongenases ADH1B and ADH1C, and gluthathione-S-transferases GSTM1 and GSTT1, *Pharmakogenetics*, 13, 225–230, 2003.

48. Brennan, E. et al., Pooled analysis of alcohol dehydrogenase genotypes and head and neck cancer: a huge review, *Am J Epidemiol*, 159, 1–16, 2004.

49. Visapää, J.P. et al., Increased cancer risk in heavy drinkers with the alcohol dehydrogenase 1C*1 allele, possibly due to salivary acetaldehyde, *Gut*, 53, 871–876, 2004.

50. Maier, H. et al., The effect of chronic ethanol consumption on salivary gland morphology and function in the rat, *Alcohol Clin Exp Res*, 10, 425–427, 1986.

51. Maier, H. et al., Effect of chronic alcohol consumption on the morphology of the oral mucosa, *Alcohol Clin Res*, 18, 387–391, 1994.

52. Stickel, F. et al., Genetic predisposition for alcohol-associated upper aerodigestive tract cancer and hepatocellular carcinoma in heavy drinkers with the alcohol dehydrogenase 3*1 allele, *Gastroenterology* (abstract), 124, A547, 2003.

53. Jokelainen, K. et al., Increased acetaldehyde production by mouthwashings from patients with oral cavity, laryngeal, or pharyngeal cancer, *Alcohol Clin Exp Res*, 20, 1206–1210, 1996.

54. Homann, N. et al., Increased salivary acetaldehyde levels in heavy drinkers and smokers: a microbiological approach to oral cavity cancer, *Carcinogenesis*, 21, 663–668, 2000.

55. Homann, N. et al., Poor dental status increases the acetaldehyde production from ethanol in saliva: a possible link to the higher risk of oral cancer among alcohol consumers, *Oral Oncol*, 37, 153–158, 2001.

56. Salaspuro, M.P. et al., Acetaldehyde, microbes, and cancer of the digestive tract, *Crit Rev Clin Lab Sci*, 40, 183–208, 2003.

57. Seitz, H.K. et al., Enhancement of 1,2-dimethylhydrosine induced rectal carcinogenesis following chronic ethanol consumption in the rat, *Gastroenterology*, 86, 886–891, 1984.

58. Simanowski, U.A. et al., Chronic ethanol consumption selectively stimulates rectal cell proliferation in the rat, *Gut*, 27, 278–282, 1986.

59. Vincon, P. et al., Inhibition of alcohol-associated colonic hyperregeneration by alpha-tocoperol in the rat, *Alcoholism Clin Exp Res*, 27, 100–106, 2003.

60. Deschner, E.E. et al., Differential susceptibility of AKR, C57BL/6J, and CF1 mice to 1,2-dimethylhydrazine-induced colonic tumor formation predicted by proliferative characteristics of colonic epithelial cells, *J Natl Cancer Inst*, 70, 279–282, 1983.

61. Deschner, E.E. et al., Differential susceptibility of inbred mouse strains forecast by acute colonic proliferative response to methylazoxymethanol, *J Natl Cancer Inst*, 72, 195–198, 1984.

62. Lipkin, M., Method for binary classification and risk assessment of individuals with familial polyposis based on 3H-TdR labelling of ephitelial cells in colonic crypts, *Cell Tissue Kinet*, 17, 209–222, 1984.

63. Simanowski, U.A. et al., Increased rectal cell proliferation following alcohol abuse, *Gut*, 49, 418–422, 2001.

64. Tiemersma, E.W. et al., Alcohol consumption, alcohol dehydrogenase 3 polymorphism and colorectal adenomas, *Cancer Epidemiol Biomarkers Prev*, 12, 419–425, 2003.

65. Ellison, R., et al., Exploring the relation of alcohol consumption to risk of breast cancer, *Am J Epidemiol,* 154, 740–747, 2001.

66. Longnecker, M., Alcoholic beverage consumption in relation to risk of breast cancer: meta analysis and review, *Cancer Causes Control,* 5, 73–82, 1994.

67. Rohan, T. et al., Alcohol consumption and risk of breast cancer: a cohort study, *Cancer Causes Control* 11, 239–247, 2000.

68. Smith-Warner, S. et al., Alcohol and breast cancer in women: a pooled analysis of cohort studies, *J Am Med Assoc,* 279, 535–540, 1998.

69. Coutelle, C. et al., Risk factors in alcohol associated breast cancer: alcohol dehydrogenase polymorphism and estrogens, *Int J Oncol,* 25, 1127–1132, 2004.

70. Freudenheim, J. et al., Alcohol dehydrogenase 3 genotype modification of the association of alcohol consumption with breast cancer risk, *Cancer Causes Control,* 10, 369–377, 1999.

71. Purohit, V., Can alcohol promote aromatization of androgens to estrogens? A review, *Alcohol,* 22, 123–127, 2000.

72. Sarkola, T. et al., Acute effect of alcohol on estradiol, estrone, progesterone, prolactin, cortisol, and luteinizing hormone in premenopausal women, *Alcohol Clin Exp Res,* 23, 976–982, 1999.

73. Enger, S. et al., Alcohol consumption and breast cancer oestrogen and progesteron receptor status, *Br J Cancer,* 79, 1308–1314, 1999.

74. Fan, S. et al., Alcohol stimulates estrogen receptor signaling in human breast cancer cells, *Cancer Res,* 60, 5635–5639, 2000.

75. Singletary, K., Frey, R., and Yan, W., Effect of ethanol on proliferation and estrogen receptor-alpha expression in human breast cancer cells, *Cancer Lett,* 165, 131–137, 2001.

76. Nasca, P. et al., Alcohol consumption and breast cancer: estrogen receptor status and histology, *Am J Epidemiol,* 140, 980–988, 1994.

77. Liu, C. et al., Ethanol enhances retinoic acid metabolism into metabolites in rat liver via induction of cytochrome P-4502E1, *Gastroenterology,* 120, 179–189, 2001.

78. Wang, X.D. et al., Chronic alcohol intake reduces retinoic acid concentration and enhances AP-1 (c-jun and c-fos) expression in rat liver, *Hepatology,* 28, 744–750, 1998.

79. Muti, P. et al., Alcohol consumption and total estradiol in premenopausal women, *Cancer Epidemiol Biomarkers Prev,* 7, 189–193, 1998.

80. Dorgan, J. et al., Serum hormones and the alcohol-breast cancer association in postmenopausal women, *J Natl Cancer Inst,* 93, 710–715, 2001.

81. Ginsburg, E., Estrogen, alcohol and breast cancer risk, *J Steroid Biochem Mol Biol,* 69, 299–306, 1999.

82. Sarkar, D., Liehr, J., and Singletary, K., Role of estrogen in alcohol promotion of breast cancer and prolactinomas, *Alcohol Clin Exp Res,* 25, 230–236, 2001.

10 Genetic Polymorphism of *N*-Acetyltransferase Genes as Risk Modifiers of Colorectal Cancer from Consumption of Well-Done Meat

La Creis Renee Kidd, Robert C.G. Martin, Jason H. Moore, and David W. Hein

CONTENTS

10.1 INTRODUCTION

Colorectal cancer is one of the most common cancers among men and women residing in the U.S. and worldwide.[1,2] In 2005, it is estimated that approximately 145,290 U.S. residents will be diagnosed with colorectal cancer and 56,290 will die from the disease.[1] The etiological risk factors of colorectal cancer include age, personal or family history of colorectal polyps or inflammatory bowel disease, obesity, and physical inactivity.[3,4] Colorectal neoplasms occurring in the general population may also be attributed to both environmental and genetic influences, such as fatty foods, low fiber, and cooked meat. It has been speculated that high consumption of red meat or particularly well-done meat may play a role in colorectal cancer in humans.[5,6]

Evidence for the relationship between meat-derived carcinogens such as heterocyclic amines (HAs) and colorectal tumorigenesis primarily stems from rodent assays and, to a lesser extent, epidemiological studies. In fact, mice and rats fed diets containing high levels of HAs develop tumors of the large and small intestines and other target sites.[7–13] Although some observational studies demonstrate a positive association between human consumption of meats prepared under conditions that yield high levels of HAs (e.g., pan-fried, grilled, barbecued, or broiled meats) and colorectal cancer risk,[14–18] these findings are not consistent for all reported studies.[19–21]

It has been hypothesized that dietary exposure to cooked meats containing HAs, combined with inherited variations in carcinogen metabolism genes such cytochrome P-450 (*CYP1A2*) and *N*-acetyltransferase 1 (*NAT1*) and 2 (*NAT2*), play a more important role in colorectal cancer risk than either one of these factors alone. Recently, many studies have focused on the relationship between genetic polymorphisms and the risk of developing colorectal cancer; however, the findings from these studies remain inconsistent due to a variety of factors, including misclassification of genotyping status, failure to consider other genetic factors, under- or overestimation of cooked meat and HA exposure, and limitations in sample size. With respect to sample size, we propose that investigators consider using a nonparametric statistical method (i.e., multifactor dimensionality reduction) to overcome statistical power issues associated with the use of parametric statistical methods (i.e., logistic regression analysis models) to investigate diet–gene interactions.

10.2 HETEROCYCLIC AMINES

Mutagenic HAs such as 2-aminoimidazoarenes (e.g., $MeIQ_x$, MeIQ, and IQ) and imidazopyridines (i.e., PhIP) have been identified in the charred and brown surfaces of fried or high-temperature-prepared meats (100 to 300°C).[22,23] These HAs are formed via a nonenzymatic browning reaction, involving condensation among meat-derived precursors such as reducing sugars, amino acids, and creatinine.[24,25] High-temperature cooking methods such as grilling, broiling, pan-frying, and barbecuing have higher levels of mutagenic HAs in comparison to low- and moderate-temperature cooking methods (i.e., boiling, baking, roasting, or stewing). These direct high-temperature cooking methods enable the meat surface temperatures to get well over 100°C, resulting in appreciable levels of HA mutagen formation. The two most abundant HAs detected in meats prepared under these conditions include PhIP (0.56 to 69.2 ng/g) and MeIQ$_x$ (0.8 to 12 ng/g).[7,26,27] The estimated daily intake of these carcinogens is between 43 to 110 ng/g and 14 to 47 ng/g for PhIP and MeIQx, respectively.[28] These compounds are highly mutagenic in bacterial and mammalian cell lines and induce tumors in several target organs, including the large and small intestine, in rodents.[7-11,13] In addition to HAs' ability to induce tumors in rodents, these substances have recently joined the list of carcinogens reasonably expected to be carcinogenic to humans (for details, http://ntp.niehs.nih.gov/ntp/roc/eleventh/reason.pdf). However, prior to HAs initiating tumorigenic events, they must first undergo metabolic activation and conversion to highly reactive electrophilic intermediates that cause DNA damage and mutagenesis.

10.3 METABOLISM OF HETEROCYCLIC AMINES

Metabolic activation of HAs has been shown to include hepatic *CYP1A2*-catalyzed *N*-hydroxylation followed by *O*-acetylation, to the *N*-acetoxy derivative catalyzed by hepatic or colon-derived *NAT1* and/or *NAT2*.[28,29] After formation in the liver, the *N*-hydroxylarylamines and *N*-acetoxy esters of HAs are transported to extrahepatic tissue via the bloodstream. These proximate carcinogens are then converted to ultimate reactive species, presumably a nitrenium ion that binds to DNA, leading to the formation of DNA adducts, an initiating event in colorectal tumorigenesis.[30,31]

10.4 FUNCTIONAL CONSEQUENCES OF VARIANT METABOLIC ACTIVATION GENES

Numerous investigations suggest that individuals who have a high capacity to rapidly convert these compounds to their ultimate reactive forms may have increased susceptibility to colorectal cancer. Thus, a review of investigations on the functional consequences of variations in *CYP1A2*, *NAT1*, and *NAT2* metabolic activation genes in various human populations, their functional consequences, and their potential role in environmentally induced colorectal cancer susceptibility are summarized in Table 10.1 to Table 10.5. In brief, the principal mechanisms in which genetic polymorphisms influence the expression of the gene products or catalytic activity of the respective enzyme are summarized as follows: (1) nucleotide variations in the coding region of the gene, resulting in amino acid substitutions and subsequent alterations in enzyme activity or substrate binding, (2) polymorphisms in the noncoding region may affect transcriptional regulatory factors involved in enzyme expression or induction, and (3) variations in the polyadenylation signal of a gene may affect mRNA stability, which may in turn influence the quantity of the enzyme and colorectal cancer susceptibility. These aforementioned genetic variations may ultimately result in alterations in colorectal cancer risk, as detailed in the upcoming paragraphs.

10.5 CYP1A2

Cytochrome P-450 1A2 is involved in the metabolic activation of a broad range of drugs as well as environmental carcinogens, including aromatic and heterocyclic amines. In humans, there is a wide interindividual variation in *CYP1A2* activity.[32–36] For instance, Butler and coworkers demonstrated that study participants from three subpopulations (e.g., Arkansas, Italy, and China) were categorized as slow (12 to 13%), intermediate (51 to 67%), and rapid (20 to 37%) metabolizers.[37] The interindividual variability in *CYP1A2* activity is attributed to induction of this enzyme by various substances (i.e., polycyclic aromatic hydrocarbons, HAs, and cigarette-derived mutagens) and genetic polymorphisms. To date, a variety of variant *CYP1A2* alleles have been identified (www.imm.ki.se/CYPalleles/cyp1a2.htm); however, little is known about their functional consequences on enzyme activity and levels and their association with colorectal cancer risk. *CYP1A2* metabolic activity may be estimated by the capacity to biotransform caffeine, as this enzyme is involved in the initial major step of caffeine metabolism (i.e., 3-demethylation). Methods to assess *CYP1A2* activity based on caffeine metabolites and several urinary metabolite ratios have been reported in different populations.[32,37–39]

10.6 N-ACETYLTRANSFERASE 1 (NAT1)

NAT1 is highly polymorphic and includes a reference allele (*NAT1*4*) and over 25 variant alleles[29] (Table 10.1). A common variant allele, *NAT1*10*, defined by two single nucleotide polymorphisms in the 3' untranslated region ($T^{1088}A$ and $C^{1095}A$) may cause a shift in the position of the mRNA polyadenylation signal, resulting in a potential increase in mRNA stability.[40] Two studies show that the *NAT1*10* configuration may represent a rapid acetylator allele, as it was associated with increased *N*-acetylation activity (*p*-amino benzoic acid activity assay) in human bladder and colonic mucosa and higher DNA adduct formation in the urinary bladder.[40–42] However, these findings have not been replicated and remain controversial.[43,44] Among population controls, the frequency of *NAT1*10* is more common than another putative rapid acetylator allele, namely *NAT1*11*.[40,45] Additional variant *NAT1* alleles, such as slow *NAT1*14B, *15, *17, *19*, and *22* alleles are less common, particularly among Caucasians,[45] exhibit negligible levels of *NAT1* protein expression, and have lower catalytic activity toward *N*-hydroxy PhIP,[46] a well-established carcinogenic HA. The association of these slow acetylator *NAT1* genotypes with reduced metabolic activation of *N*-hydroxy-PhIP suggests that *NAT1* polymorphism may play a role in HA-induced colorectal tumorigenesis. However, this relationship has not been confirmed within observational studies, as detailed in Table 10.3.

10.7 N-ACETYLTRANSFERASE 2 (NAT2)

Polymorphism in the *NAT2* gene has led to the identification of a *NAT2*4* (reference allele) and over 25 variant alleles[29] (Table 10.1). Several single nucleotide polymorphisms (SNPs) (e.g., $G^{191}A$, $T^{341}C$, $G^{590}A$, and $G^{857}A$) result in *NAT2* alleles with reduced activity (e.g., *NAT2*5, *6, *7, *14*), as depicted in Table 10.1. However,

TABLE 10.1
Role of Polymorphic Xenobiotic Metabolizing Genes on Nucleotide/Amino Acid Sequence, Enzyme Function, and Potential Role in Colorectal Cancer Susceptibility[a]

Gene/ Protein	Selected Alleles[b]	Selected Nucleotide Change[b]	Amino Acid Change	Enzyme Activity/Level	Proposed Influence on Colorectal Cancer Risk
NAT1[c]	*4	None		Reference	
	*3	$C^{1095}A$	3′UTR		
	*10	$T^{1088}A$, $C^{1095}A$	3′UTR, 3′UTR	Rapid?	Increase?
	*11	$G^{445}A$, $C^{1095}A$, $T^{640}G$	Val^{149}Ile, Ser^{214}Ala	Rapid?	Increase?
	*14 (A or B)	$G^{560}A$, $T^{1088}A$, $C^{1095}A$	Arg^{187}Gln	Slow	
	*15	$C^{559}T$	Arg^{187}Stop	Slow	
	*17	$C^{190}T$	Arg^{64}Tyr	Slow	
	*19	$C^{97}T$	Arg^{33}Stop	Slow	
	*22	$A^{752}T$	Asp^{251}Val	Slow	
NAT2[d]	*4	None		Reference (Rapid)	Increase
	*5A	$T^{341}C$, $C^{481}T$	Ile^{114}Thr	Slow	
	*5B	$T^{341}C$, $C^{481}T$, $A^{803}G$	Ile^{114}Thr, Lys^{268}Arg	Slow	
	*5C	$T^{341}C$, $A^{803}G$	Ile^{114}Thr, Lys^{268}Arg	Slow	
	*6A	$C^{282}T$, $G^{590}A$	Arg^{197}Gln	Slow	
	*6B	$G^{590}A$	Arg^{197}Gln	Slow	
	*7A	$G^{857}A$	Gly^{286}Glu	Slow	
	*7B	$C^{282}T$, $G^{857}A$	Gly^{286}Glu	Slow	
	*12A	$A^{803}G$	Lys^{268}Arg	Rapid	Increase
	*12B	$C^{282}T$, $A^{803}G$	Lys^{268}Arg	Rapid	Increase
	*13	$C^{282}T$	None	Rapid	Increase
	*14A	$G^{191}A$	Arg^{64}Gln	Slow	
	*14B	$G^{191}A$, $C^{282}T$	Arg^{64}Gln	Slow	

[a] Adapted from Hein et al., 2000.[29]
[b] In addition to the aforementioned selected *NAT1* and *NAT2* alleles, additional single nucleotide polymorphisms have been identified and characterized, as described at www.louisville.edu/medschool/pharmacology/NAT.html.

polymorphism found in the *NAT2*5* ($T^{341}C$) and *NAT2*14* ($G^{191}A$) clusters, respectively, resulted in the greatest reduction in *N*- and *O*-acetylation activity when compared to the reference genotype.[47] Moreover, *NAT2*5B* and *NAT2*5D* alleles have lower protein expression relative to the *NAT2*4* allele.[48] In contrast, *NAT2*12* and **13* alleles are rapid *N*-acetylation alleles.[47] The prevalence of both rapid and slow *NAT2* genotype varies with ethnic group.[29]

10.8 VARIANT *CYP1A2* AND *N*-ACETYLTRANSFERASE GENES AND THEIR EFFECT ON COLORECTAL CANCER RISK IN RODENTS AND HUMANS

It has long been known that administration of heterocyclic amines such as PhIP induces colon tumors in rats.[12,13,49] The morphology and multistep progression of the PhIP-induced colon tumors in rats show similarity to human colon tumors.[50] In both rats and humans, aberrant crypt foci serve as preneoplastic markers of colon cancer.[50–53]

The role of *NAT2* acetylator genotype on PhIP-induced colorectal tumors has been investigated in rodent models, as they enable investigators to control for certain experimental variables such as carcinogen exposure and genetic variability. In a congenic Syrian hamster model in which rapid and slow acetylators are genetically identical, except at the *NAT2* locus,[54] colon *O*-acetyltransferase activity levels were significantly higher in rapid than slow acetylators.[55–56] Consistent with the enzyme expression data, aberrant crypt foci were significantly higher in rapid than slow acetylator rats following administration of PhIP.[57] These data lend mechanistic support to the epidemiological studies reporting a higher incidence of colorectal cancer in humans with rapid *NAT2* acetylator phenotype and genotype.

Individuals may be categorized as rapid or slow *N*-oxidizers or acetylators based on their phenotype (i.e., urinary excretion of caffeine metabolites following a caffeine dose or sulfamethazine metabolism, respectively) or genotype.[37] It has been hypothesized that rapid *N*-oxidizers and acetylators may have an increased capacity to metabolically activate HAs detected in well-done meat and, as a consequence, may experience an increased susceptibility to colorectal cancer. In support of this hypothesis, three out of six phenotype studies demonstrated a 1.8 (OR = 1.8; 95% CI = 1.0 to 3.3) to 3.7 (OR = 3.73; 95% CI = 1.4 to 9.6) increase in colorectal cancer among individuals who possessed the rapid *NAT2* phenotype when compared to slow acetylators, as depicted in Table 10.2.[58–62] However, this positive link between *NAT2* and colorectal cancer has not been consistently reported across all genetic epidemiology studies, as shown in Table 10.2. In terms of the rapid *NAT1* genotype, two out of five investigations observed a statistically significant increase in colorectal cancer susceptibility among individuals who possessed the putative *NAT1*10* rapid allele relative to slow acetylators, as shown in Table 10.3.[40,63–66]

Inconsistencies in the data regarding these carcinogen-metabolizing genes and colorectal cancer may arise for a variety of reasons, including sample size limitations or failure to consider whether inheritance of multiple genetic variations (i.e., rapid-rapid *CYP1A2/NAT2* genotypes) and/or environmental exposure (i.e., well-done/cooked meat or HA intake) play a role in the risk of developing colorectal cancer. In an attempt to overcome sample size issues presented by many epidemiological studies, Chen and coworkers[67] conducted a meta-analysis consisting of 39 observational studies evaluating the relationship between colorectal cancer risk and phenotypic/genotypic

TABLE 10.2
Association between Polymorphic *N*-Acetyltransferase 2 and Colorectal Cancer Susceptibility

Risk Genotype/ Phenotype Status	Method of Phenotyping/ Alleles Evaluated	Ethnicity/ Country	No. of Cases/ No. of Controls	Genotype Frequency% Cases/Controls	OR (95% CI)	References
		Positive Reports				
Rapid *NAT2*	SMZ[a]	U.S. (Arkansas)	43/41			Lang et al., 1986[58]
	Slow			46.5/68.0	1.0 (Reference value)	
	Rapid			53.5/32.0	2.37 (1.0–5.9)	
Rapid *NAT2*	SMZ[a]	Caucasian	110/110			Roberts-Thompson et al., 1996[59]
	Slow			—	1.0 (Reference value)	
	Rapid			—	1.8 (1.0–3.3)	
Rapid *NAT2*	SMZ[a]	—	49/41			Ilett et al., 1987[60]
	Slow			45.0/76.0	1.0 (Reference value)	
	Rapid			55.0/24.0	3.73 (1.4–9.6)	
		Null Reports				
Rapid/intermediate *NAT2*	SMZ[a]	Spanish	109/96			Ladero et al., 1991[61]
	Slow			45.0/41.7	1.0 (Reference value)	
	Rapid			55.0/58.3	NS[i]	

(continued)

TABLE 10.2 (continued)
Association between Polymorphic N-Acetyltransferase 2 and Colorectal Cancer Susceptibility

Risk Genotype/Phenotype Status	Method of Phenotyping/Alleles Evaluated	Ethnicity[c]/Country	No. of Cases/No. of Controls	Genotype Frequency% Cases/Controls	OR (95% CI)	References
Rapid NAT2	Caffeine metabolism[b]	88% EA 12% AA	75[f]/205			Lang et al., 1994[33]
Slow				48.0/55.0	1.0 (Reference value)	
Rapid				52.0/45.0	NS	
Rapid NAT2	Caffeine metabolism[b]	60.2% Japanese 25.9% Caucasian 13.9% Hawaiian	349/467			Le Marchand et al., 2001[66]
Slow				29.8/33.4	1.0 (Reference value)	
Intermediate				38.7/33.2	1.4 (0.9–2.0)	
Rapid				31.5/33.4	1.0 (0.6–1.5)	
Rapid/intermediate NAT2	Rapid (*4/*12) vs. slow (*5ABC/*6/*7)	88% Caucasian 12% other	143/208			Ishibe et al., 2002[63]
Slow (two slow alleles)				55.2/52.9	(Reference value)	
Rapid (≥ one *4/*12 allele)				44.8/47.1	0.91 (0.57–1.45)	
Rapid NAT2	Rapid (*4/*12/*13) vs. slow (*5ABC, *6AB, *7AB)	60.2% Japanese 25.9% Caucasian 13.9% Hawaiian	543/654			Le Marchand et al., 2001[66]
Slow (two slow alleles)				22.8/24.0	1.0 (Reference value)	
Intermediate (one slow allele)				41.1/41.3	1.1 (0.8–1.5)	
Rapid (other)				36.1/34.7	1.1 (0.7–1.5)	

Rapid/intermediate *NAT2*	Rapid (*4) vs. slow (*5ABC, *6AB, *7AB)	—	433/433	38.0/41.1	0.89 (0.67, 1.17)	Barrett et al., 2003[80]
	Slow (two slow alleles)					
	Rapid (≥ one *4 allele)					
Rapid/intermediate *NAT2*	Rapid (WT) vs. slow (M1, M2, M3)[c]	75% EA 25% AA	44/28	54.5/53.5 45.5/46.5	1.0 (Reference value) NS	Rodriguez et al., 1993[81]
	Slow (two slow alleles)					
	Rapid (≥ one WT allele)					
Rapid/intermediate *NAT2*	—	Japanese	36/36	8.4/8.3 91.6/91.7	1.0 (Reference value) 1.2 (0.15–8.9)	Oda et al., 1994[70]
	Slow					
	Rapid/intermediate					
Rapid/intermediate *NAT2*	—	Japanese	234/329	11.1/9.6 88.9/90.5	1.3 (0.6–2.9)	Shibuta et al., 1994[82]
	Slow					
	Rapid/intermediate					
Rapid/intermediate *NAT2*	Rapid (WT) vs. slow (M1, M2, M3, M4)[d]	Caucasian	202/112	52.0/55.0 48.0/45.0	1.0 (Reference value) 1.1 (0.7–1.8)	Bell et al., 1995[40]
	Slow (two slow alleles)					
	Rapid/intermediate (≥ one WT allele)					
Rapid/intermediate *NAT2*	Rapid (*4) vs. slow (*5, *6B, *7A)	Caucasian	275/343	63.6/59.2 36.4/40.8	1.0 (Reference value) NS	Hubbard et al., 1997[83]
	Slow (two slow alleles)					
	Rapid/intermediate (≥ one *4)					

-(continued)

TABLE 10.2 (continued)
Association between Polymorphic N-Acetyltransferase 2 and Colorectal Cancer Susceptibility

Risk Genotype/Phenotype Status	Method of Phenotyping/Alleles Evaluated	Ethnicity/Country	No. of Cases/No. of Controls	Genotype Frequency% Cases/Controls	OR (95% CI)	References
Rapid NAT2	Rapid (*4 *12ABC) vs. slow (*5ABCDE, *6AB, 7AB, 14ABC)	Spanish	120#/258			Agundez et al., 2000[84]
	Slow (two slow alleles)					
	Rapid (≥ one *4/*12)			50.0/53.9	1.0	
				50.0/46.1	NS	
Rapid NAT2	Rapid (*4, *12AB) vs. *5ABC, *6AB, *7AB, *14)	EA 91.4% AA 4.2% Hispanic 4.4%	1611/1955			Slattery et al., 1998[85]
	Slow (other)	Men	531/602	58.7/58.3	1.0 (Reference value)	
		Women	391/550	55.3/59.7	1.0 (Reference value)	
	Intermediate (one *4/*12 allele)	Men	321/359	35.5/34.7	1.0 (0.8–1.2)	
		Women	279/320	39.5/34.7	1.2 (1.0–1.5)	
	Rapid (two *4/*12 alleles)	Men	52/72	5.8/7.0	0.9 (0.6–1.2)	
		Women	37/52	5.2/5.6	1.0 (0.7–1.6)	
	Rapid/intermediate (≥ one *4/*12)	Men	373/431	41.3/41.7	1.0 (0.8–1.2)	
		Women	316/372	44.7/40.3	1.2 (1.0–1.5)	

		Population	N	%	OR (95% CI)	Reference
Rapid NAT2	Rapid vs. slow (*4, *12)	Netherlands	258/857	44/42		van der Hel et al., 2003[86]
	Slow (no *4/*12 alleles)			56/58	1.00 (Reference value)	
	Rapid (≥ one *4/*12)			44/42	1.06 (0.8–1.41)	
Rapid NAT2	Rapid (*4) vs. slow (*5ABC, *6AB, *7B)	Caucasians	490/593	—		Sachse et al., 2002[87]
	Slow (two slow alleles)		304/348	62.0/58.9	1.00 (Reference value)	
	intermediate (*4/other)		186/243	38.0/41.1	0.88 (0.69–1.12)	
	Rapid (*4/*4)		—	—	—	
Rapid/intermediate NAT2	Rapid (*4) vs. slow (*5, *6, *7)	Caucasian	219/200		1.00 (Reference value)	Butler et al., 2001[88]
	Slow (two slow alleles)					
	Rapid/intermediate (≥ one *4 allele)				1.01 (0.68–1.5)	
Rapid NAT2	*4, *5, *6, *7, *12	Netherlands	431[b]/433			Tiemersma et al., 2004[65]
	Slow (no *4/*12)			60.7/58.6	1.00 (Reference value)	
	intermediate (one *4/*12)			33.7/33.8	0.96 (0.72–1.29)	
	Rapid (two *4/*12 alleles)			5.6/7.6	0.71 (0.41–1.24)	
Rapid NAT2	Rapid (*4) vs. slow (*5, *6, *7, *14)	Japanese	103[b]/122			Katoh et al., 2000[64]
	Slow (2 slow alleles)			63.1/62.3	1.00 (Reference value)	
	Rapid/intermediate (≥ one *4 allele)			36.9/37.7	1.06 (0.61–1.83)	

(continued)

TABLE 10.2 (continued)
Association between Polymorphic N-Acetyltransferase 2 and Colorectal Cancer Susceptibility

Risk Genotype/ Phenotype Status	Method of Phenotyping/ Alleles Evaluated	Ethnicity[e]/ Country	No. of Cases/ No. of Controls	Genotype Frequency% Cases/Controls	OR (95% CI)	References
Rapid NAT2	Rapid (*4) vs. slow (*5AB, *6A, *7B)	Caucasian	174/174			Welfare et al., 1997[68]
	Slow (two slow alleles)			—	1.00 (Reference value)	
	Rapid/intermediate (≥ one *4 allele)			—	0.95 (0.61–1.49)	

[a] N-acetylator activity was determined by the rate of acetylation of sulphamethazine given orally.

[b] N-acetylation activity was determined by the urinary ratio of caffeine metabolites (AFMU:1X).

[c] N-acetylation alleles were designated as follows: WT, wildtype; M1, $C^{481}T$; M2, $C^{282}T$; M3, $C^{282}T$ and $G^{857}A$.

[d] N-acetylation alleles were designated as follows: WT, wildtype; M1, $C^{481}T$; M2, $C^{282}T$; M3, $C^{282}T$ and $G^{857}A$; M4, $G^{191}A$.

[e] EA, European American; AA, African American.

[f] Cases were diagnosed with either colorectal cancer (n = 34) or polyps (n = 41).

[g] Cases were diagnosed with nonsigmoid (n = 40), sigmoid (n = 41), and rectum (n = 39) colon cancer.

[h] Cases were diagnosed with colorectal adenocarcinoma.

[i] NS, not statistically significant.

TABLE 10.3
**Relationship between Polymorphic *N*-Acetyltransferase 1 (*NAT1*)
and Colorectal Cancer Susceptibility**

Risk Genotype/ Phenotype	Method of Phenotyping/ Alleles Evaluated	Ethnicity/ Country	No. of Cases/ No. of Controls	Genotype Frequency (% cases/ controls)	OR (95% CI)	Refs.
Rapid *NAT1*10*	Rapid (*10*) vs. slow (*3, *4, *11*)	Caucasian	202/112			Bell et al., 1995[40]
	Slow (2 slow alleles) Rapid/interme diate (≥ one *10*)			55.4/70.5 44.6/29.5	1.0 1.92 (1.2–3.2)	
Rapid/ intermediate *NAT1*10*	*3, *4, *10, *11, *14AB, *15, *17, *22*	88% Caucasian 12% Other	132/192			Ishibe et al., 2002[63]
	No *10* alleles *10/*10, *10/other*		77[a]/126 55/66	58.3/65.6 41.7/34.4	1.00 1.43 (0.86–2.36)	
Rapid *NAT1*10*	*3, *4, *10, *11, *14, *15, *17*	Japanese	103/122			Katoh et al., 2000[64]
	Slow (2 slow alleles) Intermediate (*10/other) Rapid (*10/*10)	38/46 43/50 22/26	38/46 43/50 22/26	34.2/37.7 41.7/41.0 21.4/21.3	1.00 1.05 (0.57–1.91) 1.05 (0.51–2.17)	
Rapid *NAT1*10*	*4, *3, *10, *11*	Netherlands	427[a]/431			Tiermersa et al., 2004[65]
	Slow (≥ one *11* allele) Normal (no *10/*11) Rapid (*10/*10)		11/23 248/259 168/149	2.6/5.3 58.1/60.1 39.3/34.6	1.00 2.00 (0.96–4.19) 2.36 (1.11–5.00)	

TABLE 10.3 (continued)
Relationship between Polymorphic N-Acetyltransferase 1 (NAT1)
and Colorectal Cancer Susceptibility

Risk Genotype/ Phenotype	Method of Phenotyping/ Alleles Evaluated	Ethnicity/ Country	No. of Cases/ No. of Controls	Genotype Frequency (% cases/ controls)	OR (95% CI)	Refs.
Rapid NAT1*10	*4,*10	60.2% Japanese	539/649			Le Marchand et al., 2001[66]
	Slow (*4/*4)	25.9% Caucasian	249/268	46.2/41.3	1.0 (Reference value)	
	Intermediate (*10/*4)	13.9% Hawaiian	189/269	35.1/41.4	0.8 (0.6–1.0)	
	Rapid (*10/*10)		101/112	18.7/17.2	1.0 (0.7–1.4)	

[a] Cases were diagnosed with colorectal adenoma.

variations in *NAT1* and *NAT2*. However, this investigation resulted in mixed findings, as depicted in Table 10.4. In this meta-analysis, Chen and coworkers[67] demonstrated a 1.25-fold increase in colorectal cancer risk associated with the rapid *NAT1* acetylator genotype among 520 cumulative cases and 433 controls. In addition, they revealed a 5 to 15%-fold increased risk among individuals who had the rapid *NAT2* phenotype or genotype within 8 and 10 observation studies, respectively. However, this link was only statistically significant in 8 phenotype alone (2182 cumulative

TABLE 10.4
Meta-Analysis of NAT1(2) Polymorphisms and Risk
for Colorectal Cancer[a]

Risk Allele	# Studies	No. of Cases/ No. of Controls	OR (95% CI)	P-value
Rapid NAT1*10	3	520/433	1.25 (0.96–1.63)	> 0.10
Rapid NAT2 (P & G)[b]	18	6741/8015	1.08 (1.00–1.16)	< 0.05
Rapid NAT2 (P)[c]	8	2182/2861	1.15 (1.02–1.31)	< 0.05
Rapid NAT2 (G)[d]	10	4559/5154	1.05 (0.94–1.14)	> 0.20

[a] Reviewed in Chen, K., Jiang, Q.T., and He, H.Q., Relationship between metabolic enzyme polymorphism and colorectal cancer, *World J. Gastroenterol.*, 11, 331, 2005.
[b] P&G, *N*-acetyltransferase phenotype and genotype.
[c] P, *N*-acetyltransferase phenotype.
[d] G, *N*-acetyltransferase genotype.

cases and 2861 cumulative controls) and 10 phenotype combined with genotype studies (6741 cumulative cases and 8015 cumulative controls).

10.9   *CYP1A2* AND *N*-ACETYLTRANSFERASE GENE POLYMORPHISMS, ALONE OR IN COMBINATION, AND THEIR EFFECT ON COLORECTAL CANCER RISK AMONG CONSUMERS OF WELL-DONE MEAT

Several investigators evaluated whether consumption of high levels of well-done and cooked meat in combination with one or two polymorphic metabolic activation genes plays a role in colorectal cancer risk in humans. Moreover, Lang and coworkers[33] designed a case–control study to evaluate the roles of metabolic phenotype and dietary exposure to HAs. In terms of gene–gene interactions, Lang and coworkers observed a 2.8-fold higher (OR = 2.79; 1.69 to 2.81) colorectal cancer susceptibility among individuals with the rapid–rapid *CYP1A2–NAT2* phenotype in comparison to those who were slow–slow metabolizers, as depicted in Table 10.5. In order to assess whether indirect surrogates of HA exposure influenced the association between the rapid–rapid *CYP1A2–NAT2* activity and colorectal cancer, a modified Block dietary questionnaire was used to ascertain detailed information on meat-cooking practices. Interestingly, the risk of developing colorectal cancer (OR = 6.45) increased even further among individuals who had the same rapid–rapid phenotype and consumed well-done meat. In another case–control study (349 cases and 467 controls), Le Marchand and coworkers ascertained information on dietary practices, including a question on whether the subject ate red meat and, if so, did they have a preference toward rare, medium-rare, medium, well-done, or very well done meat.[66] Consistent with Lang's findings, Le Marchand et al. demonstrated that individuals who had a preference toward well done meat and possessed the rapid–rapid *CYP1A2–NAT2* status had a threefold increased risk of developing colorectal cancer (OR = 3.3; 95% CI = 1.69–2.81), as depicted in Table 10.5. Moreover, in a prospective case–control study, Welfare and coworkers used a food frequency questionnaire that focused on foods known to have a high HA content combined with *NAT2* genotyping to evaluate the role of fried meat consumption and acetylator status in colorectal cancer.[68] In this prospective case–control study, individuals who consumed fried meat more than twice a week and possessed the rapid *NAT2* genotype had a 6-fold increased risk of developing colorectal cancer when compared to slow acetylators who consumed fried meat less frequently. In addition, Ishibe and coworkers only revealed a link between the putative *NAT1*10* rapid allele and colorectal cancer among individuals who consumed very high levels of PhIP (63.0 ng/day), as shown in Table 10.5.[63] In a larger study, consisting of 952 cases and 1205 controls, Murtaugh and coworkers revealed a nonsignificant relationship between colorectal cancer and well-done red meat (OR = 1.63; 95% CI = 1.03–2.59) and red meat mutagen index (OR = 1.67; 95% CI = 1.00–2.80) among men, but not women.[69] Lastly, out of five reported studies that investigated gene–diet interactions, only one study did not observe any significant relationship between indicators of HA exposure (i.e., high consumption of very dark meat) and colorectal cancer risk.[65] Thus, polymorphisms

TABLE 10.5

Multiple Carcinogen Metabolism Genes, Alone or in Combination with Heterocyclic Amine Exposure/Surrogate, and Their Effect on Colorectal Cancer Susceptibility

Risk Genotype/Phenotype	Method of Phenotyping/Alleles Evaluated	Exposure	No. of Cases/No. of Controls	OR (95% CI)	References
Rapid CYP1A2[a]	Caffeine metabolism		75 [b]/205	1.91 (1.20–2.87)	Lang et al., 1994[33]
Rapid CYP1A2	Caffeine metabolism	Well-done meat	75 [b]/201	6.45	
Rapid–rapid CYP1A2–NAT2				2.79 (1.69–4.47)	
Rapid CYP1A2[a]	Caffeine metabolism		349/467		Le Marchand et al., 2001[66]
Intermediate vs. slow		None	112/155	1.1 (0.7–1.6)	
Rapid vs. slow		None	133/156	1.3 (0.9–1.8)	
Rapid–rapid CYP1A2–NAT2	Caffeine metabolism	Well-done meat	349/467	3.3 (1.3–8.1)	
Rapid CYP1A2[a]	Caffeine metabolism	None	140/210	1.46 (0.76–2.81)	Ishibe et al., 2002[63]
Rapid CYP1A2[a]		> 27 ng MeIQ$_x$		NS	
Rapid–rapid CYP1A2–NAT2[a]		None		NS	
Rapid–rapid CYP1A2–NAT2 [a]		> 27 ng MeIQ$_x$		NS	
Rapid NAT2		> 27 ng MeIQ$_x$		NS	
Rapid NAT1*10	*3, *4, *10, *11, *14AB, *15, *17, *22	> 27 ng MeIQ$_x$ 63.0 ng PhIP	132/192	7.67 (0.73–9.02) 2.81 (1.33–5.92)	
Rapid NAT2*4	*4, *5AB, *6A, *7B	Fried meat > twice/week	72/72	6.04 (1.6–26.0)	Welfare et al., 1997[68]
Rapid NAT2*4/*12	*4, *5, *6, *7, *12	Very dark meat	427/432	0.6 (0.3–1.1)	Tiemersma et al., 2004[65]
Rapid NAT2	$C^{481}T$, $G^{590}A$, $G^{857}A$		952/1205		Murtaugh et al., 2004[69]
		Well-done red meat		1.63 (1.03–2.59), men 0.87 (0.5–1.5), women	
		Red meat mutagen index		1.67 (1.00–2.80), men 0.62 (0.31–1.23), women	

TABLE 10.5 (continued)
Multiple Carcinogen Metabolism Genes, Alone or in Combination with Heterocyclic Amine Exposure/Surrogate, and Their Effect on Colorectal Cancer Susceptibility

Risk Genotype/ Phenotype	Method of Phenotyping/ Alleles Evaluated	Exposure	No. of Cases/ No. of Controls	OR (95% CI)	References
		White meat mutagen index		1.04 (0.61–1.78), men 0.54 (0.27–1.08), women	

[a] *N*-oxidation and *N*-acetylation activity was determined by the urinary ratio of caffeine metabolites, namely (17U + 17X):137X and (AFMU:1X), respectively.
[b] Cases consisted of participants diagnosed with colorectal cancer (n = 34) and polyps (n = 41).

in the aforementioned carcinogen metabolism genes (i.e., *CYP1A2*, *NAT1*, and *NAT2*) may increase colorectal cancer risk only when dietary exposure to HAs is also taken into consideration.

10.10 LIMITATIONS OF GENE–DIET INTERACTION STUDIES

The controversy over whether one or more variant carcinogen metabolism genes alone or in combination with consumption of well-done meat are related to colorectal cancer stem from a variety of factors. Factors that may contribute to inconsistencies in 2-way and 3-way interactions include: failure to consider the expression of *N*-acetyltransferase genes in target organs (i.e., colon); inadequate surrogates or estimates of HA exposure; failure to completely confirm that "rapid" *NAT1* and *NAT2* genotypes correlate with the "rapid" phenotype; misclassification of *N*-acetyltransferase genotype status; and insufficient sample size.

Genotyping assays performed prior to 1995 may have inaccurately categorized individuals as rapid or slow *N*-acetylators due to the unavailability of assays used to discriminate among various *NAT1* and *NAT2* variants. For instance, although Oda and coworkers[70] evaluated one reference (i.e., *NAT2*4*) and two *NAT2* slow alleles (i.e., *NAT2*5* and *6*), they did not consider other slow (i.e., *NAT2*7*AB and *14AB*) and rapid (i.e., *NAT2*12*AB and *13*) acetylation alleles, which may result in misclassification of acetylation status and a subsequent under- or overestimation of colorectal cancer risk.[71]

In terms of potential misclassification by HA exposure status, a majority of the earlier observational studies may have used inadequate estimates of HA exposure, such as cooking style preferences, well-done meat, etc., which may result in an underestimation of HA intake and an attenuation of colorectal susceptibility. In contrast to these indirect HA assessment strategies, Ishibe and coworkers used a food frequency questionnaire (FFQ) linked to a cooking module and database specifically designed to measure HAs, in order to obtain more accurate HA intake levels.[63] This HA assessment, first introduced by Sinha et al.[72] and subsequently validated,[73] involves the estimation of meat consumption, using frequency of consumption and portion sizes, for each cooking technique and "doneness" level. HA intake is derived by multiplying grams of meat consumption by HA concentration measured for each cooking technique/doneness level contribution for that meat type. HA concentration was then summed across all meat categories. In order to further elucidate the role HAs and genetic susceptibilities play in colorectal cancer, future observational studies should utilize available and validated HAA assessment tools.

In addition to limitations in assessing metabolic activation phenotype and HA intake, gene–gene and gene–gene–nutrient interaction studies are limited by insufficient sample size, which may lead to over- or underestimation of the colorectal cancer risk estimates and extremely wide 95% confidence intervals. In order to ensure adequate statistical power (P-value $\geq$ 80%), observational studies would require thousands of subjects, which may be cost-prohibitive. Strategies to overcome the limitations associated with traditional genetic epidemiology studies evaluating the aforementioned gene–gene and gene–diet interactions, including small sample size and budgetary restrictions, may involve the use of data-mining methodologies, such as multifactor dimensionality reduction, to investigate higher-order interaction studies.

10.11 FUTURE DIRECTIONS: STRATEGIES TO OVERCOME SAMPLE SIZE LIMITATIONS OF DIET–GENE INTERACTION STUDIES

Multifactor dimensionality reduction (MDR) is a model-free (i.e., it does assume a specified genetic model) and nonparametric (i.e., it does not estimate parameters) method for detecting and characterizing high-order gene–gene–diet interactions in case–control studies, even in the presence of relatively small sample sizes (i.e., $\geq$ 200 cases and 200 controls).[74] With MDR, multilocus genotypes are pooled into high-risk and low-risk groups, reducing high-dimensional data to a single dimension, permitting an investigation of gene–gene–diet interactions. This one dimensional multilocus genotype variable is evaluated for its ability to classify and predict disease susceptibility through cross-validation and permutation testing. Information on the application of MDR to gene–gene–diet interactions (i.e., polymorphic carcinogen metabolism genes and HA exposure) is detailed below.

10.12 THE MULTIFACTOR DIMENSIONALITY REDUCTION (MDR) METHOD

The multifactor dimensionality reduction (MDR) method is a data-mining approach that may be used to assess the role single nucleotide polymorphisms in N-acetyltransferase genes combined with dietary exposure to HAs plays in colorectal cancer.

This software is available at www.epistasis.org. The advantage of this approach is its ability to detect high-order interactions in a variety of genetic and epidemiological study designs when traditional methods such as logistic regression are underpowered. The theoretical and empirical details of the MDR method have been described previously.[74-78] The MDR method for case–control studies involves the following four steps: (1) selection of a set of alleles, haplotypes, or genotypes (i.e., *CYP1A2*, *NAT1*, and *NAT2*), and HA exposure status categories (e.g., lowest vs. highest tertiles of HA consumption); (2) calculation of case–control ratios for each exposure–genotype combination; for example, for two loci with three genotypes each combined with three HA exposure levels (i.e., low, medium, and high), MDR would calculate nine different ratios; and (3) categorization of each multiloci cell as either a "high-risk" if the case:control ratio exceeds 1.0 or "low-risk"; and (4) calculation of the prediction error of each model is estimated by tenfold cross validation. In order to calculate the prediction error (i.e., the proportion of subjects for which an incorrect prediction was made), the genotyping data is first randomly divided into 10 equal parts, of which nine-tenths of the data is used to develop an MDR model that is used to make predictions about the case status of the remaining one-tenth of the data. The aforementioned steps are repeated for all possible diet–gene combinations. Among all of the diet–gene combinations, a single model that minimizes prediction error is selected. Assessment of prediction error using cross-validation plays a very important role in limiting the possibility of false-positives as has been demonstrated by Coffey et al.[79] This data-mining approach may help to minimize the budget required to assess whether variations in a selected pathway (e.g., meat-derived carcinogens combined with genes involved in their metabolic activation of HAs) is involved in the modification of colorectal cancer risk in humans. Ultimately, MDR may be used to enhance traditional molecular epidemiology approaches to assessing gene–gene–diet interactions.

10.13 SUMMARY

In summary, several investigators have studied the relationship between colorectal cancer risk and susceptibility in genes involved in carcinogen metabolism alone or in combination with direct/indirect surrogates of HA exposure. Although genetic polymorphisms in genes that play a role in the metabolic activation of HAs may be slightly linked to colorectal cancer, these susceptibilities appear to play a more vital role in colorectal tumorigenesis when at least two polymorphic genes (e.g., *CYP1A2* and *NAT2*) and HA exposure are taken into consideration. Inconsistencies in gene–gene and gene–gene–diet interactions may be partially attributed to relatively small observational studies and inadequate estimates of HA exposure. In order to further address these limitations, future interaction studies should utilize available nonparametric data-mining strategies (i.e., multifactor dimensionality reduction, MDR) and available food frequency questionnaires that are linked to a HA database, specifically designed to assess human exposure to HAs. Application of the available HA exposure assessment tools and appropriate statistical strategies may help to further elucidate the role HAs combined with polymorphisms in metabolic activation genes may play in the risk of developing colorectal cancer in humans.

REFERENCES

1. American Cancer Society (ACS), *Cancer Facts and Figures,* Publication number 5008.05, ACS, Atlanta, GA, 1, 2005.
2. World Health Organization, *The World Health Report,* Geneva, 1997.
3. Giovannucci, E., Diet, body weight, and colorectal cancer: a summary of the epidemiologic evidence, *J. Womens Health (Larchmt.),* 12, 173, 2003.
4. Sandler, R.S., Epidemiology and risk factors for colorectal cancer, *Gastroenterol. Clin. N. Am.,* 25, 717, 1996.
5. Chen, J. et al., A prospective study of N-acetyltransferase genotype, red meat intake, and risk of colorectal cancer, *Cancer Res.,* 58, 3307, 1998.
6. Gil, J.P. and Lechner, M.C., Increased frequency of wild-type arylamine-N-acetyltransferase allele NAT2*4 homozygotes in Portuguese patients with colorectal cancer, *Carcinogenesis,* 19, 37, 1998.
7. Wakabayashi, K. et al., Food-derived mutagens and carcinogens, *Cancer Res.,* 52, 2092S, 1992.
8. Shirai, T. et al., The prostate: a target for carcinogenicity of 2-amino-1-methyl-6-phenylimidazo[4,5-b]pyridine (PhIP) derived from cooked foods, *Cancer Res.,* 57, 195, 1992.
9. Esumi, H. et al., Induction of lymphoma in CDF1 mice by the food mutagen, 2-amino-1-methyl-6-phenylimidazo[4,5-b]pyridine, *Jpn. J. Cancer Res.,* 80, 1176, 1989.
10. Kato, T. et al., Carcinogenicity in rats of a mutagenic compound, 2-amino-3,8-dimethylimidazo[4,5-f]quinoxaline, *Carcinogenesis,* 9, 71, 1988.
11. Ohgaki, H. et al., Carcinogenicity in mice of a mutagenic compound, 2-amino-3,8-dimethylimidazo[4,5-f]quinoxaline (MeIQx) from cooked foods, *Carcinogenesis,* 8, 665, 1987.
12. Ito, N. et al., Carcinogenicity of 2-amino-1-methyl-6-phenylimidazo[4,5-b]pyridine (PhIP) in the rat, *Mutat. Res.,* 376, 107, 1997.
13. Ito, N. et al., A new colon and mammary carcinogen in cooked food, 2-amino-1-methyl-6-phenylimidazo[4,5-b]pyridine (PhIP), *Carcinogenesis,* 12, 1503, 1991.
14. de Verdier, G. et al., Meat, cooking methods and colorectal cancer: a case-referent study in Stockholm, *Int. J. Cancer,* 49, 520, 1991.
15. Nowell, S. et al., Analysis of total meat intake and exposure to individual heterocyclic amines in a case-control study of colorectal cancer: contribution of metabolic variation to risk, *Mutat. Res.,* 506–507, 175, 2002.
16. Sinha, R. et al., Well-done, grilled red meat increases the risk of colorectal adenomas, *Cancer Res.,* 59, 4320, 1999.
17. Butler, L.M. et al., Heterocyclic amines, meat intake, and association with colon cancer in a population-based study, *Am. J. Epidemiol.,* 157, 434, 2003.
18. Probst-Hensch, N.M. et al., Meat preparation and colorectal adenomas in a large sigmoidoscopy-based case-control study in California (United States), *Cancer Causes Control,* 8, 175, 1997.
19. Augustsson, K. et al., Dietary heterocyclic amines and cancer of the colon, rectum, bladder, and kidney: a population-based study, *Lancet,* 353, 703, 1999.
20. Kampman, E. et al., Meat consumption, genetic susceptibility, and colon cancer risk: a United States multicenter case-control study, *Cancer Epidemiol. Biomarkers Prev.,* 8, 15, 1999.
21. Muscat, J.E. and Wynder, E.L., The consumption of well-done red meat and the risk of colorectal cancer, *Am. J. Public Health,* 84, 856, 1994.

22. Felton, J.S. et al., The isolation and identification of a new mutagen from fried ground beef: 2-amino-1-methyl-6-phenylimidazo[4,5-b]pyridine (PhIP), *Carcinogenesis*, 7, 1081, 1986.

23. Turesky, R.J. et al., Analysis of mutagenic heterocyclic amines in cooked beef products by high-performance liquid chromatography in combination with mass spectrometry, *Food Chem. Toxicol.*, 26, 501, 1988.

24. Jagerstad, M. et al., Effects of meat composition and cooking conditions on the formation of mutagenic imidazoquinoxalines (MeIQx and its methyl derivatives), *Princess Takamatsu Symp.*, 16, 87, 1985.

25. Overvik, E. et al., A. Influence of creatine, amino acids and water on the formation of the mutagenic heterocyclic amines found in cooked meat, *Carcinogenesis*, 10, 2293, 1989.

26. Sinha, R. et al., High concentrations of the carcinogen 2-amino-1-methyl-6-phenylim-idazo-[4,5-b]pyridine (PhIP) occur in chicken but are dependent on the cooking method, *Cancer Res.*, 55, 4516, 1995.

27. Gross, G.A. et al., Heterocyclic aromatic amine formation in grilled bacon, beef and fish and in grill scrapings, *Carcinogenesis*, 14, 2313, 1993.

28. Cross, A.J. and Sinha, R., Meat-related mutagens/carcinogens in the etiology of colorectal cancer, *Environ. Mol. Mutagen.*, 44, 44, 2004.

29. Hein, D.W. et al., Molecular genetics and epidemiology of the NAT1 and NAT2 acetylation polymorphisms, *Cancer Epidemiol. Biomarkers Prev.*, 9, 29, 2000.

30. Hein, D.W. et al., Metabolic activation and deactivation of arylamine carcinogens by recombinant human NAT1 and polymorphic NAT2 acetyltransferases, *Carcinogenesis*, 14, 1633, 1993.

31. Minchin, R.F., Kadlubar, F.F., and Ilett, K.F., Role of acetylation in colorectal cancer, *Mutat. Res.*, 290, 35, 1993.

32. Kalow, W. and Tang, B.K., Use of caffeine metabolite ratios to explore CYP1A2 and xanthine oxidase activities, *Clin. Pharmacol. Ther.*, 50, 508, 1991.

33. Lang, N.P. et al., Rapid metabolic phenotypes for acetyltransferase and cytochrome P4501A2 and putative exposure to food-borne heterocyclic amines increase the risk for colorectal cancer or polyps, *Cancer Epidemiol. Biomarkers Prev.*, 3, 675, 1994.

34. Nakajima, M. et al., Phenotyping of CYP1A2 in Japanese population by analysis of caffeine urinary metabolites: absence of mutation prescribing the phenotype in the CYP1A2 gene, *Cancer Epidemiol. Biomarkers Prev.*, 3, 413, 1994.

35. Schrenk, D. et al., A distribution study of CYP1A2 phenotypes among smokers and non-smokers in a cohort of healthy Caucasian volunteers, *Eur. J. Clin. Pharmacol.*, 53, 361, 1998.

36. Ou-Yang, D.S. et al., Phenotypic polymorphism and gender-related differences of CYP1A2 activity in a Chinese population, *Br. J. Clin. Pharmacol.*, 49, 145, 2000.

37. Butler, M.A. et al., Determination of CYP1A2 and NAT2 phenotypes in human populations by analysis of caffeine urinary metabolites, *Pharmacogenetics*, 2, 116, 1992.

38. Campbell, M.E., Spielberg, S.P., and Kalow, W., A urinary metabolite ratio that reflects systemic caffeine clearance, *Clin. Pharmacol. Ther.*, 42, 157, 1987.

39. Grant, D.M., Tang, B.K., and Kalow, W., Variability in caffeine metabolism, *Clin. Pharmacol. Ther.*, 33, 591, 1983.

40. Bell, D.A. et al., Polyadenylation polymorphism in the acetyltransferase 1 gene (NAT1) increases risk of colorectal cancer, *Cancer Res.*, 55, 3537, 1995.

41. Badawi, A.F. et al., Role of aromatic amine acetyltransferases, NAT1 and NAT2, in carcinogen-DNA adduct formation in the human urinary bladder, *Cancer Res.*, 55, 5230, 1995.

42. Yang, M. et al., Relationship between NAT1 genotype and phenotype in a Japanese population, *Pharmacogenetics*, 10, 225, 2000.

43. de Leon, J.H., Vatsis, K.P., and Weber, W.W., Characterization of naturally occurring and recombinant human N-acetyltransferase variants encoded by NAT1, *Mol. Pharmacol.*, 58, 288, 2000.

44. Hein, D.W., Molecular genetics and function of NAT1 and NAT2: role in aromatic amine metabolism and carcinogenesis, *Mutat. Res.*, 506–507, 65, 2002.

45. Doll, M.A. and Hein, D.W., Rapid genotype method to distinguish frequent and/or functional polymorphisms in human N-acetyltransferase-1, *Anal. Biochem.*, 301, 328, 2002.

46. Fretland, A.J. et al., Functional characterization of nucleotide polymorphisms in the coding region of N-acetyltransferase 1, *Pharmacogenetics*, 11, 511, 2001.

47. Fretland, A.J. et al., Functional characterization of human N-acetyltransferase 2 (NAT2) single nucleotide polymorphisms, *Pharmacogenetics*, 11, 207, 2001.

48. Leff, M.A. et al., Novel human N-acetyltransferase 2 alleles that differ in mechanism for slow acetylator phenotype, *J. Biol. Chem.*, 274, 34519, 1999.

49. Hasegawa, R. et al., Dose-dependence of 2-amino-1-methyl-6-phenylimidazo[4,5-b]-pyridine (PhIP) carcinogenicity in rats, *Carcinogenesis*, 14, 2553, 1993.

50. Nakagama, H. et al., A rat colon cancer model induced by 2-amino-1-methyl-6-phenylimidazo[4,5-b]pyridine, PhIP, *Mutat. Res.*, 506–507, 137, 2002.

51. Tudek, B., Bird, R.P., and Bruce, W.R., Foci of aberrant crypts in the colons of mice and rats exposed to carcinogens associated with foods, *Cancer Res.*, 49, 1236, 1989.

52. Pretlow, T.P. et al., Aberrant crypts: putative preneoplastic foci in human colonic mucosa, *Cancer Res.*, 51, 1564, 1991.

53. Takayama, T. et al., Aberrant crypt foci of the colon as precursors of adenoma and cancer, *N. Engl. J. Med.*, 339, 1277, 1998.

54. Hein, D.W., A new model for toxic risk assessments: construction of homozygous rapid and slow acetylator congenic Syrian hamster lines, *Toxicol. Methods*, 1, 44, 1991.

55. Hein, D.W. et al., Metabolic activation of N-hydroxy-2-aminofluorene and N-hydroxy-2-acetylaminofluorene by monomorphic N-acetyltransferase (NAT1) and polymorphic N-acetyltransferase (NAT2) in colon cytosols of Syrian hamsters congenic at the NAT2 locus, *Cancer Res.*, 53, 509, 1993.

56. Fretland, A.J. et al., DNA adduct levels and absence of tumors in female rapid and slow acetylator congenic hamsters administered the rat mammary carcinogen 2-amino-1-methyl-6-phenylimidazo[4,5-b] pyridine, *J. Biochem. Mol. Toxicol.*, 15, 26-33, 2001.

57. Purewal, M. et al., 2-Amino-1-methyl-6-phenylimidazo[4,5-b]pyridine induces a higher number of aberrant crypt foci in Fischer 344 (rapid) than in Wistar Kyoto (slow) acetylator inbred rats, *Cancer Epidemiol. Biomarkers Prev.*, 9, 529, 2000.

58. Lang, N.P. et al., Role of aromatic amine acetyltransferase in human colorectal cancer, *Arch. Surg.*, 121, 1259, 1986.

59. Roberts-Thomson, I.C. et al., Diet, acetylator phenotype, and risk of colorectal neoplasia, *Lancet*, 347, 1372, 1996.

60. Ilett, K.F., David, B.M., Detchon, P., Castleden, W.M., and Kwa, R., Acetylation phenotype in colorectal carcinoma, *Cancer Res.*, 47, 1466, 1987.

61. Ladero, J.M. et al., Acetylator polymorphism in human colorectal carcinoma, *Cancer Res.*, 51, 2098, 1991.

62. Kirlin, W.G. et al., Acetylator genotype-dependent expression of arylamine N-acetyltransferase in human colon cytosol from non-cancer and colorectal cancer patients, *Cancer Res.*, 51, 549, 1991.

63. Ishibe, N. et al., Genetic polymorphisms in heterocyclic amine metabolism and risk of colorectal adenomas, *Pharmacogenetics*, 12, 145, 2002.
64. Katoh, T. et al., Inherited polymorphism in the N-acetyltransferase 1 (NAT1) and 2 (NAT2) genes and susceptibility to gastric and colorectal adenocarcinoma, *Int. J. Cancer*, 85, 46, 2000.
65. Tiemersma, E.W. et al., Risk of colorectal adenomas in relation to meat consumption, meat preparation, and genetic susceptibility in a Dutch population, *Cancer Causes Control*, 15, 225, 2004.
66. Le Marchand, L. et al., Combined effects of well-done red meat, smoking, and rapid N-acetyltransferase 2 and CYP1A2 phenotypes in increasing colorectal cancer risk, *Cancer Epidemiol. Biomarkers Prev.*, 10, 1259, 2001.
67. Chen, K., Jiang, Q.T., and He, H.Q., Relationship between metabolic enzyme polymorphism and colorectal cancer, *World J. Gastroenterol.*, 11, 331, 2005.
68. Welfare, M.R. et al., Relationship between acetylator status, smoking, and diet and colorectal cancer risk in the north-east of England, *Carcinogenesis*, 18, 1351, 1997.
69. Murtaugh, M.A. et al., Meat consumption patterns and preparation, genetic variants of metabolic enzymes, and their association with rectal cancer in men and women, *J. Nutr.*, 134, 776, 2004.
70. Oda, Y., Tanaka, M., and Nakanishi, I., Relation between the occurrence of K-ras gene point mutations and genotypes of polymorphic N-acetyltransferase in human colorectal carcinomas, *Carcinogenesis*, 15, 1365, 1994.
71. Deitz, A.C. et al., Impact of misclassification in genotype-exposure interaction studies: example of N-acetyltransferase 2 (NAT2), smoking, and bladder cancer, *Cancer Epidemiol. Biomarkers Prev.*, 13, 1543, 2004.
72. Sinha, R. and Rothman, N., Role of well-done, grilled red meat, heterocyclic amines (HCAs) in the etiology of human cancer, *Cancer Lett.*, 143, 189, 1999.
73. Cantwell, M. et al., Relative validity of a food frequency questionnaire with a meat-cooking and heterocyclic amine module, *Cancer Epidemiol. Biomarkers Prev.*, 13, 293, 2004.
74. Ritchie, M.D. et al., Multifactor-dimensionality reduction reveals high-order interactions among estrogen-metabolism genes in sporadic breast cancer, *Am. J. Hum. Genet.*, 69, 138, 2001.
75. Ritchie, M.D., Hahn, L.W., and Moore, J.H., Power of multifactor dimensionality reduction for detecting gene–gene interactions in the presence of genotyping error, missing data, phenocopy, and genetic heterogeneity, *Genet. Epidemiol.*, 24, 150, 2003.
76. Hahn, L.W., Ritchie, M.D., and Moore, J.H., Multifactor dimensionality reduction software for detecting gene–gene and gene–environment interactions, *Bioinformatics*, 19, 376, 2003.
77. Hahn, L.W. and Moore, J.H., Ideal discrimination of discrete clinical endpoints using multilocus genotypes, *In Silico Biol.*, 4, 183, 2004.
78. Moore, J.H., Computational analysis of gene-gene interactions using multifactor dimensionality reduction, *Expert. Rev. Mol. Diagn.*, 4, 795, 2004.
79. Coffey, C.S. et al., An application of conditional logistic regression and multifactor dimensionality reduction for detecting gene–gene interactions on risk of myocardial infarction: the importance of model validation, *BMC Bioinformatics*, 5, 49, 2004.
80. Barrett, J.H. et al., Investigation of interaction between N-acetyltransferase 2 and heterocyclic amines as potential risk factors for colorectal cancer, *Carcinogenesis*, 24, 275, 2003.

81. Rodriguez, J.W. et al., Human acetylator genotype: relationship to colorectal cancer incidence and arylamine N-acetyltransferase expression in colon cytosol, *Arch. Toxicol.*, 67, 445, 1993.

82. Shibuta, K. et al., Molecular genotyping for N-acetylation polymorphism in Japanese patients with colorectal cancer, *Cancer*, 74, 3108, 1994.

83. Hubbard, A.L. et al., N-acetyltransferase 2 genotype in colorectal cancer and selective gene retention in cancers with chromosome 8p deletions, *Gut*, 41, 229, 1997.

84. Agundez, J.A.G. et al., N-acetyltransferase 2 (NAT2) genotype and colorectal carcinoma: risk variability according to tumour site, *Scand. J. Gastroenterol.*, 35, 1087, 2000.

85. Slattery, M.L. et al., NAT2, GSTM-1, cigarette smoking, and risk of colon cancer, *Cancer Epidemiol. Biomarkers Prev.*, 7, 1079, 1998.

86. van der Hel, O.L. et al., Rapid N-acetyltransferase 2 imputed phenotype and smoking may increase risk of colorectal cancer in women (Netherlands), *Cancer Causes Control*, 14, 293, 2003.

87. Sachse, C. et al., A pharmacogenetic study to investigate the role of dietary carcinogens in the etiology of colorectal cancer, *Carcinogenesis*, 23, 1839, 2002.

88. Butler, W.J., Ryan, P., and Roberts-Thomson, I.C., Metabolic genotypes and risk for colorectal cancer, *J. Gastroenterol. Hepatol.*, 16, 631, 2001.

11 Ferritin and Serine Hydroxymethyltransferase

Patrick J. Stover

CONTENTS

11.1 PHYSIOLOGICAL ROLE AND REGULATION OF FOLATE-MEDIATED ONE-CARBON METABOLISM

Tetrahydrofolate (THF) is an enzyme cofactor that chemically activates and carries single carbons on N^5 and/or N^{10} at three different oxidation states (Figure 11.1). This cofactor family donates and accepts one-carbons in a metabolic network known as one-carbon metabolism. Folate-mediated one-carbon metabolism occurs in the mitochondrial and cytoplasmic compartments of cells (Figure 11.2).[1] In the cytoplasm, 10-formyl THF cofactors carry activated formate that becomes the C^2 and C^8 of the purine ring, methylene THF carries activated formaldehyde for the methylation

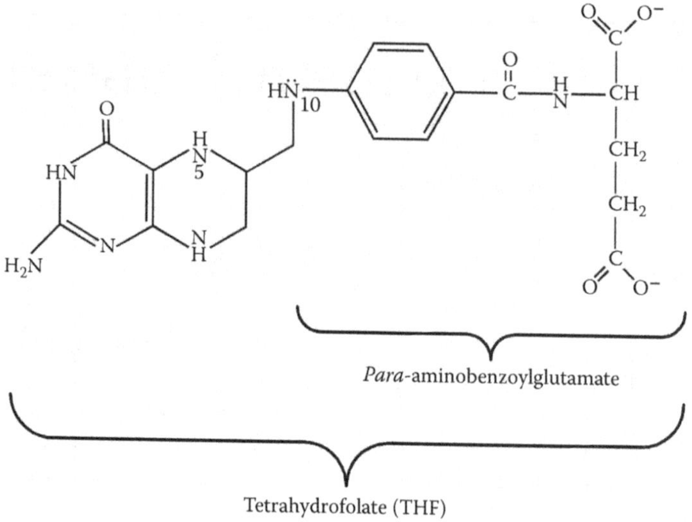

Para-aminobenzoylglutamate

Tetrahydrofolate (THF)

FIGURE 11.1 Structure of tetrahydrofolate. Tetrahydrofolate (THF) is a metabolic cofactor that carries and chemically activates single carbons on the N^5 or N^{10} position for one-carbon transfer reactions.

of 2′-deoxyuridine 5′-monophosphate (dUMP) to deoxythymidylate (dTMP), and 5-methyl THF carries activated methanol that is required for the folate-dependent methylation of homocysteine to methionine (Figure 11.2).[2] Methionine can be adenylated subsequently to form S-adenosylmethionine (AdoMet), which serves as a methyl-group donor for numerous methylation reactions.[3,4] This cytoplasmic network generates precursors for DNA and RNA synthesis, protein synthesis, DNA and protein methylation, phospholipids, and cell-signaling molecules and, therefore, is fundamental for cell growth and proliferation.[5] Almost immediately following the discovery of folate as a required metabolic cofactor for DNA synthesis, folate analogs or antifolates were developed that proved to be effective antimicrobial and antineoplasic agents.[6–9]

The primary function of mitochondrial folate metabolism is to generate formate from the catabolism of amino acids; it also generates 10-formyl-THF for mitochondrial fMet-tRNA$_i^{met}$ synthesis, although this function may not be essential.[10] Mitochondria-derived formate traverses to the cytoplasm where it is a major source of one-carbon units for cytoplasmic one-carbon metabolism (Figure 11.2).[1,11] The hydroxymethyl group of serine is a primary source of formate in most mammalian cells;[12] formate can also be generated in liver mitochondria from the folate-dependent catabolism of the amino acids glycine, sarcosine, and dimethylglycine.[11,13] Glycine is also a source of formate in kidney and astrocyte mitochondria, as well as in neurogenic regions of the brain.[13–17] Although the products of folate metabolism are required for all cells, folate metabolism is uniquely tailored in each cell type with respect to the source of single-carbon units, the mechanisms of folate import, and the expression of proteins that regulate folate metabolism.[18]

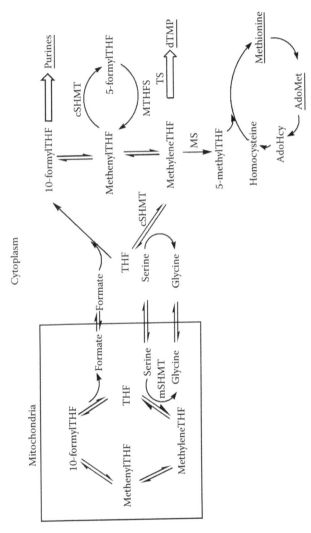

FIGURE 11.2 Folate-dependent one-carbon metabolism. Folate metabolism is required for the synthesis of purines and dTMP, and for the remethylation of homocysteine to methionine in the cytoplasm. Methionine can be adenylated to AdoMet, which serves as a cofactor for numerous methylation reactions. One-carbons are generated in the mitochondria primarily from the amino acid serine. mSHMT, mitochondrial serine hydroxymethyltransferase; cSHMT, cytoplasmic serine hydroxymethyltransferase; MTHFS, methenyltetrahydrofolate synthetase; TS, thymidylate synthase; MS, methionine synthase.

There is increasing evidence that folate-dependent biosynthetic pathways must compete for a limiting pool of folate cofactors and that the flux through any individual folate-dependent anabolic pathway may not be fully saturated.[18–21] The cellular concentration of folate-binding proteins exceeds that of folate derivatives, therefore, the concentration of free folate in the cell is negligible.[18,20,22] This metabolic competition is most pronounced for the two enzymes that utilize methylene THF: thymidylate synthase (TS) and methylenetetrahydrofolate reductase (MTHFR).[23] TS catalyzes the methylene THF-dependent synthesis of dTMP for DNA synthesis; MTHFR catalyzes the synthesis of 5-methyl THF from methylene THF, a reaction that commits one-carbon units to the methionine cycle (and AdoMet synthesis). Based on observations of monkeys rendered vitamin B_{12}-deficient through long-term nitrous oxide administration, Scott et al. proposed that limited methyl-group availability, caused either by folate or methionine deficiency, shifts the flux of one-carbon units among folate-dependent pathways that enables folate cofactors to be preferentially shuttled to the methionine cycle to protect methylation reactions and consequently suppress DNA synthesis.[21] A kinetic model that assumed MTHFR and TS compete directly for a common cellular pool of methylene THF reached similar conclusions; the model predicted that folate coenzymes are preferentially directed towards AdoMet synthesis at low cellular folate concentrations and that metabolic flux through the MTHFR enzyme would be insensitive to changes in methylene THF availability, whereas TS activity would be highly sensitive.[24] Such evidence indicates that dTMP and methionine synthesis are competitive reactions that coordinately regulate each other and that AdoMet synthesis may have priority over dTMP synthesis. Less understood is the effect of other folate-utilizing enzymes on this metabolic competition; especially those that display tissue-specific or inducible modes of regulation and thereby tailor one-carbon metabolism for cell-specific metabolism or enable homeostatic responses to metabolic or environmental stimuli.

11.2 IMPAIRMENTS IN FOLATE-MEDIATED ONE-CARBON METABOLISM

Disruptions in folate metabolism lead to pathologies that are specific for an individual tissue, including megaloblastic anemia, neural tube defects,[25,26] cardiovascular disease,[27–29] cancer,[30–34] and the inborn error, nonketotic hyperglycinaemia.[35,36] Folate metabolism can be impaired by folate and other B-vitamin deficiencies and/or genetic mutations and polymorphisms.[25,37–39]

Folate is essential for the synthesis, repair, and expression of the genome. Although the mechanism underlying folate-related pathologies are not well understood, impaired folate metabolism compromises both genome stability and genome expression, both of which are sensitive to the supply of methylene THF. Genome stability is compromised by increased mutation rates that can result from increased uracil content in DNA[30] and alterations in genome methylation patterns that disrupt chromatin structure. Folate deficiency depresses deoxythymidine triphosphate (dTTP) synthesis in humans,[30] which results in DNA with elevated uracil content because of the misincorporation of uracil into DNA during replication and repair.[30,40] Folate deficiency also impairs methionine synthesis, leading to elevations in homocysteine in serum and elevated cellular S-adenosylhomocysteine (AdoHcy) levels because the equilibrium for this hydrolysis reaction favors AdoHcy synthesis[3,23] (Figure 11.2). AdoHcy is a potent inhibitor of AdoMet-dependent methylation reactions, including DNA and protein methyltransferases,[3] leading to hypomethylated DNA and protein (including histones).[41,42] Alterations in DNA methylation alter chromatin structure leading to changes in gene expression, gene imprinting, and mutation rate.[43,44] Other established biomarkers of whole-body folate deficiency include low red blood cell folate concentrations, DNA hypomethylation, elevated formininoglutamate in urine, megaloblastic anemia, and neutrophil hypersegmentation.[29,45] However, biochemical mechanisms that detail the role of altered folate metabolism in the initiation or progression of these pathologies remain elusive.

Several penetrant single nucleotide polymorphisms (SNPs) have been identified in genes that encode enzymes involved in the one-carbon network and that modify the risk for folate-related pathologies. Allelic variants of the methylene THF gene, *MTHFR* (A222V), and methylene THF dehydrogenase gene, *MTHFD1* (R653Q), are associated with increased risk for neural tube defects, whereas the *MTHFR* A222V variant is protective against colon cancer in the absence of folate deficiency.[46,47] These polymorphisms are not in the Hardy–Weinberg equilibrium[5,46,48–50] (the percentage of individuals homozygous for the allelic variants is less than what is expected based on their allelic frequency), consistent with data indicating that the *MTHFR* A222V polymorphism is a risk factor for spontaneous miscarriage and decreased fetal viability.[48,51] The *MTHFR* A222V polymorphism is prevalent in Caucasian and Asian populations but is absent in most African populations.[52,53] The molecular mechanisms that account for the risk modification of neural tube defects and cancer by these allelic variants are unknown.

The *MTHFR* A222V is the most studied allelic variant that modifies folate metabolism.[54] The allelic variant encodes an enzyme that has reduced affinity for riboflavin cofactors, is thermolabile and, therefore, is associated with decreased MTHFR activity.[55] Carriers of the *MTHFR* A222V tend to display lower red blood cell folate levels and require higher dietary folate intake to reduce serum homocysteine levels.[56] Carriers of the *MTHFR* A222V variant exhibit DNA hypomethylation, which is a biomarker for impaired AdoMet-dependent methylation reactions.[41,57] However, because MTHFR and TS compete for methylene THF, carriers of the *MTHFR* A222V variant also exhibit increased flux of single-carbons through the dTMP synthesis pathway.[58] Either or both of these metabolic alterations could account for their risk modification of folate-related pathologies.

11.3 SERINE HYDROXYMETHYLTRANSFERASE

The best experimental evidence indicates that folate-associated pathologies result from impairments in the regulation and/or utilization of methylene THF. The enzyme, serine hydroxymethyltransferase (SHMT) is an important regulator of methylene THF. SHMT catalyzes the pyridoxal-phosphate-dependent and reversible interconversion of serine and THF to glycine and methylene THF:

$$\text{serine} + \text{THF} \leftrightarrow \text{glycine} + 5,10\text{-methylene THF}$$

The SHMT reaction is fully reversible *in vitro*, and under physiological concentrations of serine, glycine, THF, and methylene THF, the cSHMT enzymatic reaction is predicted to be freely reversible. The law of mass action predicts that the serine/glycine and THF/methylene THF ratios are critical in determining the directionality and, hence, the metabolic function of the enzyme. When catalyzing serine cleavage, this reaction generates one-carbon units for folate-dependent anabolic reactions and is the major source of one-carbon units in mammals (Figure 11.2).[58,59] When catalyzing serine synthesis, it can deplete the pool of folate-activated one-carbons for the one-carbon network. SHMT exists in both the mitochondria (mSHMT) and cytoplasm (cSHMT). The two proteins are encoded by distinct genes, have similar kinetic properties,[59–61] but display vastly different expression profiles and have distinct intracellular functions.[1,23]

11.3.1 Mitochondrial SHMT

The mSHMT isozyme is expressed at similar levels in human tissue and appears to function as a housekeeping gene.[59,60] Chinese hamster ovary (CHO) cells that lack mSHMT are auxotrophic for glycine[23,62,63] and display a one-carbon deficit in the cytoplasm, suggesting that the mSHMT enzyme is responsible for glycine synthesis and the generation of one-carbon units in these cells.[59]

11.3.2 Cytoplasmic SHMT

The cSHMT isozyme cannot compensate for the loss of mSHMT activity in CHO cells[62] and does not appear to be the primary source of glycine or one-carbon units in the cytoplasm.[23,60] Unlike the mSHMT expression profile, cSHMT mRNA is enriched only in the adult human liver, skeletal muscle, and kidney,[60] but it also appears to be present in lymphocytes and tumor cell lines.[23,64,65] Other adult tissues contain less than 5% of the levels found in liver,[60] which is consistent with previous studies that examined the level of SHMT activity in tissues. *In vivo* isotope studies indicate that cSHMT contributes one-carbon units for cytoplasmic metabolism in rats[66] and humans[12] (Figure 11.2), whereas other studies indicate that cSHMT catalyzes serine synthesis.[65,67] Therefore, cSHMT can perform different functions depending on the directionality of its reaction. Several metabolic functions have been ascribed to cSHMT as outlined in the following subsections.

11.3.2.1 Serine Synthesis for Gluconeogenesis

The high levels of cSHMT activity in liver and kidney indicate a role for cSHMT and cytoplasmic serine synthesis in gluconeogenesis, as glycine is a glucogenic amino acid.[17] Hepatic cSHMT may be required to meet fetal demands for serine during gestation; serine is not transported from the placenta to the fetus.[68]

11.3.2.2 Regulation of Methylene THF Pools

When the cSHMT enzyme catalyzes serine synthesis, it competes with MTHFR for methylene THF and depletes the supply of one-carbon units in the cytoplasm[23]

(Figure 11.2). Elevations in cellular glycine and/or methylene THF are necessary to drive the SHMT-catalyzed reaction toward serine synthesis. Consistent with this expectation, Fowler et al. demonstrated that human fibroblasts isolated from patients with decreased MTHFR activity displayed increased rates of cytoplasmic serine synthesis from glycine.[67] Furthermore, in nonketotic hyperglycinaemia, affected individuals lack a functional glycine cleavage system and exhibit elevated tissue and serum glycine concentrations. These patients also exhibit impaired utilization of methylene THF for methionine synthesis, as evidenced by marked elevations of homocysteine in the cerebrospinal fluid.[35] In cultured neuroblastoma cells, the directionality of the cSHMT catalyzed reaction is dependent upon glycine concentrations in the culture medium.[65] When glycine concentrations in the medium exceed 1 mM, the enzyme catalyzes serine synthesis and competes with MTHFR for methylene THF cofactors. Exogenous glycine availability also depletes both 5-methyl THF and AdoMet levels in MCF-7 cells.[23] It has also been proposed that SHMT-catalyzed serine synthesis may serve to enhance purine biosynthesis by shunting methylene THF derivatives away from homocysteine remethylation and regenerating THF for purine biosynthesis.[67]

The cSHMT-catalyzed serine synthesis may also serve to prevent the accumulation cellular 5-methyl THF levels by limiting the supply of methylene THF. 5-Methyl THF can accumulate in cells because its synthesis from methylene THF, catalyzed by MTHFR, is essentially irreversible *in vivo*; therefore, only the remethylation of homocysteine to methionine, catalyzed by methionine synthase, can deplete 5-methyl THF once it accumulates. In the most extreme case, inhibition of methionine synthase by nitric oxide results in the accumulation of intracellular folate as 5-methyl THF.[21,69] The accumulation of 5-methyl THF occurs at the expense of all other folate cofactors, which in turn inhibits purine and dTMP biosynthesis due to the depletion of 10-formyl THF and methylene THF cofactors. Therefore, inhibition of a single folate biosynthetic pathway and subsequent imbalances in the folate one-carbon pool has the potential to compromise all folate biosynthetic pathways. Feedback mechanisms exist to prevent the trapping of folate as 5-methyl THF, including the allosteric inhibition of MTHFR by AdoMet.[4] These mechanisms are important to maintain folate cofactor supply for all folate-dependent reactions. Although feedback inhibition of MTHFR activity by AdoMet plays a role in preventing the accumulation of 5-methyl THF, this mechanism alone may not be sufficient. The cSHMT enzyme may also contribute to the prevention of 5-methyl THF accumulation.

11.3.2.3   cSHMT as a Metabolic Switch

Stable isotope tracer studies have supported a role for cSHMT as a mediator of the competition for methylene THF through the dTMP and methionine biosynthetic pathways.[23] This switch function by cSHMT occurs by two independent mechanisms (Figure 11.3). First, methylene THF that is generated through the activity of cSHMT is preferentially shunted to the dTMP synthesis. Second, cSHMT inhibits the homocysteine remethylation pathway by sequestering 5-methyl THF, making it unavailable for the enzyme methionine synthase. *In vitro*, cSHMT binds 5-methyl THF tightly, and this binding activity inhibits its one-carbon transfer activity.[23,70] A

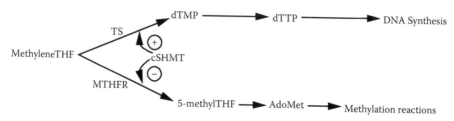

FIGURE 11.3 cSHMT as a metabolic switch. cSHMT serves as a metabolic switch by directing methylene THF to the dTMP pathway and by inhibiting AdoMet synthesis by sequestering 5-methyl THF and thereby making it unavailable for MTHFR.

twofold increase in cSHMT protein in MCF-7 cells resulted in a 90% reduction in intracellular AdoMet concentrations resulting from the sequestration of 5-methyl THF and the creation of a methyl trap similar to that seen in vitamin B_{12} deficiency[23] (Figure 11.2). Therefore, in systems where *cSHMT* is not highly expressed, methylene THF is preferentially directed towards AdoMet synthesis at the expense of dTMP synthesis.[21,23,24,71] Enhancement of *cSHMT* expression favors dTMP synthesis over AdoMet synthesis.[23] The metabolic changes observed in MCF-7 cells result from as little as twofold increases in cSHMT protein levels and are associated with dramatic alterations in the MCF-7 cell proteome profile,[72] indicating that small changes in *cSHMT* expression can have dramatic effects on metabolism (AdoMet levels) and the expression of many genes.[72] Collectively, these data support the hypothesis that homocysteine remethylation and nucleotide biosynthesis are competitive pathways for the substrate methylene THF, and that this metabolic competition is mediated in part by changes in cSHMT expression (Figure 11.3).

11.3.2.4 Biosynthesis of 5-Formyl THF

SHMT also catalyzes the hydrolysis of 5,10-methenyl THF to 5-formyl THF in the presence of glycine *in vitro* and *in vivo* (Figure 11.2). Yeast strains that completely lack SHMT activity have undetectable levels of 5-formyl THF, and *E. coli* and *Neurospora crassa* deficient in SHMT activity do not accumulate 5-formyl-THF.[10,73,74] 5-Formyl THF is the most chemically stable form of reduced folate,[75] and clinically, 5-formyl THF is known as *leucovorin*. It is administered to patients to elevate intracellular folate concentrations. 5-Formyl THF is unique as compared to other one-carbon-substituted forms of folate. It does not serve as a cofactor or one-carbon donor for one-carbon transfer reactions but, rather, is a powerful inhibitor of several folate-dependent enzymes including mammalian phosphoribosyl amino-imidazole-carboxamide (AICAR) transformylase (which is involved in the *de novo* purine biosynthesis pathway[76]), the cytoplasmic and mitochondrial isozymes of SHMT,[70] the glycine cleavage system (Stover, unpublished results) and, potentially, other folate-dependent enzymes.[75] Therefore, SHMT synthesizes its own endogenous slow-binding inhibitor, 5-formyl THF.[70,74] Neuroblastomas depleted of 5-formyl THF have increased cSHMT activity, suggesting that 5-formyl-THF is an effective inhibitor *in vivo*[65] and that 5-formyl THF regulates one-carbon metabolism *in vivo*.[75]

The enzyme 5,10-methenyltetrahydrofolate synthetase (MTHFS) (EC 6.3.3.2) is the only enzyme that uses 5-formyl THF as a substrate and catalyzes its irreversible conversion to methenyl THF in an ATP-requiring reaction (Figure 11.2). MTHFS activity is required to reintroduce 5-formyl THF back into the metabolically useful one-carbon cofactor pool; and deletion of the *MTHFS* gene in *S. cerevisiae* results in the accumulation of cellular folate as 5-formyl THF.[10] MTHFS is found exclusively in the cytoplasm of rabbit liver and human cell-culture lines;[65] one study of human liver indicated that 85% of MTHFS activity is cytoplasmic and 15% is mitochondrial.[76–78] Therefore, cellular concentrations of 5-formyl THF are regulated by a futile cycle involving the enzymes SHMT and MTHFS that functions in the cytoplasm and perhaps the mitochondria (Figure 11.2). The presence of MTHFS in many organisms ranging from bacteria and plants to mammals indicates that it plays an important role in one-carbon metabolism.[79,80] Because 5-formyl THF is the most stable reduced folate derivative, it may function as the primary storage form of folate in the cell.[75] Dormant cells such as *Neurospora crassa* spores and soy beans have high concentrations of 5-formyl THF, suggesting that 5-formyl THF may indeed function as the storage form of folate.[73] Therefore, MTHFS may play a critical role in regulating one-carbon metabolism through the modulation of 5-formyl THF levels. However, 5-formyl THF is not known to accumulate in mammalian cells and typically represents less than 5 to 10% of total cellular folate, which suggests that MTHFS tightly controls cellular 5-formyl THF levels.

11.4 REGULATION OF *cSHMT* EXPRESSION

Because the cSHMT enzyme functions as a metabolic switch that regulates both the methylene THF pool size as well as its partitioning between the dTMP and methionine synthesis pathways, it is an excellent candidate to investigate the etiology of folate associated pathologies. Furthermore, the regulation of cSHMT expression is expected to be a primary determinant of one-carbon flux through the folate-mediated one-carbon network (Figure 11.3). Studies to date indicate that cSHMT gene expression appears to be stringent and complex. The enzyme displays a wide range of tissue-specific expression and the mRNA undergoes alternative splicing patterns within the open reading frame and 5′ untranslated region.[60,81,82] The cSHMT enzyme may also autoregulate its own translation by binding to the 5′-untranslated region of its mRNA and inhibit translation[81] in a manner similar to what has been observed for other folate-dependent enzymes.[83–85]

The expression of *cSHMT* is also sensitive to nutrients, including zinc and retinoic acid. One study demonstrated that *cSHMT* mRNA levels were depleted in embryonic carcinoma cells that were stimulated to differentiate with retinoic acid;[86] no other studies have followed up this observation. However, the mechanism for the regulation of *cSHMT* expression by zinc has been demonstrated. Iron chelators inhibit transcription of the *cSHMT* gene in MCF-7 cells;[72] cells exposed to mimosine or deferoxamine lack cSHMT protein and mRNA after 24 h of exposure to these chelators. This effect is cell-specific; cSHMT protein levels are not affected by iron chelators in human neuroblastoma or hepatoma cells.[72] Mimosine-responsive elements were identified and characterized in the *cSHMT* promoter of MCF-7 cells and found to be *cis*-elements that bind the zinc-finger transcription factors MTF-1 and Sp1.[87] Iron chelators bind zinc with high affinity and can deplete the labile intracellular zinc pool in cultured murine thymocytes.[88,89] In humans, chronic deferiprone treatment for iron overload is associated with zinc deficiency,[89,90] which may account for thymocyte apoptosis during therapy.[89] The effect of iron chelators on *cSHMT* expression could be recapitulated by removal of zinc from the culture medium, indicating that iron chelators impair *cSHMT* expression by chelating zinc. The cell-specific regulation of *cSHMT* transcription by the zinc-sensing transcription factor MTF-1 indicates that the one-carbon network is sensitive to zinc status, and this has been demonstrated in an animal study. Rats fed zinc-deficient diets displayed 65% lower plasma homocysteine concentrations and had reduced hepatic 5-methyl THF concentrations relative to animals on a control, zinc-replete diet.[91] Although the mechanism for this observation in animals has not been established, the effects of zinc depletion on one-carbon metabolism are consistent with cell-culture studies that demonstrate an attenuation of *cSHMT* expression during zinc depletion[87] and subsequent derepression of the homocysteine remethylation cycle.[23] Collectively, these studies suggest that cSHMT activity plays specialized regulatory functions in different tissues, and its expression and activity are responsive to environmental stimuli.

11.5 IRON–FOLATE RELATIONSHIPS

Over the past 40 years, iron deficiency (ID) has been demonstrated to impair folate metabolism in cell-culture models, animal models, and in humans, but the underlying biochemical mechanisms that account for these effects have never been established.[45,92,93] Iron deficient rats display elevated secretion of formiminoglutamate, a clinical index of 5-methyl THF trapping or folate deficiency.[45,94,95] In humans, ID, in the absence of frank whole-body folate deficiency, can result in morphological alterations in granulocytes that are similar to those observed in folate deficiency[96] as well as neutrophil hypersegmentation, which is indicative of cobalamin and/or folate deficiency.[97] Folate- or cobalamin-deficiency induced megaloblastosis results from impaired DNA synthesis; neutrophil hypersegmentation has been proposed to result from accumulation or trapping of cellular folate as 5-methyl THF.[96]

In addition, maternal iron deficiency decreases secretion of folate into milk by up to 75%[45,94,95,98,99] without decreasing maternal serum or red blood cell folate levels in rats. Although no mechanism has been established that accounts for the effects of iron deficiency on milk folate content, the best evidence indicates that the mammary secretary cells are unable to accumulate folate and therefore do not secrete adequate levels of folate into milk.[45,94] However, the biochemical mechanisms underlying the influence of iron deficiency on folate metabolism are only beginning to be elucidated.[18,19,72]

11.6 FERRITIN

Ferritin is a heterogeneous spherical oligomer, composed of 24 heavy (HCF) and light chain (LCF) subunits,[100,101] that functions to chelate and store cellular iron.

HCF has ferroxidase activity; it binds cellular Fe^{++} and catalyzes its oxidation to Fe^{+++} for storage in the mineral core of the sphere.[100,102,103] LCF does not contain the ferroxidase activity but may function to promote iron mineralization at the core.[100] The relative ratio of heavy and light chain subunits in the ferritin polymer exhibits tissue-specific variation. Liver ferritin is composed mostly of LCF subunits, whereas heart contains mostly HCF subunits.[100] The cellular concentration of HCF predicts the rate of iron uptake into ferritin, and increased expression of *HCF* in cells depletes the labile or free iron pool in cells.[104,105] Free iron catalyzes the Fenton reaction, the generation of hydroxyl radicals (OH·) from hydrogen peroxide (H_2O_2) and superoxide O_2^-.[106] Iron chelation by ferritin reduces the intracellular concentration of reactive oxygen species, including the OH· and thereby protects the cell from oxidative damage.[105,107]

11.7 FOLATE–FERRITIN INTERACTIONS

11.7.1 REGULATION OF CELLULAR FOLATE ACCUMULATION

Folate catabolism refers to the irreversible oxidative degradation of folate cofactors. *In vitro*, folates are unstable and sensitive to oxidative degradation with the exception of 5-formyl THF.[108,109] Until recently, *in vivo* folate catabolism was believed to result from the nonregulated, nonenzymatic degradation of labile folate cofactors. Folate catabolism often results in the formation of the degradation product *para*-aminobenzoylglutamate (*p*-ABG) or its acetylated form acetyl*p*ABG (A*p*ABG) (Figure 11.1). Urinary A*p*ABG is indicative of folate catabolism and is a indicator of folate status[110] and turnover in rats[111,112] and humans.[113] Accelerated rates of folate catabolism or turnover are observed during certain physiological states, including cancer and perhaps pregnancy;[18] increased rates of folate catabolism can deplete cellular folate concentrations in a tissue-specific manner[19] and may account for differences in rates of folate turnover among tissues.[114,115]

Cellular folate accumulation is a function of uptake, polyglutamylation, export, and turnover.[8,11,18,116] Carrier proteins[117] and/or folate receptors[116] transport folate monoglutamates into cells, which must be converted polyglutamate forms of folate to accumulate in the cytoplasm.[11] The addition of the polyglutamate polypeptide to folate derivatives increases its affinity for folate-binding proteins and aids in cellular retention of the cofactor.[2] Alternatively, folate monoglutamates are transported into mitochondria[118] and converted to polyglutamate cofactors in that compartment which accounts for about 50% of total cellular folate.[119,120] Disruption of folate transport and polyglutamylation impairs folate accumulation in all cells,[121] but tissue-specific folate deficiencies can occur in the absence of dietary or whole-body deficiency.

A protein capable of catalyzing the formation of *p*ABG from 5-formyl THF was isolated from rat liver extracts.[19] The protein was identified to be HCF and is the only protein identified to date that catalyzes the catabolism of folate. HCF was shown to play a major role in regulating intracellular folate concentrations in cell cultures; it determined the upper level of folate accumulation independent of folate availability in the culture medium.[18,19] Increased expression of rat HCF two- to fourfold over endogenous HCF concentrations in CHO cells increased rates of folate turnover and reduced intracellular folate concentrations by 15% relative to control cells when cultured with medium containing pharmacological levels of folic acid (2 µM), and by 40% when cultured in folate-depleted medium for 48 h. Folate becomes less susceptible to HCF-mediated catabolism with increased residency time in the cell, indicating that newly imported monoglutamate folates are most vulnerable to degradation. This indicates that HCF-mediated folate catabolism can prevent newly imported folate entering into "stable pools," and that folate derivatives are protected from HCF-mediated catabolism once they enter a stable pool. The identification of the HCF-mediated folate-catabolism pathway in cell cultures may account for observations of tissue-specific folate deficiencies that occur in the absence of systemic folate deficiency in patients and animals.[18]

Physiological states associated with increased folate catabolism correlate with increased *HCF* expression. *HCF* message levels are markedly elevated during the implantation stage of pregnancy in the rat.[122] Compared to levels of *HCF* mRNA normally found in the uteri of nonpregnant (estrous cycle) rats, *HCF* mRNA increased eight- to tenfold in pregnant rats. The *HCF* mRNA and protein-expression profiles parallel progesterone concentrations, which are low in the estrous cycle, surge after fertilization, and remain high until parturition, when they drop sharply. *HCF* mRNA also declines rapidly after parturition.[122] Increased *HCF* expression during pregnancy was localized primarily in the cytoplasm of endometrial stromal cells whereas *LCF* mRNA expression did not change appreciably. Progesterone alone can induce *HCF* message levels in male and female rats.[122]

There is also evidence that increased rates of folate catabolism occur in cancer and lead to folate deficiency. Tumor cells exhibit increased rates of folate uptake,[34] and large doses of folate in well-established cancers lead to accelerated proliferation whereas folate deprivation leads to reduced or delayed growth.[34] Tumor cells also display increased rates of folate catabolism. Folate catabolism is increased by 50% in mice with ascitic tumors as measured by the urinary catabolites, [^{3}H]pABG and [^{3}H]N-ApABG.[123] Cancer patients with active or metastatic malignancies exhibit folate deficiency without evidence of malnourishment, malabsorption, or increased intact folate excretion.[34] Localized tissue deficiency has been observed in patients with colorectal adenoma whose normal mucosa had significantly lower folate levels in comparison to patients with nonneoplastic polyps, in the absence of significantly low serum or red blood cell folate concentrations.[124] In other studies, the folate content of neoplastic cells was significantly lower than that in adjacent normal cells.[125] Increased folate catabolism in cancerous tissue correlates with elevated HCF levels. Increased ferritin expression has been observed in leukemic cells,[126] kidney cancer,[127,128] and mammary carcinomas[129,130] relative to normal tissue. Patients with malignant breast carcinoma showed a sevenfold increase in tissue cytosol ferritin compared to those with benign breast disease.[131] Increased ferritin levels in cancer cells may be influenced by expression of the oncogene *c-myc*. *HCF* and *c-myc* message levels are elevated in rats with chemically induced hepatocellular carcinoma. In this same model, the expression of *HCF* increased tenfold as the tumor progressed.[132] The relationship between *c-myc* and *HCF* expression was validated in cell culture. Transfection of nontumorigenic clones with the *c-myc* cDNA increased expression of *HCF* mRNA in clones that acquired a tumorigenic phenotype.[133] Wu et al.[132] found increased *HCF* mRNA expression in patients with hepatocellular carcinoma but not in patients with benign tumors (adenomas), cirrhosis, or in healthy patients. *HCF* mRNA levels were two- to twelvefold higher in tumors as compared to adjacent nontumor tissues in 70% of patients and were highly correlated with *c-myc* mRNA levels in most of the patients.[134] Therefore, these studies indicate that HCF plays an important role in regulating folate concentrations, and that the increased rates of folate catabolism and folate deficiency seen in tumors may result from increased HCF synthesis.

Increased rates of folate catabolism, as occurs during cancer and pregnancy, suggest that folate turnover may be a regulated process. The biochemical advantages associated with increased rates of folate catabolism during states of rapid cell division, including cancer and pregnancy, are not obvious. Maintaining low cellular folate concentrations may be advantageous by promoting (a) metabolic channeling of folate cofactors among folate-dependent enzymes and (b) enabling competitive regulation of folate metabolic pathways. Channeling of folate cofactors has been shown to increase enzyme activities by decreasing K_m and increasing k_{cat} values relative to transfer by diffusion,[20,135] and *in vitro* reconstituted folate-dependent metabolic pathways function optimally when folate levels are present in subsaturating concentrations, such that the receiving enzyme active site is open and unliganded.[135] Maintaining subsaturating levels of cellular folate enables metabolic competition for folate cofactors among the metabolic pathways within the one-carbon network, and this competition may serve a regulatory function as proposed by Scott.[136]

11.7.2 REGULATION OF *cSHMT* EXPRESSION BY FERRITIN

Expression of the *HCF* cDNA in human cell cultures increases cSHMT protein levels without affecting *cSHMT* mRNA levels by increasing the *cSHMT* translation rate through the *cSHMT* 5′ untranslated region.[72] *LCF* expression does not influence cSHMT levels.[72] Ferritin induced elevations in cSHMT protein leads to increased rates of dTMP synthesis and impaired AdoMet synthesis, consistent with a role for cSHMT as an HCF-responsive metabolic switch.[23] The mechanisms for HCF activation of *cSHMT* translation are not known, but it has been established that HCF is an mRNA-binding protein.[137]

11.8 FOLATE AND CARCINOGENESIS

Numerous studies have established a role for dietary folate in cancer susceptibility and prevention.[32,47,138–142] Results from epidemiological, genetic, biochemical, and animal studies are revealing that impairments in folate metabolism contribute to the initiation and progression of epithelial and other cancers, especially colon cancer.[32,34,47,140–142] Two general mechanisms have been proposed to account for the many associations between altered folate metabolism and colon cancer. All of the proposed mechanisms are speculative[32] and have not been rigorously validated in experimental animal models.

11.8.1 Mechanism 1: Alteration of DNA Methylation

Approximately 4% of cytosine bases within the mammalian genome are modified by methylation, and both genome-wide and allele-specific DNA methylation is influenced by folate metabolism.[143] Methylated cytosine residues are located in CpG islands, which are dinucleotide repeat sequences commonly found in the 5′ promoter regions of genes. Up to 90% of cytosine bases are methylated within CpG islands.[144] The association between DNA methylation and carcinogenesis represents a paradox. Genome-wide DNA hypomethylation occurs in nearly all cancers and precedes mutational and chromosomal abnormalities that occur as cancer progresses (the so-called hypermutable phenotype),[34] whereas allelic-specific hypermethylation and gene silencing occur concurrently.[139,144] That is, global DNA hypomethylation proceeds and may trigger allelic-specific DNA hypermethylation.[34] DNA hypomethylation, which can be induced by folate-deficiency, has two primary effects on the mammalian genome. First, folate deficiency-induced DNA hypomethylation (and, potentially, histone hypomethylation) can influence the expression of genes regulated by methylation.[41,145,146] Second, DNA hypomethylation relaxes chromatin structure[147] and thereby may enhance the accessibility of DNA to damaging agents, resulting in increased genomic mutation (hypermutable phenotype), particularly in "hot spots" that are associated with cancers.[44,148] In support of this mechanism, rodents fed diets deficient in folate and other sources of methyl groups were shown to be more susceptible to chemically induced hepatocarcinoma,[149,150] although other similar studies did not observe any protective effect for folate in chemically induced tumors.[151–153]

Two lines of evidence support a role for genetic modulation of DNA methylation in folate-associated cancer risk. Reduced expression and activity of cytosine DNA methyltransferase (*dmnt1*) dramatically decreases the number of adenomas that occur from loss of p53 activity in mouse models,[154] indicating that loss of DNA methylation by some mechanisms can protect against colon cancer. Furthermore, humans with the *MTHFR* A222V variant have a much lower specific activity of this enzyme and, subsequently, a reduced capacity to remethylate homocysteine and generate AdoMet.[47,155] Homozygotes for this polymorphism have a 40% decreased incidence of colorectal cancer compared to those with heterozygous or normal genotypes, in the absence of folate deficiency. However, it must be emphasized that the protection afforded by the polymorphism is lost with folate deficiency.[47] Therefore, it is unlikely that genome-wide hypomethylation resulting from folate deficiency alone is protective against cancer, but DNA hypomethylation resulting from reduced DNMT1 or MTHFR activity may be protective or is merely associated with the protection. In summary, the relationships between alterations in DNA methylation and risk for colon cancer are not understood and mechanisms are not established.

11.8.2 Mechanism 2: Increased Mutation Rates

Folate deficiency in cell cultures results in imbalances in the dNTP pools and increases uracil concentration in DNA and the number of chromosomal breaks.[156,157] All of these abnormalities can be reversed by folate repletion of the culture medium.

Tumors also display these biochemical characteristics.[34] In humans and rodents, folate status correlates inversely with uracil content in DNA, presumably resulting from impaired dTMP synthesis and subsequent elevations in dUTP pools. Once uracil is incorporated into DNA, excision repair of uracil from DNA has the potential to result in strand breaks if the residues are in close proximity and are located on opposite strands of the helix. *In vitro* studies have demonstrated that a linearization of plasmid DNA occurs when uracil residues are placed within circular plasmid DNA following addition of the repair enzyme, uracil DNA glycosylase.[158] Imbalances in the dNTP pool may increase the error associated with DNA polymerase activity, as well as excision repair enzymes. This mechanism may be consistent with associational studies that demonstrate a protective effect of the *MTHFR* A222V variant in human colon cancer.[47] Because both DNA synthesis and homocysteine remethylation compete for a limited pool of folate cofactors,[21,23,67,159] impairment of homocysteine remethylation, as occurs with the *MTHFR* variant allele, will increase the availability of methylene THF for conversion of dUTP to dTTP, thereby lowering uracil content in DNA.[32] However, direct proof of this mechanism is lacking.

Impairments in folate metabolism can result in the simultaneous mutation of DNA and epigenetic alterations in genome expression induced by hypomethylation. Hypomethylation may also create an environment that permits increased rates of DNA mutation and these alterations in methylation density may be loci specific. Therefore, both increased DNA mutation rates and alterations in genome methylation may function in concert during cellular transformation and cannot be considered in isolation during experimentation.

11.9 FUTURE PROSPECTS: HCF AND cSHMT INTERACTIONS IN CANCER PREVENTION

There is increasing evidence that the interactions between HCF and cSHMT may play an important role in both the initiation and progression of cellular transformation, and that this interaction may be an attractive target for nutritional prevention of cancer. Elevated *HCF* expression in cancers have been established and, although less studied, SHMT activity has been shown to be increased in human and rat colonic tumors,[160] and a prevalent single-nucleotide polymorphism in the *cSHMT* gene (L474F) has been shown to be associated with protection against leukemia[161] and lymphoma.[162]

The physiological functions of may prevent cancer initiation, but enable growth of established tumors and, therefore, exhibit both pro- and anticarcinogenic properties. The induction of *cSHMT* expression provides a second mechanism whereby HCF may prevent the initiation of cellular transformation. Increased expression of *cSHMT*, induced by HCF or other stimuli, has the same metabolic consequences on the one-carbon network as the *MTHFR* A222V polymorphism that is protective against colon cancer; it suppresses methionine (AdoMet) biosynthesis and enhances dTMP synthesis. HCF-mediated alterations in folate metabolism may function in concert with HCF-mediated reduction in reactive oxygen species to lower DNA mutation rates. In support of this hypothesis, *HCF* is a Nrf2-regulated gene and its expression is induced by chemoprotective dithiolethiones.[163,164] Furthermore, *HCF* expression, and subsequent reduction in the labile iron pool, is induced by NF-κB through TNF-α. Increased *HCF* expression and reduction in reactive oxygen species is critical to the antioxidant and antiapoptotic activities of NF-κB[105,107] and to the acute-phase response to stress, injury, and infection. In established tumors, increased *HCF*-expression is associated with aggressive tumors and resistance to anticancer therapies; the same functions that prevent cellular transformation have been proposed to contribute to NF-κB-dependent chemoresistance.[105] The roles of HCF-induced alterations in folate metabolism during apoptosis, the acute-phase response, cancer initiation, and tumor growth are virtually unknown. However, continued investigation of the many functions of HCF and its coordinated regulation of oxidative stress, apoptosis, and folate metabolism (including impact on genome integrity, mutation rate, and methylation) will open new avenues for understanding the mechanisms of cellular transformation and the nutritional and metabolic etiology of cancer; these advances will ultimately lead to more informed approaches for cancer prevention.

REFERENCES

1. Appling, D.R. Compartmentation of folate-mediated one-carbon metabolism in eukaryotes. *FASEB J* 5, 2645, 1991.
2. Shane, B. Folylpolyglutamate synthesis and role in the regulation of one-carbon metabolism. *Vitam Horm* 45, 263, 1989.
3. Clarke, S. and Banfield, K. S-adenosylmethionine-dependent methyltransferases, in *Homocysteine in Health and Disease*. Eds., Carmel, R. and Jacobson, D.W. Cambridge University Press, Cambridge, 2001.
4. Finkelstein, J.D. Pathways and regulation of homocysteine metabolism in mammals. *Semin Thromb Hemost* 26, 219, 2000.
5. Stover, P.J. Physiology of folate and vitamin B12 in health and disease. *Nutr Rev* 62, S3, 2004.
6. Kisliuk, R.L. Synergistic interactions among antifolates. *Pharmacol Ther* 85, 183, 2000.
7. Kisliuk, R.L. Deaza analogs of folic acid as antitumor agents. *Curr Pharm Des* 9, 2615, 2003.
8. Moran, R.G. Roles of folylpoly-gamma-glutamate synthetase in therapeutics with tetrahydrofolate antimetabolites: an overview. *Semin Oncol* 26, 24, 1999.
9. Zhao, R. and Goldman, I.D. Resistance to antifolates. *Oncogene* 22, 7431, 2003.
10. Holmes, W.B. and Appling, D.R. Cloning and characterization of methenyltetrahydrofolate synthetase from *Saccharomyces cerevisiae*. *J Biol Chem* 277, 20205, 2002.
11. Shane, B. Folate chemistry and metabolism, in *Folate in Health and Disease*. Ed., Bailey, L.B., Marcel Dekker, New York, 1995.
12. Davis, S.R. et al. Tracer-derived total and folate-dependent homocysteine remethylation and synthesis rates in humans indicate that serine is the main one-carbon donor. *Am J Physiol Endocrinol Metab* 286, E272, 2004.
13. Wagner, C. Biochemical role of folate in cellular metabolism, in *Folate in Health and Disease*. Ed., Bailey, L.B., Marcel Dekker, New York, 1995.
14. Ichinohe, A. et al. Glycine cleavage system in neurogenic regions. *Eur J Neurosci* 19, 2365, 2004.

15. Sato, K., Yoshida, S., Fujiwara, K., Tada, K., and Tohyama, M. Glycine cleavage system in astrocytes. *Brain Res* 567, 64, 1991.

16. Kure, S., Koyata, H., Kume, A., Ishiguro, Y., and Hiraga, K. The glycine cleavage system: the coupled expression of the glycine decarboxylase gene and the H-protein gene in the chicken. *J Biol Chem* 266, 3330, 1991.

17. Cowin, G.J., Willgoss, D.A., and Endre, Z.H. Modulation of glycine-serine interconversion by TCA and glycolytic intermediates in normoxic and hypoxic proximal tubules. *Biochim Biophys Acta* 1310, 41, 1996.

18. Suh, J.R., Herbig, A.K., and Stover, P.J. New perspectives on folate catabolism. *Annu Rev Nutr* 21, 255, 2001.

19. Suh, J.R., Oppenheim, E.W., Girgis, S., and Stover, P.J. Purification and properties of a folate-catabolizing enzyme. *J Biol Chem* 275, 35646, 2000.

20. Schirch, V. and Strong, W.B. Interaction of folylpolyglutamates with enzymes in one-carbon metabolism. *Arch Biochem Biophys* 269, 371, 1989.

21. Scott, J.M., Dinn, J.J., Wilson, P., and Weir, D.G. Pathogenesis of subacute combined degeneration: a result of methyl group deficiency. *Lancet* 2, 334, 1981.

22. Strong, W.B., Tendler, S.J., Seither, R.L., Goldman, I.D., and Schirch, V. Purification and properties of serine hydroxymethyltransferase and C1-tetrahydrofolate synthase from L1210 cells. *J Biol Chem* 265, 12149, 1990.

23. Herbig, K. et al. Cytoplasmic serine hydroxymethyltransferase mediates competition between folate-dependent deoxyribonucleotide and S-adenosylmethionine biosyntheses. *J Biol Chem* 277, 38381, 2002.

24. Green, J.M., MacKenzie, R.E., and Matthews, R.G. Substrate flux through methylenetetrahydrofolate dehydrogenase: predicted effects of the concentration of methylenetetrahydrofolate on its partitioning into pathways leading to nucleotide biosynthesis or methionine regeneration. *Biochemistry* 27, 8014, 1988.

25. van der Put, N.M. and Blom, H.J. Neural tube defects and a disturbed folate dependent homocysteine metabolism. *Eur J Obstet Gynecol Reprod Biol* 92, 57, 2000.

26. Scott, J.M. Evidence of folic acid and folate in the prevention of neural tube defects. *Bibl Nutr Dieta*, 192, 2001.

27. Ueland, P.M., Refsum, H., Beresford, S.A., and Vollset, S.E. The controversy over homocysteine and cardiovascular risk. *Am J Clin Nutr* 72, 324, 2000.

28. Gerhard, G.T. and Duell, P.B. Homocysteine and atherosclerosis. *Curr Opin Lipidol* 10, 417, 1999.

29. Lindenbaum, J. and Allen, R.H. Clinical spectrum and diagnosis of folate deficiency, in *Folate in Health and Disease*. Ed., Bailey, L.B. Marcel Dekker, New York, 1995.

30. Blount, B.C. et al. Folate deficiency causes uracil misincorporation into human DNA and chromosome breakage: implications for cancer and neuronal damage. *Proc Natl Acad Sci U S A* 94, 3290, 1997.

31. Ames, B.N. DNA damage from micronutrient deficiencies is likely to be a major cause of cancer. *Mutat Res* 475, 7, 2001.

32. Choi, S.W. and Mason, J.B. Folate and carcinogenesis: an integrated scheme. *J Nutr* 130, 129, 2000.

33. Pogribny, I.P. et al. Breaks in genomic DNA and within the p53 gene are associated with hypomethylation in livers of folate/methyl-deficient rats. *Cancer Res* 55, 1894, 1995.

34. Kim, Y.I. Folate and cancer prevention: a new medical application of folate beyond hyperhomocysteinemia and neural tube defects. *Nutr Rev* 57, 314, 1999.

35. Van Hove, J.L. et al. One-methyl group metabolism in non-ketotic hyperglycinaemia: mildly elevated cerebrospinal fluid homocysteine levels. *J Inherit Metab Dis* 21, 799, 1998.

36. Tada, K. and Kure, S. Non-ketotic hyperglycinaemia: molecular lesion, diagnosis and pathophysiology. *J Inherit Metab Dis* 16, 691, 1993.

37. Bailey, L.B. Folate requirements and dietary recommendations, in *Folate in Health and Disease.* Ed., Bailey, L.B. Marcel Dekker, New York, 1995.

38. McNulty, H. Folate requirements for health in different population groups. *Br J Biomed Sci* 52, 110, 1995.

39. Scott, J.M. How does folic acid prevent neural tube defects? *Nat Med* 4, 895, 1998.

40. Ames, B.N. Micronutrient deficiencies: a major cause of DNA damage. *Ann N Y Acad Sci* 889, 87, 1999.

41. Friso, S. et al. A common mutation in the 5,10-methylenetetrahydrofolate reductase gene affects genomic DNA methylation through an interaction with folate status. *Proc Natl Acad Sci U S A* 99, 5606, 2002.

42. Friso, S., Choi, S.W., Dolnikowski, G.G., and Selhub, J. A method to assess genomic DNA methylation using high-performance liquid chromatography/electrospray ionization mass spectrometry. *Anal Chem* 74, 4526, 2002.

43. Jubb, A.M., Bell, S.M., and Quirke, P. Methylation and colorectal cancer. *J Pathol* 195, 111, 2001.

44. Kim, M., Trinh, B.N., Long, T.I., Oghamian, S., and Laird, P.W. Dnmt1 deficiency leads to enhanced microsatellite instability in mouse embryonic stem cells. *Nucleic Acids Res* 32, 5742, 2004.

45. O'Connor, D.L. Interaction of iron and folate during reproduction. *Prog Food Nutr Sci* 15, 231, 1991.

46. Brody, L.C. et al. A polymorphism, R653Q, in the trifunctional enzyme methylenetetrahydrofolate dehydrogenase/methenyltetrahydrofolate cyclohydrolase/formyltetrahydrofolate synthetase is a maternal genetic risk factor for neural tube defects: report of the birth defects research group. *Am J Hum Genet* 71, 1207, 2002.

47. Ma, J. et al. Methylenetetrahydrofolate reductase polymorphism, dietary interactions, and risk of colorectal cancer. *Cancer Res* 57, 1098, 1997.

48. Nelen, W.L. et al. Homocysteine and folate levels as risk factors for recurrent early pregnancy loss. *Obstet Gynecol* 95, 519, 2000.

49. Nelen, W.L. et al. Methylenetetrahydrofolate reductase polymorphism affects the change in homocysteine and folate concentrations resulting from low dose folic acid supplementation in women with unexplained recurrent miscarriages. *J Nutr* 128, 1336, 1998.

50. Reyes-Engel, A. et al. Implications on human fertility of the 677C→T and 1298A→C polymorphisms of the MTHFR gene: consequences of a possible genetic selection. *Mol Hum Reprod* 8, 952, 2002.

51. Nelen, W.L., Blom, H.J., Steegers, E.A., den Heijer, M., and Eskes, T.K. Hyperhomocysteinemia and recurrent early pregnancy loss: a meta-analysis. *Fertil Steril* 74, 1196, 2000.

52. Shi, M., Caprau, D., Romitti, P., Christensen, K., and Murray, J.C. Genotype frequencies and linkage disequilibrium in the CEPH human diversity panel for variants in folate pathway genes MTHFR, MTHFD, MTRR, RFC1, and GCP2. *Birth Defects Res A Clin Mol Teratol* 67, 545, 2003.

53. Mutchinick, O.M., Lopez, M.A., Luna, L., Waxman, J., and Babinsky, V.E. High prevalence of the thermolabile methylenetetrahydrofolate reductase variant in Mexico: a country with a very high prevalence of neural tube defects. *Mol Genet Metab* 68, 461, 1999.

54. Goyette, P. et al. Human methylenetetrahydrofolate reductase: isolation of cDNA mapping and mutation identification. *Nat Genet* 7, 551, 1994.

55. Guenther, B.D. et al. The structure and properties of methylenetetrahydrofolate reductase from *Escherichia coli* suggest how folate ameliorates human hyperhomocysteinemia. *Nat Struct Biol* 6, 359, 1999.

56. Bailey, L.B. Folate, methyl-related nutrients, alcohol, and the MTHFR 677C→T polymorphism affect cancer risk: intake recommendations. *J Nutr* 133, 3748S, 2003.

57. Yi, P. et al. Increase in plasma homocysteine associated with parallel increases in plasma S-adenosylhomocysteine and lymphocyte DNA hypomethylation. *J Biol Chem* 275, 29318, 2000.

58. Quinlivan, E.P. et al. Methylenetetrahydrofolate reductase 677C→T polymorphism and folate status affect one-carbon incorporation into human DNA deoxynucleosides. *J Nutr* 135, 389, 2005.

59. Stover, P.J. et al. Molecular cloning, characterization, and regulation of the human mitochondrial serine hydroxymethyltransferase gene. *J Biol Chem* 272, 1842, 1997.

60. Girgis, S. et al. Molecular cloning, characterization and alternative splicing of the human cytoplasmic serine hydroxymethyltransferase gene. *Gene* 210, 315, 1998.

61. Garrow, T.A. et al. Cloning of human cDNAs encoding mitochondrial and cytosolic serine hydroxymethyltransferases and chromosomal localization. *J Biol Chem* 268, 11910, 1993.

62. Pfendner, W. and Pizer, L.I. The metabolism of serine and glycine in mutant lines of Chinese hamster ovary cells. *Arch Biochem Biophys* 200, 503, 1980.

63. Chasin, L.A., Feldman, A., Konstam, M., and Urlaub, G. Reversion of a Chinese hamster cell auxotrophic mutant. *Proc Natl Acad Sci U S A* 71, 718, 1974.

64. Elsea, S.H. et al. Haploinsufficiency of cytosolic serine hydroxymethyltransferase in the Smith-Magenis syndrome. *Am J Hum Genet* 57, 1342, 1995.

65. Girgis, S., Suh, J.R., Jolivet, J., and Stover, P.J. 5-Formyltetrahydrofolate regulates homocysteine remethylation in human neuroblastoma. *J Biol Chem* 272, 4729, 1997.

66. Martinez, M., Cuskelly, G.J., Williamson, J., Toth, J.P., and Gregory, J.F., III. Vitamin B-6 deficiency in rats reduces hepatic serine hydroxymethyltransferase and cystathionine beta-synthase activities and rates of in vivo protein turnover, homocysteine remethylation and transsulfuration. *J Nutr* 130, 1115, 2000.

67. Fowler, B., Whitehouse, C., Wenzel, F., and Wraith, J.E. Methionine and serine formation in control and mutant human cultured fibroblasts: evidence for methyl trapping and characterization of remethylation defects. *Pediatr Res* 41, 145, 1997.

68. Narkewicz, M.R., Moores, R.R., Jr., Battaglia, F.C., and Frerman, F.F. Ontogeny of serine hydroxymethyltransferase isoenzymes in fetal sheep liver, kidney, and placenta. *Mol Genet Metab* 68, 473, 1999.

69. Herbert, V. and Zalusky, R. Interrelations of vitamin B12 and folic acid metabolism: folic acid clearance studies. *J Clin Invest* 41, 1263, 1962.

70. Stover, P. and Schirch, V. 5-Formyltetrahydrofolate polyglutamates are slow tight binding inhibitors of serine hydroxymethyltransferase. *J Biol Chem* 266, 1543, 1991.

71. Green, J.M., Ballou, D.P., and Matthews, R.G. Examination of the role of methylenetetrahydrofolate reductase in incorporation of methyltetrahydrofolate into cellular metabolism. *FASEB J* 2, 42, 1988.

72. Oppenheim, E.W., Adelman, C., Liu, X., and Stover, P.J. Heavy chain ferritin enhances serine hydroxymethyltransferase expression and de novo thymidine biosynthesis. *J Biol Chem* 276, 19855, 2001.

73. Kruschwitz, H.L., McDonald, D., Cossins, E.A., and Schirch, V. 5-Formyltetrahydropteroylpolyglutamates are the major folate derivatives in *Neurospora crassa* conidiospores. *J Biol Chem* 269, 28757, 1994.

74. Stover, P. and Schirch, V. Serine hydroxymethyltransferase catalyzes the hydrolysis of 5,10-methenyltetrahydrofolate to 5-formyltetrahydrofolate. *J Biol Chem* 265, 14227, 1990.

75. Stover, P. and Schirch, V. The metabolic role of leucovorin. *Trends Biochem Sci* 18, 102, 1993.

76. Bertrand, R. and Jolivet, J. Methenyltetrahydrofolate synthetase prevents the inhibition of phosphoribosyl 5-aminoimidazole 4-carboxamide ribonucleotide formyltransferase by 5-formyltetrahydrofolate polyglutamates. *J Biol Chem* 264, 8843, 1989.

77. Maras, B., Stover, P., Valiante, S., Barra, D., and Schirch, V. Primary structure and tetrahydropteroylglutamate binding site of rabbit liver cytosolic 5,10-methenyltetrahydrofolate synthetase. *J Biol Chem* 269, 18429, 1994.

78. Bertrand, R., Beauchemin, M., Dayan, A., Ouimet, M., and Jolivet, J. Identification and characterization of human mitochondrial methenyltetrahydrofolate synthetase activity. *Biochim Biophys Acta* 1266, 245, 1995.

79. Anguera, M.C., Liu, X., and Stover, P.J. Cloning, expression, and purification of 5,10-methenyltetrahydrofolate synthetase from Mus musculus. *Protein Expr Purif* 35, 276, 2004.

80. Anguera, M.C. et al. Methenyltetrahydrofolate synthetase regulates folate turnover and accumulation. *J Biol Chem* 278, 29856, 2003.

81. Liu, X., Reig, B., Nasrallah, I.M., Stover, P.J. Human cytoplasmic serine hydroxymethyltransferase is an mRNA binding protein. *Biochemistry* 39, 11523, 2000.

82. Liu, X., Szebenyi, D.M., Anguera, M.C., Thiel, D.J., and Stover, P.J. Lack of catalytic activity of a murine mRNA cytoplasmic serine hydroxymethyltransferase splice variant: evidence against alternative splicing as a regulatory mechanism. *Biochemistry* 40, 4932, 2001.

83. Chu, E. and Allegra, C.J. The role of thymidylate synthase as an RNA binding protein. *Bioessays* 18, 191, 1996.

84. Chu, E., Grem, J.L., Johnston, P.G., and Allegra, C.J. New concepts for the development and use of antifolates. *Stem Cells* 14, 41, 1996.

85. Chu, E. and Allegra, C.J. The role of thymidylate synthase in cellular regulation. *Adv Enzyme Regul* 36, 143, 1996.

86. Nakshatri, H., Bouillet, P., Bhat-Nakshatri, P., and Chambon, P. Isolation of retinoic acid-repressed genes from P19 embryonal carcinoma cells. *Gene* 174, 79, 1996.

87. Perry, C., Sastry, R., Nasrallah, I.M., and Stover, P.J. Mimosine attenuates serine hydroxymethyltransferase transcription by chelating zinc: implications for inhibition of DNA replication. *J Biol Chem*, 280, 396, 2005.

88. Hider, R.C., Bittel, D., and Andrews, G.K. Competition between iron(III)-selective chelators and zinc-finger domains for zinc(II). *Biochem Pharmacol* 57, 1031, 1999.

89. Maclean, K.H., Cleveland, J.L., and Porter, J.B. Cellular zinc content is a major determinant of iron chelator-induced apoptosis of thymocytes. *Blood* 98, 3831, 2001.

90. al-Refaie, F.N. et al. Zinc concentration in patients with iron overload receiving oral iron chelator 1,2-dimethyl-3-hydroxypyrid-4-one or desferrioxamine. *J Clin Pathol* 47, 657, 1994.

91. Hong, K.H., Keen, C.L., Mizuno, Y., Johnston, K.E., and Tamura, T. Effects of dietary zinc deficiency on homocysteine and folate metabolism in rats(1). *J Nutr Biochem* 11, 165, 2000.

92. Vitale, J.J., Streiff, R.R., and Hellerstein, E.E. Folate metabolism and iron deficiency. *Lancet* 12, 393, 1965.

93. O'Connor, D.L., Green, T., and Picciano, M.F. Maternal folate status and lactation. *J Mammary Gland Biol Neoplasia* 2, 279, 1997.

94. O'Connor, D.L., Picciano, M.F., Tamura, T., and Shane, B. Impaired milk folate secretion is not corrected by supplemental folate during iron deficiency in rats. *J Nutr* 120, 499, 1990.

95. O'Connor, D.L., Picciano, M.F., Sherman, A.R., and Burgert, S.L. Depressed folate incorporation into milk secondary to iron deficiency in the rat. *J Nutr* 117, 1715, 1987.

96. Das, K.C., Herbert, V., Colman, N., and Longo, D.L. Unmasking covert folate deficiency in iron-deficient subjects with neutrophil hypersegmentation: dU suppression tests on lymphocytes and bone marrow. *Br J Haematol* 39, 357, 1978.

97. Westerman, D.A., Evans, D., and Metz, J. Neutrophil hypersegmentation in iron deficiency anaemia: a case-control study. *Br J Haematol* 107, 512, 1999.

98. O'Connor, D.L., Moriarty, P., and Picciano, M.F. The impact of iron deficiency on the flux of folates within the mammary gland. *Int J Vitam Nutr Res* 62, 173, 1992.

99. O'Connor, D.L., Picciano, M.F., Roos, M.A., and Easter, R.A. Iron and folate utilization in reproducing swine and their progeny. *J Nutr* 119, 1984, 1989.

100. Harrison, P.M. and Arosio, P. The ferritins: molecular properties, iron storage function and cellular regulation. *Biochim Biophys Acta* 1275, 161, 1996.

101. Yewdall, S.J. et al. Structural studies on recombinant human ferritins. *Biochem Soc Trans* 18, 1028, 1990.

102. Lawson, D.M. et al. Identification of the ferroxidase centre in ferritin. *FEBS Lett* 254, 207, 1989.

103. Levi, S. et al. Evidence of H- and L-chains have co-operative roles in the iron-uptake mechanism of human ferritin. *Biochem J* 288 (Pt. 2), 591, 1992.

104. Kakhlon, O., Gruenbaum, Y., and Cabantchik, Z.I. Repression of the heavy ferritin chain increases the labile iron pool of human K562 cells. *Biochem J* 356, 311, 2001.

105. Bubici, C., Papa, S., Pham, C.G., Zazzeroni, F., and Franzoso, G. NF-kappaB and JNK: an intricate affair. *Cell Cycle* 3, 1524, 2004.

106. Stohs, S.J. and Bagchi, D. Oxidative mechanisms in the toxicity of metal ions. *Free Radic Biol Med* 18, 321, 1995.

107. Pham, C.G. et al. Ferritin heavy chain upregulation by NF-kappaB inhibits TNFalpha-induced apoptosis by suppressing reactive oxygen species. *Cell* 119, 529, 2004.

108. Lewis, G.P. and Rowe, P.B. Oxidative and reductive cleavage of folates — a critical appraisal. *Anal Biochem* 93, 91, 1979.

109. Maruyama, T., Shiota, T., and Krumdieck, C.L. The oxidative cleavage of folates: a critical study. *Anal Biochem* 84, 277, 1978.

110. Kownacki-Brown, P.A., Wang, C., Bailey, L.B., Toth, J.P., and Gregory, J.F., III. Urinary excretion of deuterium-labeled folate and the metabolite p-aminobenzoylglutamate in humans. *J Nutr* 123, 1101, 1993.

111. Geoghegan, F.L., McPartlin, J.M., Weir, D.G., and Scott, J.M. Para-cetamidobenzoylglutamate is a suitable indicator of folate catabolism in rats. *J Nutr* 125, 2563, 1995.

112. Wang, C., Song, S., Bailey, L.B., and Gregory, J.F., III. Relationship between urinary excretion of p-aminobenyolyglutamate and folate statusin the growing rat. *Nutr Res* 14, 875, 1994.

113. Gregory, J.F., III, Williamson, J., Liao, J.F., Bailey, L.B., and Toth, J.P. Kinetic model of folate metabolism in nonpregnant women consuming [2H2]folic acid: isotopic labeling of urinary folate and the catabolite para-acetamidobenzoylglutamate indicates slow, intake-dependent, turnover of folate pools. *J Nutr* 128, 1896, 1998.

114. Scott, K.C. and Gregory, J.F., III. The fate of [3H]folic acid in folate adequate rats. *J. Nutr. Biochem.* 7, 261, 1996.

115. Eisenga, B.H., Collins, T.D., and McMartin, K.E. Incorporation of 3H-label from folic acid is tissue-dependent in folate-deficient rats. *J Nutr* 122, 977, 1992.

116. Antony, A.C. Folate receptors. *Annu Rev Nutr* 16, 501, 1996.

117. Sirotnak, F.M. and Tolner, B. Carrier-mediated membrane transport of folates in mammalian cells. *Annu Rev Nutr* 19, 91, 1999.

118. Titus, S.A. and Moran, R.G. Retrovirally mediated complementation of the glyB phenotype: cloning of a human gene encoding the carrier for entry of folates into mitochondria. *J Biol Chem* 275, 36811, 2000.

119. Lin, B.F., Huang, R.F., and Shane, B. Regulation of folate and one-carbon metabolism in mammalian cells. III. Role of mitochondrial folylpoly-gamma-glutamate synthetase. *J Biol Chem* 268, 21674, 1993.

120. Lin, B.F. and Shane, B. Expression of *Escherichia coli* folylpolyglutamate synthetase in the Chinese hamster ovary cell mitochondrion. *J Biol Chem* 269, 9705, 1994.

121. Finnell, R.H., Greer, K.A., Barber, R.C., and Piedrahita, J.A. Neural tube and craniofacial defects with special emphasis on folate pathway genes. *Crit Rev Oral Biol Med* 9, 38, 1998.

122. Zhu, L.J., Bagchi, M.K., and Bagchi, I.C. Ferritin heavy chain is a progesterone-inducible marker in the uterus during pregnancy. *Endocrinology* 136, 4106, 1995.

123. Kelly, D.A., Scott, J.M., and Weir, D.G. Increased folate catabolism in mice with ascitic tumours. *Clin Sci (Lond)* 65, 303, 1983.

124. Kim, Y.I. et al. Colonic mucosal concentrations of folate correlate well with blood measurements of folate status in persons with colorectal polyps. *Am J Clin Nutr* 68, 866, 1998.

125. Meenan, J., O'Hallinan, E., Scott, J., and Weir, D.G. Epithelial cell folate depletion occurs in neoplastic but not adjacent normal colon mucosa. *Gastroenterology* 112, 1163, 1997.

126. White, G.P., Worwood, M., Parry, D.H., and Jacobs, A. Ferritin synthesis in normal and leukaemic leukocytes. *Nature* 250, 584, 1974.

127. Kirkali, Z., Esen, A.A., Kirkali, G., and Guner, G. Ferritin: a tumor marker expressed by renal cell carcinoma. *Eur Urol* 28, 131, 1995.

128. Kirkali, Z., Guzelsoy, M., Mungan, M.U., Kirkali, G., and Yorukoglu, K. Serum ferritin as a clinical marker for renal cell carcinoma: influence of tumor size and volume. *Urol Int* 62, 21, 1999.

129. Guner, G., Kirkali, G., Yenisey, C., and Tore, I.R. Cytosol and serum ferritin in breast carcinoma. *Cancer Lett* 67, 103, 1992.

130. Marcus, D.M. and Zinberg, N. Isolation of ferritin from human mammary and pancreatic carcinomas by means of antibody immunoadsorbents. *Arch Biochem Biophys* 162, 493, 1974.

131. Weinstein, R.E. et al. Tissue ferritin concentration and prognosis in carcinoma of the breast. *Breast Cancer Res Treat* 14, 349, 1989.

132. Wu, C.G. et al. Increased hepatic ferritin-H messenger RNA levels correlate with those of c-myc in human hepatocellular carcinoma. *Int J Oncol* 11, 187, 1997.

133. Modjtahedi, N. et al. Increased expression of cytokeratin and ferritin-H genes in tumorigenic clones of the SW 613-S human colon carcinoma cell line. *Exp Cell Res* 201, 74, 1992.

134. Wu, C.G. et al. Rat ferritin-H: cDNA cloning, differential expression and localization during hepatocarcinogenesis. *Carcinogenesis* 18, 47, 1997.

135. Strong, W.B. and Schirch, V. In vitro conversion of formate to serine: effect of tetrahydropteroylpolyglutamates and serine hydroxymethyltransferase on the rate of 10-formyltetrahydrofolate synthetase. *Biochemistry* 28, 9430, 1989.

136. Scott, J.M. and Weir, D.G. The methyl folate trap: a physiological response in man to prevent methyl group deficiency in kwashiorkor (methionine deficiency) and an explanation for folic-acid induced exacerbation of subacute combined degeneration in pernicious anaemia. *Lancet* 2, 337, 1981.

137. Heise, T., Nath, A., Jungermann, K., and Christ, B. Purification of a RNA-binding protein from rat liver: identification as ferritin L chain and determination of the RNA/protein binding characteristics. *J Biol Chem* 272, 20222, 1997.

138. Glynn, S.A. et al. Colorectal cancer and folate status: a nested case-control study among male smokers. *Cancer Epidemiol Biomarkers Prev* 5, 487, 1996.

139. Kim, Y.I. Methylenetetrahydrofolate reductase polymorphisms, folate, and cancer risk: a paradigm of gene-nutrient interactions in carcinogenesis. *Nutr Rev* 58, 205, 2000.

140. Chen, J. et al. A methylenetetrahydrofolate reductase polymorphism and the risk of colorectal cancer. *Cancer Res* 56, 4862, 1996.

141. Giovannucci, E. et al. Alcohol, low-methionine–low-folate diets, and risk of colon cancer in men. *J Natl Cancer Inst* 87, 265, 1995.

142. Kato, I. et al. Serum folate, homocysteine and colorectal cancer risk in women: a nested case-control study. *Br J Cancer* 79, 1917, 1999.

143. Jaenisch, R. and Bird, A. Epigenetic regulation of gene expression: how the genome integrates intrinsic and environmental signals. *Nat Genet* 33 (Suppl.), 245, 2003.

144. Zingg, J.M. and Jones, P.A. Genetic and epigenetic aspects of DNA methylation on genome expression, evolution, mutation and carcinogenesis. *Carcinogenesis* 18, 869, 1997.

145. Balaghi, M. and Wagner, C. DNA methylation in folate deficiency: use of CpG methylase. *Biochem Biophys Res Commun* 193, 1184, 1993.

146. Cooney, C.A., Dave, A.A., and Wolff, G.L. Maternal methyl supplements in mice affect epigenetic variation and DNA methylation of offspring. *J Nutr* 132, 2393S, 2002.

147. Antequera, F., Boyes, J., and Bird, A. High levels of de novo methylation and altered chromatin structure at CpG islands in cell lines. *Cell* 62, 503, 1990.

148. Kim, Y.I. et al. Folate deficiency in rats induces DNA strand breaks and hypomethylation within the p53 tumor suppressor gene. *Am J Clin Nutr* 65, 46, 1997.

149. Newberne, P.M. and Rogers, A.E. Labile methyl groups and the promotion of cancer. *Annu Rev Nutr* 6, 407, 1986.

150. Rogers, A.E. Methyl donors in the diet and responses to chemical carcinogens. *Am J Clin Nutr* 61, 659S, 1995.

151. Steele, V.E. et al. Preclinical efficacy evaluation of potential chemopreventive agents in animal carcinogenesis models: methods and results from the NCI Chemoprevention Drug Development Program. *J Cell Biochem Suppl* 20, 32, 1994.

152. Shivapurkar, N., Tang, Z., Frost, A., and Alabaster, O. Inhibition of progression of aberrant crypt foci and colon tumor development by vitamin E and beta-carotene in rats on a high-risk diet. *Cancer Lett* 91, 125, 1995.

153. Wargovich, M.J. et al. Aberrant crypts as a biomarker for colon cancer: evaluation of potential chemopreventive agents in the rat. *Cancer Epidemiol Biomarkers Prev* 5, 355, 1996.

154. Laird, P.W. et al. Suppression of intestinal neoplasia by DNA hypomethylation. *Cell* 81, 197, 1995.

155. van der Put, N.M. et al. Decreased methylene tetrahydrofolate reductase activity due to the 677C→T mutation in families with spina bifida offspring. *J Mol Med* 74, 691, 1996.

156. Melnyk, S. et al. Uracil misincorporation, DNA strand breaks, and gene amplification are associated with tumorigenic cell transformation in folate deficient/repleted Chinese hamster ovary cells. *Cancer Lett* 146, 35, 1999.

157. Branda, R.F. and Blickensderfer, D.B. Folate deficiency increases genetic damage caused by alkylating agents and gamma-irradiation in Chinese hamster ovary cells. *Cancer Res* 53, 5401, 1993.

158. Salganik, R.I. and Dianov, G.L. Molecular mechanisms of the formation of DNA double-strand breaks and induction of genomic rearrangements. *Mutat Res* 266, 163, 1992.

159. Champion, K.M., Cook, R.J., Tollaksen, S.L., and Giometti, C.S. Identification of a heritable deficiency of the folate-dependent enzyme 10-formyltetrahydrofolate dehydrogenase in mice. *Proc Natl Acad Sci U S A* 91, 11338, 1994.

160. Snell, K., Natsumeda, Y., Eble, J.N., Glover, J.L., and Weber, G. Enzymic imbalance in serine metabolism in human colon carcinoma and rat sarcoma. *Br J Cancer* 57, 87, 1988.

161. Skibola, C.F. et al. Polymorphisms in the thymidylate synthase and serine hydroxymethyltransferase genes and risk of adult acute lymphocytic leukemia. *Blood* 99, 3786, 2002.

162. Hishida, A. et al. Associations between polymorphisms in the thymidylate synthase and serine hydroxymethyltransferase genes and susceptibility to malignant lymphoma. *Haematologica* 88, 159, 2003.

163. Pietsch, E.C., Chan, J.Y., Torti, F.M., and Torti, S.V. Nrf2 mediates the induction of ferritin H in response to xenobiotics and cancer chemopreventive dithiolethiones. *J Biol Chem* 278, 2361, 2003.

164. Thimmulappa, R.K. et al. Identification of Nrf2-regulated genes induced by the chemopreventive agent sulforaphane by oligonucleotide microarray. *Cancer Res* 62, 5196, 2002.

12 Brassica–Gene Interactions and Cancer Risk

Jay H. Fowke

CONTENTS

12.1 INTRODUCTION

Not all vegetables are created equal, at least in regard to cancer prevention. Vegetables in the class Brassicaceous, genus *Brassica*, include broccoli, cabbage, cauliflower, and Brussels sprouts. Table 12.1 contains a more complete list of *Brassica* vegetables. According to several recent reviews, the protective association between *Brassica* vegetable consumption and cancer risk is one of the most consistent in the nutritional epidemiological literature. In humans, these vegetables are the dominant, if not the only, source of glucosinolates, a family of nonnutrient phytochemicals. Once ingested, glucosinolates induce several critical metabolic enzyme systems responsible for carcinogen metabolism and excretion. Many of the genes encoding these enzymes are reported to have functionally significant variations in their nucleotide sequence. Thus, genetic markers of metabolic function may provide important clues to the mechanisms relating *Brassica* to cancer risk and guide the identification of those persons who might benefit the most from *Brassica* intake.

TABLE 12.1
Common Members of the Genus *Brassica*

Common Name	Species (Variety)[a]
Turnip or turnip greens	*rapa (rapifera)*
Mustard or mustard greens	*juncea*
Rutabaga or swede	*napus*
Collard greens	*oleracea (acephala)*
Kale	*oleracea (acephala)*
Cauliflower	*oleracea (botrytis)*
Red or white cabbage	*oleracea (capitata)*
Brussels sprouts	*oleracea (gemmifera)*
Kohlrabi	*oleracea (gorgylodes)*
Broccoli	*oleracea (botrytis)*
Chinese cabbage	*pekinensis (capitata)*
Bok choy	*chinensis*

[a] Combined listing from Nugon-Baudon, L. and Rabot, S. Glucosinolates and glucosinolate derivatives: implications for protection against chemical carcinogenesis. *Nutr. Res. Rev.*, 7: 205–231, 1994; Beecher, C.W. Cancer preventive properties of varieties of *Brassica oleracea*: a review. *Am. J. Clin. Nutr.*, 59: 1166S–1170S, 1994; Kristal, A.R. and Lampe, J.W. Brassica vegetables and prostate cancer risk: a review of the epidemiological evidence. *Nutr. Cancer*, 42: 1–9, 2002.

Only recently have cancer epidemiologists started to describe the importance of genetic susceptibility markers in this association between *Brassica* consumption and cancer risk. Although the available investigations have limitations, the pattern of results from these studies suggests that several detoxifying enzymes play an important role in the *Brassica* and cancer relationship. This chapter is intended as an introduction to the areas of nutritional epidemiology, molecular epidemiology, molecular biology, and plant physiology underpinning research on *Brassica*–gene interactions with cancer risk. The summary includes a description of the purported functional pathways by which glucosinolates may inhibit carcinogenesis, current approaches to measure *Brassica* intake in epidemiological studies, interpretation of *Brassica* and cancer associations in light of these different methods of measurement, and the available epidemiological studies investigating the interaction between *Brassica* intake, genetic markers of metabolic activity, and cancer risk. References quoted in this broad description are intended to guide the reader to more detailed data and analyses within a particular area of interest. As this is a relatively new area of investigation, gaps in the literature are indicated throughout the chapter.

12.2 NUTRITIONAL EPIDEMIOLOGY

Differences in cancer risk and mortality between countries are greater than racial or ethnic differences observed within the U.S.[1] For example, prostate cancer incidence varies by as much as 65-fold between the U.S. and Asian populations and risks for breast, colon, and several other cancers are substantially lower in China than in most Western nations.[2] Perhaps a portion of these cross-national differences can be attributed to differences in dietary practices, including differences in *Brassica* intake. Cabbage and broccoli are the predominant *Brassica* vegetables produced in the U.S. (Table 12.2), China, and Japan.[3] However, China produces approximately 12-fold more cabbage and broccoli and about 20-fold more cauliflower than the U.S.[3] Japan produces roughly the same amount of cabbage and broccoli as the U.S., although the number of people living in Japan is less than half the number living in the U.S. Interestingly, large numbers of Japanese men and women have migrated to the U.S., and cancer risk among these Japanese migrants has quickly approached the risk of

TABLE 12.2
U.S. Production[a] and Use of Commonly Consumed *Brassica*

Common Name	U.S. Supply (Millions of Kg)[b]	Per Capita Use (Grams per Day)[c]
Cauliflower	194.2	1.8
Cabbage	1083.9	10.3
Brussels sprouts	29.2	0.3
Broccoli	653.3	6.2

[a] From Economic Research Service, U.S. Department of Agriculture, 2002.

[b] Supply = total U.S. production + imports − exports.

[c] Per capita use = supply/total population of 2002.

the U.S. population.[1] Breast and prostate cancer rates among Japanese-Americans approaches the overall U.S. cancer rates within two or three generations. The rapid rise in colorectal cancer risk is particularly striking. Colorectal cancer risk among Japanese-Americans reached cancer rates of the U.S. population within one generation. That this increase could occur within simply a matter of several years since migration suggests that lifestyle factors, such as a decrease in *Brassica* vegetable intake, act late in life to increase colon cancer risk.[1]

Several cohort and case–control studies of diet and cancer risk have included an analysis of *Brassica* consumption. In a comprehensive review of the research literature through 1996, Verhoven and colleagues found that approximately 70% of case–control studies reported a protective association between *Brassica* and cancer.[4] No study reported a statistically significant increase in cancer risk with greater *Brassica* vegetable consumption. Since this review, several prospective cohort studies reported that *Brassica* intake was associated with reduced risk of benign tumors,[5,6] lymphatic,[7] renal,[8] bladder,[9] urothelial,[10] prostate,[11,12] lung,[13–15] breast,[16] or colon[17] cancers and overall cancer risk among male smokers. However, several prospective cohort studies found no association (positive or negative) between *Brassica* intake and the risk of colon,[18,19] prostate,[20] lung,[21] or breast[22] cancers. Such null effects are not unusual across a large number of nutritional epidemiological studies, and differences in study results may be attributable to the lifestyle characteristics of the study populations, the measurement and analysis methods, or the amounts or types of *Brassica* consumed in the study population. Furthermore, variability in the genetic susceptibility to *Brassica* may contribute to variability in results across epidemiological studies, and none of the above described studies evaluated potential gene–*Brassica* interactions in cancer risk.

12.3 *BRASSICA* GLUCOSINOLATES

12.3.1 GLUCOSINOLATES

The effects of *Brassica* consumption on carcinogenesis have been attributed to the glucosinolates (GSLs). The GSLs include several families of β-thioglucose *N*-hydroxysulfates, consisting of a common S–C=N structural backbone and a variable side-chain (R′) (Figure 12.1). Hundreds of GSL R′ side-chain structures have been identified and, for convenience, GSLs are often grouped by the alkyl, aromatic, or indolyl moiety at R′ (Table 12.3).[23] Most *Brassica* species express only a limited number of GSLs, perhaps around 15 or fewer, across these categories;[23,24] and the general GSL pattern varies by species. For example, glucobrassicin and other indole GSLs account for 35% to 60% of the total glucosinolate content in mature broccoli and cabbage,[24,25] whereas indole GSLs comprise less than 20% of total GSLs in rutabaga or turnip.[26] The remaining GSLs consist of alkyl and aromatic GSLs.

Within each species, plant age is one of the most important determinants of the GSL content. The GSL concentration decreases as the plant grows, with a redistribution of GSLs to the leaves and other vulnerable regions of the plant. Also, the composition of GSLs within the plant changes with age. For example, broccoli

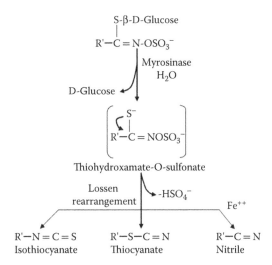

FIGURE 12.1 Degradation of aliphatic or aromatic glucosinates. Plant myrosinase or myrosinase-like activity in the gut releases the glucose moiety. Rearrangement of the resulting sulfonate leads to isothiocyanates, thiocyanates, and nitriles. Most research activity has focused on the ability of the isothiocyanates to induce Phase II enzyme activity or apoptosis.

sprouts do not express indole GSLs in any appreciable level, whereas the mature broccoli plant expresses high indole GSL amounts.[24,27–29] Other environmental factors, such as the mineral and sulfur content of the soil, water availability, and sun exposure are also significant determinants of GSL levels in *Brassica* plants.[30]

12.3.2 BREAKDOWN OF GLUCOSINOLATES

Intact GSLs must be cleaved to induce a physiological effect associated with carcinogenesis. The enzyme myrosinase (a β-thioglucosidase) and the GSLs coexist in the plant but remain physically separated under normal conditions. Any physical damage to the plant during processing, chewing, or cutting potentially releases GSLs and myrosinase from their respective storage sites. Myrosinase cleaves the thioglucoside bond, and the glucose is hydrolyzed from the S–C=N moiety (Figure 12.2 and Figure 12.3). GSLs are not detected in human urine, suggesting that uncleaved GSLs are not absorbed across the intestinal wall.[31] Any GSLs not cleaved by myrosinase during food preparation or chewing serve as substrates for myrosinase-like enzymes found in the gut microflora.[31–33] This is significant to human research studies because most *Brassica* vegetables are cooked prior to eating, and intense heat will deactivate myrosinase. To the extent that GSLs are cleaved in the gut to produce biologically active derivatives, overcooked *Brassica* vegetable consumption may continue to affect cancer risk.

After deglucosylation, alkyl or aromatic GSLs undergo a Lossen rearrangement, releasing the sulfate moiety and yielding isothiocyanates (ITC: $R'-N=C=S$), nitriles (R–C=N), and thiocyanates (R-S=CN) (Figure 12.2).[34] The relative amount of these analytes is, in part, pH dependent and also depends on the presence of required

TABLE 12.3
Examples Representing Common Glucosinolates (GSLs) and Their Biologically Active Hydrolysis Projects

GSL category	Common (Trivial) name	R'name	ITC or indole hydrolysis product[a]
Aliphatic	Glucoraphanin	4-methyl-sulphinylbutyl	Sulforaphane
	Sinigrin	Prop-2-enyl or allyl	Allyl isothiocyanate $CH_2=CH-CH_2-N=C=S$
Aromatic	Gluconasturtiin	2-phenethyl	Phenethylisothio-cyanate
	Glucotropaeolin	Benzyl-	Benzyl isothiocyanate
Indole	Glucobrassicin	3-indolylmethyl	Indole-3-carbinol
	Neoglucobrassicin	1-methoxy-3-indolylmethyl	N-methoxy-indole-3-carbinol

For Sulforaphane: $CH_3\text{-}\overset{\displaystyle O}{\underset{\displaystyle \|}{S}}\text{-}CH_2\text{-}CH_2\text{-}CH_2\text{-}CH_2\text{-}N\text{=}C\text{=}S$

For Phenethylisothiocyanate: phenyl ring–$CH_2\text{-}CH_2\text{-}N=C=S$

For Benzyl isothiocyanate: phenyl ring–$CH_2\text{-}N=C=S$

[a] Hydrolysis products also include nitriles and thiocyanate ions (see Figure 12.2 and Figure 12.3).

cofactors (e.g., iron).[23] Although certain nitrile compounds such as crambene ($NC\equiv CH_2\text{-}CHOH\text{-}CH=CH_2$) are of growing interest,[34] the majority of health research has focused on the ITC compounds produced following GSL degradation.

The composition of ITCs that humans are exposed to following *Brassica* consumption is complex. Glucoraphinin cleavage and rearrangement leads to sulphoraphane exposure, gluconasturin cleavage leads to phenethyl ITC (PEITC) exposure and, of course, other ITCs are created as determined by the GSL pattern in the plant. Myrosinase action on indole GSLs adds to this complexity because cleavage of indole GSLs produces a highly unstable ITC derivative. As shown in Figure 12.2, the thiocyanate ion is hydrolyzed rapidly to yield indole-3-carbinol (I3C).[35] The indole GSL also may be converted to indole-3-acetonitrile (not shown), although this appears to be a minor pathway.[35] I3C alone has little biological activity, and I3C may act as a stable reserve in the form of ascorbigen via reversible conjugation with ascorbic acid. Most research has focused on the biological activity of the I3C self-condensation products, including known dimers [e.g., 3,3′-diindolylmethane (DIM), indolo-3,2,b-carbazole (ICZ)), trimers (LT, CTr)], and tetramers[36–38] (Figure 12.3). Thus, an array of biologically active compounds is released following *Brassica* consumption, including a mixture of ITCs (e.g., sulphoraphane) and indoles (e.g.,

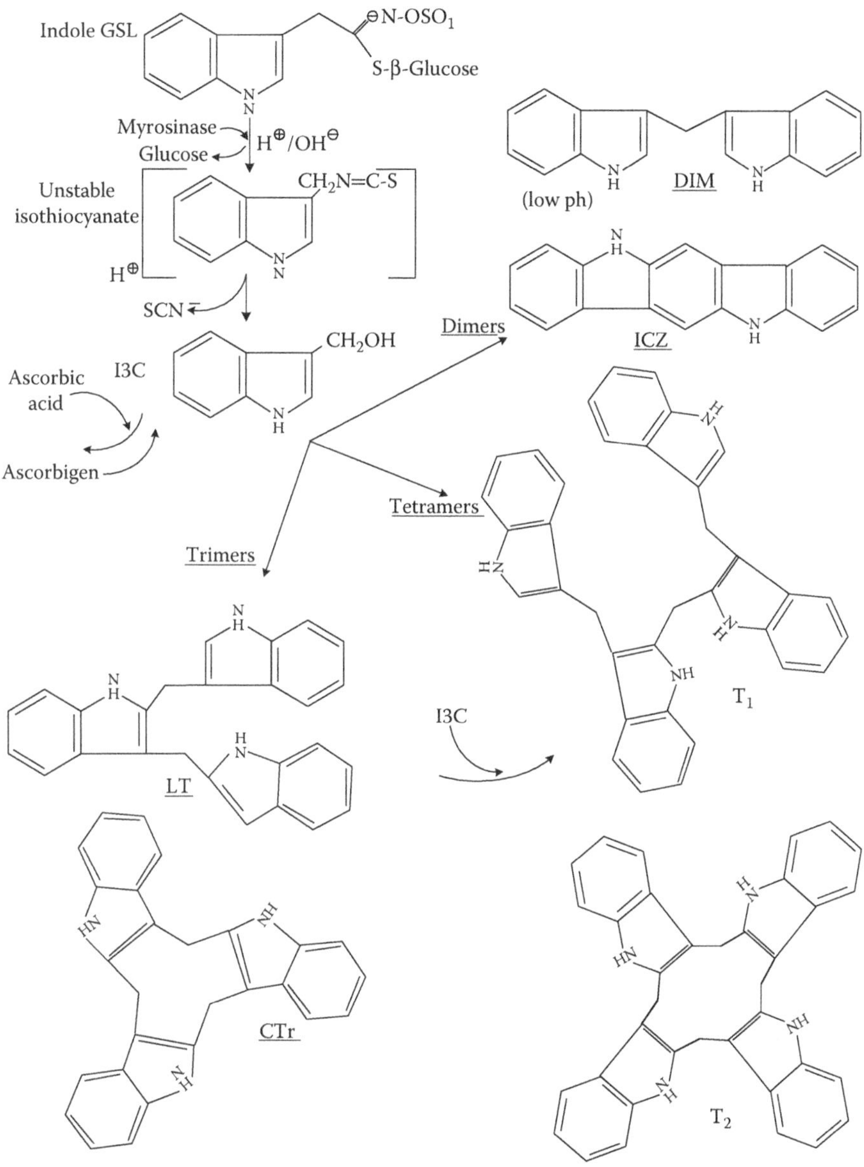

FIGURE 12.2 Indole glucosinolate degradation and the acid-condensation products of indole-3-carbinol (I3C). Plant myrosinase or myrosinase-like activity in the gut produces an unstable isothiocyanate. The SCN- moiety is lost, and the resulting I3C can reversibly bind to ascorbic acid to produce ascorbigen. Also, indole glucosinolate degradation may produce for indole acetonitriles and carbaldehydes, although these products appear to have less biologic activity. Once generated, I3C condenses under physiological conditions and low pH to form several biologically active dimers, trimers, and tetramers, including 3,3-diindolylmethane (DIM), indolo [3,2-b]carbazole (ICZ), 2-(indol-3-ylmethyl)-3,3-diindolylmethane (LT), and 5,6,11,12,17,18-hexahydrocyclona [1,2-b:4,5-b:7,8-b]tri-indole (CTr). Whereas I3C dimeric derivatives have moderate affinity for the aryl hydrocarbon receptor, I3C trimeric and tetrameric derivates appear to interact with critical cell cycle regulators and steroid hormone sensitivity.

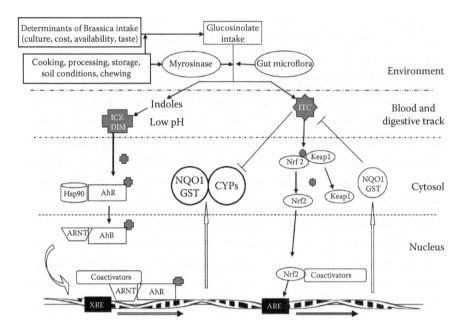

FIGURE 12.3 The protective association between *Brassica* vegetable intake and cancer risk requires a sequence of social factors, individual behaviors, and biochemical responses. The amount of *Brassica* consumed in any population, and the types and varieties of *Brassica* consumed, are determined by the economic viability of *Brassica* and cultural practices reflecting food preferences. The quantity and composition of glucosinolate within these consumed plants varies by species, plant age, soil conditions, water availability, and other environmental factors. With physical disruption of the plant cell wall, myrosinase will cleave the glucosinolates producing a range of indoles (e.g., diindoylmethane (DIM)) and isothiocyanates (ITC). Myrosinase cleavage may not occur if the vegetable is cooked under high heat, but the gut microflora also has myrosinase-like activity. Indole-3-carbinol (I3C) dimers (e.g., ICZ) bind to the aryl hydrocarbon receptor (AhR), leading to disassociation from heat shock protein 90 (hsp90), and translocates to the nucleus with the Ah receptor nuclear translocator (ARNT) with a high affinity for DNA binding at the xenobiotic response element (XRE) and induction of Phase I and Phase II enzymes. Simultaneously, isothiocyanates (ITC) disassociate NF-E2 related factor-2 (Nrf2) from Kelch-like ECH association protein 1 (Keap1), leading to induction of Phase II enzymes regulated by the antioxidant response element (ARE). Furthermore, ITCs inhibit Phase I enzymes induced by indoles, whereas Phase II enzymes conjugate ITCs leading to excretion. A break or disconnection in any step along these pathways may lead to a null-finding in an epidemiological study.

DIM). These agents are believed to be the critical components in *Brassica* that have led to the protective associations seen in prior epidemiological studies.

Work continues in an attempt to translate basic research and epidemiological investigations of *Brassica* and cancer risk into a cancer-prevention strategy. The concept that these *Brassica* phytochemicals interact with metabolic enzyme systems, and that this interaction may be a critical component of the benefits of *Brassica* consumption, derives from the seminal works of Conney, Talalay, and Wattenberg. Of course, many research groups are currently investigating the biomechanisms involved. The information presented below provides a generalized summary on the effects of ITC or of indole exposure on metabolic enzymes responsible for detoxifying carcinogens before the DNA has had the opportunity to be damaged. These pathways identify plausible targets for *Brassica*–gene interactions.

12.4 PHASE I ENZYMES AND *BRASSICA*

12.4.1 PHASE I ENZYMES

The Phase I enzyme system involves a superfamily of cytochrome P-450 mixed-function monooxygenases (CYPs). The CYPs are responsible for incorporating one atom of molecular oxygen onto an organic substrate,[39] creating a highly reactive electrophilic site. This reactive oxygen site is further targeted for conjugation with a hydrophilic moiety by Phase II enzymes (see following text), leading to excretion.

12.4.2 *BRASSICA* AND PHASE I ENZYME INDUCTION

Wattenberg first showed that rats fed a cabbage-rich diet more rapidly hydroxylated benzo-a-pyrene.[40] Since then, several studies have shown that *Brassica*-derived indoles induce CYP-dependent drug metabolism,[41,42] and *Brassica*-fed rodents have higher CYP activity in the small intestine, colon, and liver.[43–46] Preliminary human studies reported that *Brassica* consumption increased CYP1A2 activity by 12% to 19%,[47–49] and that *Brassica* consumption or I3C supplements shift estrogen metabolism in a manner consistent with CYP1A2 induction.[50,51]

The aryl hydrocarbon receptor (AhR) is the critical mediator of *Brassica*-induced Phase I enzyme induction (Figure 12.4). Indole GSL cleavage and rearrangement produces ICZ, a moderate AhR agonist.[52–56] The AhR disassociates from heat shock protein 90, and the AhR–ICZ complex translocates to the nucleus. There, it forms a heterodimer with the AhR nuclear translocator (ARNT) and induces CYP expression via the xenobiotic response elements (XRE, or the dioxin-responsive enhancer element DRE) in the 5′ regulatory region. Several CYP genes contain an XRE regulatory element, including *CYP1A1/2, CYP1B1, CYP2A, CYP2B1/2/6, CYP2C, CYP2E,* and *CYP3A*.[44,45,55]

Interestingly, the ITCs inhibit Phase I enzyme activity[57–59] (Figure 12.3), and results from Northern blot analyses were consistent with inhibition of CYP protein activity without affecting expression levels.[57] Although the overall effect of *Brassica* consumption appears to be an increase in hepatic Phase I enzyme induction, the significance of opposing action by ITCs in target tissues remains unclear but potentially very important. CYPs can activate procarcinogens, and the ITCs may moderate CYP activity to prevent carcinogen activation beyond a person's metabolic capacity to respond to this challenge. However, the relationship between ITC exposure and CYP activity has been made further unclear by research showing that ITCs induce measurable CYP activity.[57,60–63] What is clear is that the effects of *Brassica* consumption on Phase I induction will require new investigations to determine the extent to which Phase I enzymes are induced or inhibited in the target tissues. The overall effect of *Brassica* consumption on Phase I enzyme activity will depend on the

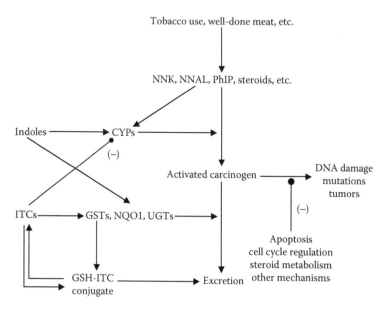

FIGURE 12.4 A model of chemical carcinogenesis, and the effects of *Brassica* indoles and isothiocyanates (ITCs) on carcinogen metabolism and excretion. Environmental or endogenous procarcinogens are able to react with DNA after oxidation by cytochrome P-450s (CYPs). Conjugation of these reactive oxygenated species by glutathione *S*-transferases (GSTs) or other Phase II enzymes may neutralize these carcinogens. *Brassica* indoles are bifunctional, inducing Phase I (CYPs) and Phase II enzyme activity. Thus, indoles may activate a procarcinogen to a reactive agent but also may facilitate conjugation and excretion. *Brassica* also provides ITCs, known Phase II enzyme inducers, that can further enhance the excretion of reactive species. ITCs are also substrates for GSTs, and Phase II enzyme induction could limit the persistence of ITCs in the body. ITCs also inhibit CYP activity and thus may prevent hydroxylation of procarcinogens. Finally, *Brassica* indoles and ITCs may inhibit tumorogenesis through inducing apoptosis in cancer cells.

balance of indoles and ITCs derived from the diet, the tissue of interest, and the individual's susceptibility to each of these agents. A number of *CYPs* are genetically polymorphic, creating functional differences in CYP metabolic activity that may be helpful in uncovering the significance of CYP activity in carcinogenesis. Unfortunately, the modification of any *Brassica* and cancer association by *CYP* genetic polymorphisms, or polymorphisms in the *AhR* or other related genes, has not been reported.

12.5 PHASE II ENZYMES AND *BRASSICA*

12.5.1 Phase II Enzyme System

Phase II enzymes include the UDP-glucuronosyltransferase (UGT), NAD(P)H:quinone oxoreductase (NQO), and glutathione *S*-transferases (GST)[27,64] enzyme systems. These systems are designed to neutralize electrophilic sites created by oxidative

(Phase I) metabolism and from other sources.[65,66] Indeed, exposure to tobacco smoke, well-done meat, sunlight, and other cancer risk factors generates reactive oxygen species that can damage DNA. Several epidemiological studies report a protective association between *Brassica* intake and tobacco-related cancers of the lung or bladder,[4] suggesting that *Brassica* consumption provides protection from oxygen reactive species. *Brassica* consumption lowers systemic oxidative stress levels, as measured by oxidative DNA adduct formation (8-oxod-G)[67,68] or lipid peroxidation (urinary F2-isoprostane).[69] The information below broadly summarizes the interactions between *Brassica* phytochemicals and the Phase II enzyme system, consistent with a defense against reactive oxygen species.[70,71]

12.5.2 *BRASSICA* PHYTOCHEMICALS AND PHASE II ENZYMES

The ITCs are well known inducers of multiple Phase II enzyme families. Several human trials have demonstrated that *Brassica* consumption induces GST enzymes in colorectal tissue or blood.[72–74] As previously reviewed, induction of these enzymes is mediated by NF-E2 related factor-2 (Nrf2) transcription factor[25,75] (Figure 12.3). ITCs disrupt the interaction between Nrf2 and the Kelch-like ECH association protein 1 (Keap1), allowing Nrf2 to translocate to the nucleus and interact with the antioxidant response element (ARE). Interestingly, GSTs, NQO, and UGT genes also contain an XRE in their regulatory region, and *Brassica* indoles are bifunctional inducers of both Phase II and Phase I enzymes.[37,75–79]

12.5.3 *GST* GENETIC POLYMORPHISMS

Many of the genes giving rise to the *GST* isoforms are polymorphic, and the response to *Brassica* intake and ITC exposure varies across individuals with different *GST* genotypes. About 50% and 40% do not have a *GSTM1* or *GSTT1* gene, respectively,[80] such that the *GST* isoform cannot be expressed (i.e., *GSTM1*-null genotype, *GSTT1*-null genotype). *Brassica* consumption did not increase GST activity in rectal biopsy specimens from subjects with the *GSTM1*-negative genotype, but *Brassica* increased total GST enzyme activity and GSTM1 protein levels in rectal tissue among subjects with the *GSTM1*-positive genotype.[81] Certain *GSTP1* single nucleotide polymorphisms (SNPs) appear to affect enzymatic activity and stability,[82,83] and *GSTP1* polymorphisms have differential specific activity toward the ITCs found in *Brassica*.[83] Also, *Brassica* intake increased GSTA levels in blood only among subjects with the *GSTM1*-null genotype,[64] illustrating that *Brassica* invokes a broad Phase II enzyme response that may, in part, compensate for a deficient early response. Thus, it is plausible that the physiological response to *Brassica* consumption appears, in part, to be determined by common genetic variations that determine an individual's Phase II enzyme activity.

12.6 ITCs AS PHASE II ENZYME SUBSTRATES

The ITCs are not only inducers of Phase II enzymes, but ITCs are also substrates for Phase II enzyme action. The ITCs are electrophilic compounds that are absorbed and excreted following glutathione (GSH) conjugation by GST enzymes.[31] In rodents, a glucoraphanin-rich diet significantly reduced GSH stores and the macrophage response associated with inflammation from reactive oxygen species.[84] Structure–function analyses suggests that the R′ group determines the rate of conjugation,[85] and ITCs are more rapidly conjugated by GSTM1 compared to the GSTA, GSTT, or GSTP superfamilies.[70,71,85] The reaction between GSTM1 and ITCs is reversible,[85] and perhaps the GSH–ITC complex circulates in the body to induce a metabolic response to reactive oxidative species in nonhepatic tissues. Ultimately, the ITC is converted to a mercapturic acid following gamma-glutamyltranspeptidase (γGTP), cysteinylglycinase (CG), and N-acetyltransferase (NAT) reactions,[85,86] and then excreted in urine.

Measurement of ITCs in human urine (as a dithiocarbamate) has enabled investigation of the significance of GST genetic polymorphisms on ITC absorption and excretion. ITCs in urine react with 1,2-benzenedithiol to form 1,3-benzodithiole-2-thione, a cyclic product with favorable properties for detection by HPLC and UV spectroscopy.[86] Seow and colleagues compared urinary ITC levels across *GST* genotypes among men and women living in Singapore.[87] Participants reported consuming *Brassica* almost daily, at an average level of 40.6 g/d. As expected, urinary ITC excretion categories and *Brassica* intake significantly increased together in a "dose–response" manner. Urinary ITC levels did not substantively vary with *GSTM1* (+/–) genotypes or the *GSTP1* (*313A→G*) polymorphism, with possible functional significance for ITC metabolism.[83] However, urinary ITC levels were significantly higher among participants with the *GSTT1*-positive genotype compared to participants with the *GSTT1*-null genotype.

Our research group evaluated urinary ITC levels across genetic polymorphisms in *GSTM1*, *GSTT1*, *GSTP1*, and *NQO1* among women living in Shanghai, China.[88] Similar to the study of Seow and colleagues,[87] average reported *Brassica* consumption increased with increasing categories of urinary ITC levels. Urinary ITC levels were higher among subjects with the *GSTT1*-null or *GSTP1*-GG genotypes, but urinary ITC levels did not vary by *GSTM1* or *NQO1* (*609C→T*) polymorphisms. Although further work is needed to understand differences between these studies, it is clear that the persistence of ITCs in the body is modified by genetic polymorphisms in Phase II enzyme systems.

12.7 *BRASSICA* AND CHEMICAL CARCINOGENESIS

As previously suggested, *Brassica*-induced Phase I or Phase II enzymes may modify cancer risk (Figure 12.3). Humans are exposed to many exogenous and endogenous agents, and many of these agents generate reactive electrophilic species leading to DNA damage and, ultimately, cancer. Well-done meat consumption and tobacco are presented as two examples of the possible interactions between *Brassica*, Phase II metabolism, and chemical carcinogenesis.

High-temperature cooking of meat creates heterocyclic amines and other carcinogenic organics.[89] Consumption of well-done meat has been associated with colon[90] and lung[91] cancer risks, however the relationship between well-done meat and human cancer is not firmly established. The procarcinogen 2-amino-1-methyl-6-phenylim-idazo[4,5-b]pyridine (PhIP) is activated by CYP hydroxylation and sulfotransferase conjugation to a highly reactive *N-O*-sulfonyl and acetyl esters.[89] Once activated, the PhIP-conjugate moiety will covalently bind to DNA and proteins to induce tumors. *Brassica* vegetable consumption increased excretion of conjugated PhiP-glucuronide metabolites in urine and decreased excretion of unmetabolized PhIP. Furthermore, ITC administration inhibited heterocyclic amine-induced DNA adduct formation,[59] suggesting that *Brassica* consumption would reduce exposure to carcinogens derived from the habitual consumption of well-done meat.

The metabolism of the tobacco-specific carcinogen 4-(Methylnitrosamino)-1-(3-pyridyl)-1-butanone (NNK) has been described in detail.[58,92] Very briefly, NNK is a procarcinogen that follows two distinct metabolic pathways. NNK may be hydroxylated, leading to DNA adduct formation and tumors in the lungs of experimental animals. Alternatively, NNK may be reduced to 4-(methylnitrosamino)-1-(3-pyridyl)-1-butanol (NNAL), another potent tobacco carcinogen. In rodents, ITC administration inhibited NNK biotransformation and lung tumors, perhaps due to CYP1A2 inhibition and an increase in NNAL excretion.[57,58,93] In humans, ITC exposure through watercress consumption increased NNAL and NNAL-glucuronide excretion.[93] Indoles from *Brassica* induced hepatic CYP1A2 activity, potentially activating tobacco carcinogens.[44,45] However, CYP1A2 hydroxylation in the liver may decrease NNK exposure in lung tissues and may shunt NNK away from the carcinogenic NNAL pathway.[94] In female tobacco smokers (U.S.), I3C administration decreased urinary NNAL and NNAL-conjugated metabolites.[95] Similarly, an analysis of smokers in Singapore found that the urinary NNAL levels significantly decreased among persons with greater estimated *Brassica* indole intake.[28]

Thus, *Brassica* ITC and indoles probably act through separate and common pathways to affect chemical carcinogenesis (Figure 12.4). Indoles are bifunctional inducers of both Phase I and Phase II enzymes, leading to the oxygenation, conjugation and, ultimately, excretion of procarcinogens. ITCs are monofunctional inducers of several Phase II detoxifying enzyme systems, and ITCs inhibit the potential activation of procarcinogens by CYP activity. The combined effects of ITCs and indoles on metabolic enzyme systems may prevent the redistribution of chemicals from the liver to other tissues and hasten the excretion of activated carcinogens. Perhaps this benefit might be evidenced most in those subjects with a lower metabolic capacity to remove these agents. Analyses of genetic polymorphisms in the metabolic enzymes responsible for mediating the effects of *Brassica* on environmental carcinogens could guide a further understanding of mechanisms of action and identify those persons who might benefit most from greater *Brassica* vegetable intake.

12.8 *BRASSICA* CONSUMPTION, PHASE II ENZYMES, AND CANCER

At this time, seven studies have investigated whether genetic variants determining Phase II enzyme response modify the *Brassica* and cancer association. Cancer sites investigated included the colon (two studies), lung (three studies), head and neck (one study), and breast (one study). All seven studies evaluated the effects of *GSTM1* genetic deletion. Furthermore, six studies included the *GSTT1* genetic deletion, two considered *GSTP1* polymorphisms, and one considered a *NQO1* polymorphism. The study population and analytic approaches are summarized below and in Table 12.4. Study results are represented as an odds ratio (OR) or relative risk (RR), with 95% confidence intervals. ORs (or RRs) greater than 1.0 indicate that *Brassica* intake was associated with greater cancer risk, whereas ORs or RRs less than 1.0 indicate that *Brassica* intake was associated with lower cancer risk. A 95% confidence interval that excludes 1.0 can be interpreted as equivalent to a *p*-value less than 0.05.

12.8.1 Modification of the *Brassica* and Cancer Association by Phase II Enzyme Genetic Polymorphisms

12.8.1.1 Colon Adenomas or Colon Cancer

Lin and colleagues compared *Brassica* vegetable consumption between patients with left-sided colon polyp and patients without a polyp on sigmoidoscopy.[96] Cases and controls were matched for gender, age, date of sigmoidoscopy, and clinical center. There were significantly fewer colon polyps among subjects reporting broccoli intake greater than one serving per week (OR = 0.47, 95% CI 0.30–0.73), and there was a significant trend (*p* = 0.04) suggesting fewer polyps among patients who consumed more kale or other greens. Colon polyp prevalence was not significantly associated with *GSTM1* genotype (*GSTM1*-positive vs. null, OR = 0.85 (0.65–1.10)). Broccoli consumption was associated with protection from colon polyps among both *GSTM1*-negative and *GSTM1*-positive subjects, but this association was stronger and statistically significant only among subjects with the *GSTM1*-null genotype (*GSTM1*-null: OR = 0.39, 95% CI 0.19–0.68; *GSTM1*-positive: OR = 0.74, 95% CI 0.40–0.99, *p* for interaction < 0.01).

Seow and colleagues prospectively investigated the association between *Brassica* consumption and colorectal cancer risk among residents of Singapore.[97] ITC exposure was estimated by weighing the habitual consumption of each *Brassica* vegetable reported on a food frequency questionnaire (FFQ) by an estimate of the ITC content of that vegetable. Estimated ITC exposure was not significantly protective for colorectal cancer risk (OR = 0.81 (0.59–1.12)). Also, colorectal cancer risk was not associated with genetic polymorphisms in *GSTM1* (positive vs. null), *GSTT1* (positive vs. null), or a *GSTP1* polymorphism (*313A→G*). Genetic polymorphisms in *GSTM1* or *GSTP1* did not substantively modify the ITC and colorectal cancer association. However, the protective association between ITC and colorectal cancer risk appeared to be stronger among subjects with the *GSTT1*-null genotype (OR = 0.63 (0.37–1.07)) compared to subjects with the *GSTT1*-positive genotype (OR = 0.97 (0.64–1.47)). In an analysis of colon cancer only, estimated ITC exposure was significantly associated with cancer risk among subjects with both *GSTM1*-null and *GSTT1*-null genotypes (OR = 0.31 (0.12–0.84), n = 24 cases), whereas estimated ITC exposure was not associated with colon cancer risk among subjects with *GSTM1*-positive and *GSTT1*-positive genotypes (OR = 1.00 (0.64–1.53)).

TABLE 12.4
Studies of *Brassica*–Gene Interactions and Cancer Risk

Cancer Site	Study Description	*Brassica* and Cancer		Genotypes and Cancer		*Brassica* — Genotype Effect		Ref.
		Brassica Measure	*Brassica* Effect	Genotype	Genotype Effect	Genotype	*Brassica* and Cancer by Genotype	
Left-side Colon Adenoma	Location: California, U.S. Design: Case–control Cases: 459 Controls: 507	Broccoli (> 1 serving/week from 126-item FFQ)	0.47 (0.30, 0.73) Adjusted for age, date, clinic, gender, saturated fat, energy, fruit, and vegetables	GSTM1 –	0.85 (0.65–1.10)	GSTM1 + GSTM1 –	0.74 (0.40–0.99) 0.36 (0.19–0.68); $P_{int} < 0.01$	96
Colorectal	Location: Singapore Design: Nested case–control Cases: 213 Controls: 1194	High ITC intake (above median intake estimated from 165-item FFQ)	0.81 (0.59–1.12) adjusted for education, BMI, smoking, physical activity, alcohol, saturated fat, gender, year of birth, and dialect	GSTM1 – GSTT1 – GSTP1AB/BB	1.22 (0.90–1.67) 0.88 (0.64–1.21) 0.94 (0.67–1.33)	GSTM1 + GSTM1 – GSTT1+ GSTT1 – GSTM1/T1 – GSTP1 AA GSTP1 AB/BB	0.71 (0.45–1.14) 0.85 (0.54–1.35) 0.97 (0.64–1.47) 0.63 (0.37–1.07) 0.31 (0.12–0.84)[a] 0.75 (0.51–1.11) 0.92 (0.50–1.69)	97
Lung	Location: Singapore Design: Case–control Cases: 233 Controls: 187	High ITC intake (above median intake estimated from FFQ)	0.63 (0.41–0.95) All subjects: adjusted for age, smoking status, years smoking, cigarettes/day	GSTM1 – GSTT1 –	1.50 (0.51–4.40) 1.95 (0.68–5.58) Ever-smokers only	GSTM1 + GSTM1 – GSTT1+ GSTT1 – GSTM1/T1 – All subjects	0.78 (0.39–1.59) 0.55 (0.33–0.93) 0.75 (0.40–1.40) 0.54 (0.31–0.95) 0.47 (0.23–0.95)	102

(continued)

TABLE 12.4 (continued)
Studies of *Brassica*–Gene Interactions and Cancer Risk

Cancer Site	Study Description	*Brassica* and Cancer		Genotypes and Cancer		*Brassica* — Genotype Effect		Ref.
		Brassica Measure	*Brassica* Effect	Genotype	Genotype Effect	Genotype	*Brassica* and Cancer by Genotype	
Lung	Location: Texas, U.S. Design: Case–control Cases: 503 Controls: 465	Low ITC intake (below median intake estimated from FFQ)	1.72 (1.13–2.62) Current smokers only	GSTM1 – GSTT1–	1.34 (0.88–2.04) 1.50 (0.89–2.53) Current smokers only; adjusted for age, gender, smoking status, and ITC intake	GSTM1 + high ITC GSTM1 + low ITC GSTM1 – high ITC GSTM1 – low ITC GSTT1 + high ITC GSTT1 + low ITC GSTT1 – high ITC GSTT1 – low ITC	1.0 (ref) 2.11 (1.15–3.85) 1.55 (0.79–3.04) 2.22 (1.20–4.10) 1.0 (ref) 1.71 (1.04–2.82) 1.31 (0.60–2.85) 3.19 (1.54–6.62) Current smokers only, adjusted for age and sex	101
	Location: Shanghai, China Design: Nested case–control Cases: 232 Controls: 710	High urine ITC (any detectable ITC level measured in prediagnostic urine samples)	0.65 (0.43–0.97) adjusted for age, age started smoking, number of cigarettes per day, years since quitting	GSTM1 – GSTT1 – GSTM1/T1 –	0.79 (0.57–1.10) 0.93 (0.67–1.30) 0.95 (0.68–1.33)	GSTM1+ GSTM1 – GSTT1 + GSTT1 – GSTM1/T1 –	1.22 (0.67–2.24) 0.36 (0.20–0.63) 0.95 (0.50–1.80) 0.28 (0.13–0.57) 0.28 (0.13–0.57)	109

Cancer	Location/Design	Brassica exposure	Effect measure	Adjustment	Genotype	Genotype effect	Gene–Brassica interaction	Ref
Head and neck	Location: N. Carolina, U.S. Design: Case–control Cases: 149 Controls: 180	High *Brassica* (any *Brassica* reported on 44-item FFQ)	1.6 (0.63–4.8)	Adjusted for age, gender, race, alcohol, tobacco	GSTM1 – GSTT1 –	0.88 (0.50–1.50) 1.20 (0.55–2.50) adjusted for age, gender, race	GSTM1 + no *Brassica* 1.0 (ref) GSTM1 + any *Brassica* 1.2 (0.25–5.9) GSTM1 – no *Brassica* 0.55 (0.07–4.2) GSTM1 – any *Brassica* 1.1 (0.23–5.4) 1.0 (ref) GSTT1 + no *Brassica* 2.1 (0.64–7.2) GSTT1 + any *Brassica* 4.4 (0.27–72.9) GSTT1 – no *Brassica* 2.2 (0.57–8.8) GSTT1 – any *Brassica*	100
Breast	Location: Shanghai, China Design: Case–control Cases: 337 Controls: 337	High urine ITC (highest quartile of urinary ITC measured in pretreatment urine samples)	0.5 (0.3–0.8)	Adjusted for soy protein, fibroadenoma, family breast cancer, leisure activity, WHR, BMI, age at menarche, number of children	GSTM1 – GSTT1 – GSTP1 AG/GG NQO1 TT	1.0 (0.7–1.3) 1.4 (1.0–1.9) 1.5 (1.0–2.0) 1.4 (0.9–2.3)	GSTM1 + 0.6 (0.3–1.4) GSTM1 – 0.5 (0.2–0.9) GSTT1 + 0.6 (0.3–1.3) GSTT1 – 0.4 (0.2–0.9) GSTP1 AA 0.6 (0.4–1.3) GSTP1 AG/GG 0.5 (0.2–1.2) NQO1 CC/CT 0.6 (0.3–1.1) NQO1 TT 0.5 (0.1–1.8)	114

Note: Effect measures include odds ratios with (95% confidence intervals) or relative risks with (95% confidence intervals).

[a] Analysis restricted to colon cancers.

12.8.1.2 Head and Neck Cancer

Tobacco and alcohol use dominate as risk factors for squamous cell carcinomas of the head and neck. Additionally, *Brassica* consumption or *Brassica* phytochemicals are among the most consistent protective factors associated with head and neck cancer.[98,99] A recent case–control study compared *Brassica* intake patterns between 149 head and neck cancer patients and 180 age- and gender-matched clinical controls with noncancerous disease of the oral cavity.[100] *Brassica* vegetable intake was not associated with head and neck cancer risk (OR = 1.6 (0.6–4.8)). Also, genetic variations in *GSTM1* and *GSTT1* (positive vs. null) were not associated with head and neck cancer risk. There was no evidence that the *Brassica* and head and neck cancer risk association was modified by *GST* genetic polymorphisms.

12.8.1.3 Lung Cancer

Spitz and colleagues compared *Brassica* intake patterns between incident lung cancer patients identified from the University of Texas M.D. Anderson Cancer Center and controls recruited from the Houston, Texas community.[101] An ITC exposure index was calculated by measuring broccoli, cauliflower, and cabbage intake by an FFQ and then weighing these intakes by vegetable-specific ITC levels[97] and daily caloric intake (mg ITC/1000 kcal). Intakes of estimated ITC, total *Brassica*, broccoli, and cauliflower or Brussels sprouts were each significantly higher among controls compared to cases. This study differs from the others in that the investigators used subjects with a high estimated ITC exposure as the reference group and evaluated the effect of low ITC exposure on lung cancer. Among current smokers, low ITC intake was significantly associated with lung cancer (OR = 1.72 (1.13–2.62)). However, *GSTT1* or *GSTM1* genotypes were not significantly associated with lung cancer risk among current smokers (OR = 1.50 (0.89–2.53); OR = 1.34 (0.88–2.04), respectively). The significant association between low ITC exposure and greater lung cancer risk was not modified by *GSTM1* genotype. However, the risk of lung cancer with low ITC exposure was 87% higher among subjects with the *GSTT1*-null genotype (Low ITC intake: *GSTT1*-null: OR = 3.19; *GSTT1*-positive: OR = 1.71; 3.19/1.71 = 1.87). *GSTT1* genotypes did not modify lung cancer risk among current smokers with high estimated ITC exposure. Similarly, lung cancer risk was only marginally higher with low ITC intake among former smokers with the *GSTT1*-null genotype (OR = 1.79 (0.95–3.37)), perhaps because former smokers reported significantly higher *Brassica* intake.

Zhao and colleagues conducted a similar case–control investigation among Chinese women living in Singapore.[102] Lung cancer cases were identified from three major hospitals within three months of diagnosis, and controls included hospital patients without a history of cancer or respiratory disease. Intake of nine common *Brassica* vegetables was measured by an FFQ, and an estimate of ITC exposure was calculated using previously measured ITC concentration in a sample of vegetables from Singapore.[103] The risk of lung cancer was lower among subjects reporting high ITC exposure (OR = 0.63 (0.41–0.95)). *GSTM1* and *GSTT1* genotypes (positive or null) were not associated with lung cancer risk. However, the lung cancer and ITC association was consistently stronger among subjects with the *GSTM1*-null (OR = 0.55 (0.33–0.93)), *GSTT1*-null (OR = 0.54 (0.31–0.91)) genotypes, or among subjects with null-genotypes for both genes (OR = 0.47 (0.23–0.95)).

12.8.2 Possible Limitations of FFQs

The five studies just described relied on FFQs to estimate habitual *Brassica* vegetable intake. Study subjects were presented with a list of food items and instructed to record the frequency, and perhaps typical portion size, for each food during a specified reference time. These responses are intended to reflect habitual diet patterns across subjects, however calibration studies have identified substantial levels of random and systematic variability in data derived from FFQs.[104] For example, the lack of a clear association between *Brassica* and head and neck cancer may reflect differential diet recall between cancer patients and noncancer controls or that there is little difference in diet between patients with different types of oral cavity disease.[100] Also, FFQs would not measure glucosinolate variability across plants or the extent of myrosinase deactivation due to food preparation.[30,105] Several reports summarize total glucosinolate levels,[106–108] indole glucosinolate levels,[28] and ITC levels[103] for specific *Brassica* species. These reviews also illustrate the tremendous variability in GSL levels within each species. Converting *Brassica* intake measured by questionnaire to an estimate of ITC exposure places more weight on those vegetables with greater ITC content but does not address the potential underlying errors in the original *Brassica* intake estimates or the within-species variability in GSL levels across the plants consumed. Indeed, estimated ITC intake and the original *Brassica* vegetable intake scores remain strongly correlated and highly comparable,[87,88] and it is unclear whether conversion to an ITC estimate substantially enhances measurement precision beyond that provided by direct measurement of *Brassica* intake. Future investigations might consider evaluating cancer risk against both *Brassica* intake and ITC exposure indices, side-by-side, to permit comparisons and to consider potential sources of error in *Brassica* intake measurement.

12.8.3 *Brassica* Intake Estimated by Urinary ITC Levels

Urinary ITC levels provide an alternative measure of *Brassica* intake. *Brassica* ITCs are usually excreted within 8 to 72 h after *Brassica* consumption[31] and, therefore, this biomarker is best used in study populations with stable and high *Brassica* intake. As described previously, urinary ITC levels are consistent with habitual *Brassica* vegetable consumption in Asian populations,[87,88] and urinary ITC levels should be independent of potential reporting errors associated with FFQs. Furthermore, urinary ITC levels may be a better index of internalized *Brassica* phytochemical exposure despite variability in GSL content, myrosinase activity, and food preparation methods. As described previously, indole GSLs do not form stable ITCs and would not be expected to contribute to the urinary ITC content (Figure 12.3).[35] However, urinary ITC levels were proportional to total GSL intake in a controlled feeding trial,[31] suggesting that urinary ITC levels capture an index of brassica phytochemical exposure across GSL categories.

12.8.4   ASSOCIATION BETWEEN URINARY ITC LEVELS AND CANCER BY *GST* POLYMORPHISMS

12.8.4.1   Lung Cancer

London and colleagues conducted a prospective investigation of *Brassica* and lung cancer risk in Shanghai, China.[109] Urinary ITC levels were measured using a conjugation reaction[110] in urine samples collected up to 12 yr prior to lung cancer diagnosis. Subjects with detectable urinary ITC levels had a significantly lower risk of lung cancer compared to subjects without detectable urinary ITC levels (OR = 0.65 (0.43–0.97)). *GSTM1* and *GSTT1* genotypes were not associated with lung cancer risk. Interestingly, the protective association between urinary ITC levels and lung cancer risk was found only among subjects with the *GSTM1*-null or *GSTT1*-null genotypes (OR = 0.36 (0.20–0.63)); (OR = 0.51 (0.30–0.86), respectively).

12.8.4.2   Breast Cancer

Established breast cancer risk factors include an early menarche, later birth of the first child, later menopause, and other reproductive factors, consistent with sustained estrogen exposure for a longer period of time. Breast cancer incidence is lower in Asian populations,[2] and several observational studies reported a protective association between *Brassica* consumption and breast cancer risk.[22,111–113] We conducted a population-based breast cancer case–control study in Shanghai, China.[114] Breast cancer cases were identified in Shanghai through a rapid-case-ascertainment system or through the Shanghai tumor registry, and urinary ITC levels were measured in pretreatment urine samples. Controls were randomly selected from the female population of Shanghai. Higher urinary ITC levels were significantly associated with a lower breast cancer risk (OR = 0.5 (0.3–0.8), p for trend < 0.01). The *GSTM1*-null genotype was not associated with breast cancer risk, however breast cancer was marginally associated ($p < 0.10$) with the *GSTT1*-null, *GSTP1* G-allele (GA or GG), or *NQO1* TT (lower functional activity) polymorphisms. The association between urinary ITC and breast cancer did not significantly differ across genotypes, although the trend between urinary ITC levels and breast cancer risk was more consistent among subjects with the *GSTM1*-null, *GSTT1*-null, and *NQO1*-T allele (CT or TT) polymorphisms.

12.8.5   *BRASSICA*–GENE INTERACTIONS: WHAT CONCLUSIONS ARE POSSIBLE AT THIS TIME?

Most observational epidemiological studies report that greater *Brassica* intake is associated with reduced cancer risk. Genetic variability in the susceptibility to *Brassica* phytochemicals may obscure a *Brassica* and cancer association, particularly when *Brassica* is measured with systematic or random error, when the study population does not consume much *Brassica* on a regular basis, or for those cancers in which the true association between *Brassica* and cancer is weak or modest. Studies that include genetic markers of metabolic enzymes known to be important in the carcinogenic pathway may confirm what we already suspect regarding a particular carcinogenic process or clarify the circumstances in which *Brassica* intake affects cancer risk. At this point in time, a few broad statements are possible from the available *Brassica*–gene investigations:

1. Genetic analyses will improve the measurement of *Brassica* vegetable exposure. Measurements of *Brassica* intake have progressed from FFQs to estimates of ITC exposure to measurement of urinary ITC levels. At this time, no single measurement can be considered superior to another. Questionnaires provide greater detail and range, whereas urinary ITC levels combined with Phase II genetic polymorphism data can provide information for a narrowly defined exposure without reporting error. Two studies have shown that urinary ITC levels vary with *GST* genotypes,[87,88] and adjusting urinary ITC levels for these genetic markers may increase the precision of future analyses. These measurement approaches are highly complementary and each compensates for the limitations of the other. Thus, future studies should employ multiple measurement approaches to evaluate the consistency across measures and, perhaps, to identify clues to the agent(s) responsible for any association.

2. The patterns of *Brassica*–gene interactions observed in the literature suggest that the genetic component is related to the persistence of ITCs in the body. Urinary ITC levels are lower among subjects with the *GSTT1*-null or the *GSTM1*-null genetic polymorphisms, suggesting that subjects with a GST-positive genotype more rapidly excrete ITCs.[87,88] Although *Brassica* consumption also induces GSTA expression among *GSTM1/T1*-null subjects, GSTA activity is less efficient at metabolizing ITCs.[64,70] Most studies found that *Brassica* was more strongly protective for cancer among subjects with a *GST*-null genotype, and perhaps the longer persistence of *Brassica* phytochemicals in the body of *GST*-null subjects leads to greater opportunities to interfere with carcinogenic processes. The specific GST enzymes involved may depend on the genetic profile of the study population, the metabolic pathways of the carcinogen, or the types of *Brassica* vegetables consumed in that population. As GSL metabolism becomes better understood, it should be possible to confirm this idea in future studies.

3. *Brassica*–gene interactions may be cancer-site specific and depend on a population's likelihood of being exposed to the carcinogens that strongly determine cancer risk. Genetic modification of the protective association between *Brassica* intake and cancer appeared to be substantial in lung and colorectal cancer research studies. Although *Brassica* and breast cancer associations also were modified by specific genetic variants, it was to a lesser degree than with lung and colon cancer. Compared to breast cancer, lung and colon cancer risks are more strongly associated with chemical carcinogenic pathways (such as tobacco) that are affected directly by metabolic enzyme activity. As illustrated in Figure 12.4, perhaps *Brassica* may increase the metabolism and excretion of chemical carcinogens from tobacco use, meat intake, or from other sources through

selective induction and inhibition of Phase II or Phase I enzymes. Accordingly, several lung cancer studies observed a stronger *Brassica*–gene interaction among current tobacco users compared to "ever-users." These same subjects may have a higher susceptibility to chemical carcinogenesis due to a lower metabolic capacity to detoxify procarcinogens.

12.9 ALTERNATIVE MECHANISMS

Alternatively, *Brassica* ITCs and indoles may reduce breast cancer risk through mechanisms that do not necessarily involve Phase II enzymes. Several studies report that *Brassica* indoles and ITCs induce apoptosis or stabilize cellular proliferation in breast, prostate, colon, blood, and other cancer cell lines.[115–125] These *Brassica* phytochemicals appear to interact directly with critical signaling pathways regulating apoptosis and proliferation.[126,127] This effect on cell cycle regulation may explain the protective associations between *Brassica* and cancer risks that are not so clearly associated with environmental carcinogens (e.g., breast cancer, prostate cancer). Of course, the effects of ITCs and indoles on cellular regulatory processes also may be relevant to lung, colon, and other cancers associated with environmental carcinogens, particularly in a situation in which the population is not highly exposed to these environmental carcinogens. At present, the effect of interaction between *Brassica* and genetic markers of variability in cell cycle regulation on cancer risk or the effect of interaction between *Brassica* and Phase II enzymes on indices of cell proliferation, have not been explored. Similarly, breast cancer risk may be associated with catechol estrogen exposure determined by several P-450 enzymes.[128] However, the interaction between *Brassica* and Phase I enzyme genetic polymorphisms have not been systematically explored.

12.10 TRANSLATING *BRASSICA*–CANCER ASSOCIATIONS TO CANCER PREVENTION

Cancer prevention utilizing a *Brassica*-based approach is somewhat controversial. Although the majority of human, animal, and cell-culture research studies have found that *Brassica* intake or exposure to related phytochemicals inhibited carcinogenesis, a minority of animal studies have reported that I3C or ITC administration increased tumor burden.[129–133] Whether these animal studies reflect the human conditions and exposure levels is unclear, and important questions remain regarding the interactions between ITC, I3C, and tumorogenesis in animals vs. humans. Nevertheless, several research groups have conducted exploratory human trials to investigate the feasibility and efficacy of, and the biomechanisms related to, a *Brassica*-based cancer prevention approach. For example, intervention studies have reported that *Brassica* vegetable consumption or I3C supplements significantly shifted estrogen metabolism in a manner consistent with reduced breast cancer risk,[50,51] or regressed cervical intraepithelial neoplasia (CIN)[134] and recurrent respiratory papillomatosis (RRP).[5,135] These preliminary studies did not report any serious adverse events associated with their respective interventions, suggesting that cancer chemoprevention based on *Brassica* phytochemicals may be possible. Clearly, research at this time is inadequate to support casual ITC or I3C supplementation. Caution and careful consideration are strongly advised before administering any high-dose ITC or I3C diet supplements to otherwise healthy people or to specific patient populations.

An alternative approach would be to promote *Brassica* vegetable consumption. *Brassica* intake combines ITCs and indoles at well-tolerated levels, at little cost or apparent toxicity. Indeed, the "dose–effect" relationship may not be linear, and the lower levels provided via food may be ideal.[136] Furthermore, greater vegetable intake is consistent with the public-health aim of promoting a healthy lifestyle and may be a feasible alternative for many subjects. In the future, it may be possible to genetically screen persons and identify those persons who may have the genetic disposition to benefit the most from adding *Brassica* to the diet.

12.11 SUMMARY

Health agencies advocate greater vegetable and fruit intakes, and *Brassica* vegetable consumption has been linked with reduced cancer risk.[2] This review provides an introduction to the available studies investigating cancer, *Brassica,* and genetic polymorphisms critical in the metabolism of *Brassica* phytochemicals or xenogenous carcinogens. *Brassica* intake appears more effective in preventing lung, colon, or breast cancers in subjects with genetic polymorphisms consistent with lower Phase II enzyme activity. However, only a handful of studies are available at this time. Cancer is a leading cause of death in the U.S., but the public-health impact of GSL exposure cannot be fully realized without additional investigations. Hopefully, this review will motivate additional research to investigate these findings across different study populations, genes, and diet assessment approaches, and to apply this information to cancer prevention or adjuvant cancer-care programs.

REFERENCES

1. Kolonel, L.N., Altshuler, D., and Henderson, B.E. The multiethnic cohort study: exploring genes, lifestyle and cancer risk. *Nat. Rev. Cancer,* 4: 1–9, 2004.
2. World Cancer Research Fund. *Food, Nutrition and the Prevention of Cancer: A Global Perspective.* Washington, D.C.: American Institute for Cancer Research, 1997.
3. United States Department of Agriculture. Per Capita Consumption. USDA/Economic Research Service, 2004.
4. Verhoeven, D.T., Goldbohm, R.A., van Poppel, G.A., Verhagen, H., and van den Brandt, P.A. Epidemiological studies of *Brassica* vegetables and cancer risk. *Cancer Epidemiol. Biomarkers Prev.,* 5: 733–748, 1996.
5. Auborn, K., Abramson, A., Bradlow, H.L., Sepkovic, D., and Mullooly, V. Estrogen metabolism and laryngeal papillomatosis: a pilot study on dietary prevention. *Anticancer Res.,* 18: 4569–4574, 1998.
6. Hung, H.C., Joshipura, K.J., Jiang, R., Hu, F.B., Hunter, D., Smith-Warner, S.A., Colditz, G.A., Rosner, B., Spiegelman, D., and Willett, W.C. Fruit and vegetable intake and risk of major chronic disease. *J. Natl. Cancer Inst. Cancer Spectrum,* 96: 1577–1584, 2004.

7. Zhang, S.M., Hunter, D.J., Rosner, B.A., Giovannucci, E.L., Colditz, G.A., Speizer, F.E., and Willett, W.C. Intakes of fruits, vegetables, and related nutrients and the risk of non-Hodgkin's lymphoma among women. *Cancer Epidemiol. Biomarkers Prev.*, 9: 477–485, 2000.

8. Rashidkhani, B., Lindblad, P., and Wolk, A. Fruits, vegetables and risk of renal cell carcinoma: a prospective study of Swedish women. *Int. J. Cancer*, 113: 451–455, 2005.

9. Michaud, D.S., Spiegelman, D., Clinton, S.K., Rimm, E.B., Willett, W.C., and Giovannucci, E.L. Fruit and vegetable intake and incidence of bladder cancer in a male prospective cohort. *J. Natl. Cancer Inst.*, 91: 605–613, 1999.

10. Zeegers, M.P.A., Goldbohm, R.A., and van den Brandt, P.A. Consumption of vegetables and fruits and urothelial cancer incidence: a prospective study. *Cancer Epidemiol. Biomarkers Prev.*, 10: 1121–1128, 2001.

11. Schuurman, A.G., Goldbohm, R.A., Dorant, E., and van den Brandt, P.A. Vegetable and fruit consumption and prostate cancer risk: a cohort study in the Netherlands. *Cancer Epidemiol. Biomarkers Prev.*, 7: 673–680, 1998.

12. Giovannucci, E., Rimm, E.B., Liu, Y., Stampfer, M.J., and Willett, W.C. A prospective study of cruciferous vegetables and prostate cancer. *Cancer Epidemiol. Biomarkers Prev.*, 12: 1403–1409, 2003.

13. Voorrips, L.E., Goldbohm, R.A., Verhoeven, D.T., van Poppel, G.A., Sturmans, F., Hermus, R.J.J., and van den Brandt, P.A. Vegetable and fruit consumption and lung cancer risk in the Netherlands cohort study on diet and cancer. *Cancer Causes Control*, 11: 101–115, 2000.

14. Neuhouser, M.L., Patterson, R.E., Thornquist, M.D., Omenn, G.S., King, I.B., and Goodman, G.E. Fruits and vegetables are associated with lower lung cancer risk only in the placebo arm of the {beta}-carotene and retinol efficacy trial (CARET). *Cancer Epidemiol. Biomarkers Prev.*, 12: 350–358, 2003.

15. Feskanich, D., Ziegler, R.G., Michaud, D.S., Giovannucci, E.L., Speizer, F.E., Willett, W.C., and Colditz, G.A. Prospective study of fruit and vegetable consumption and risk of lung cancer among men and women. *J. Natl. Cancer Inst. Cancer Spectrum*, 92: 1812–1823, 2000.

16. Flood, A., Velie, E.M., Chaterjee, N., Subar, A.F., Thompson, F.E., Lacey, J.V., Jr., Schairer, C., Troisi, R., and Schatzkin, A. Fruit and vegetable intakes and the risk of colorectal cancer in the breast cancer detection demonstration project follow-up cohort. *Am. J. Clin. Nutr.*, 75: 936–943, 2002.

17. Voorrips, L.E., Goldbohm, R.A., van Poppel, G.A., Sturmans, F., Hermus, R.J.J., and van den Brandt, P.A. Vegetable and fruit consumption and risks of colon and rectal cancer in a prospective cohort study the Netherlands cohort study on diet and cancer. *Am. J. Epidemiol.*, 152: 1081–1092, 2000.

18. Michels, K.B., Giovannucci, E., Joshipura, K.J., Rosner, B.A., Stampfer, M.J., Fuchs, C.S., Colditz, G.A., Speizer, F.E., and Willett, W.C. Prospective study of fruit and vegetable consumption and incidence of colon and rectal cancers. *J. Natl. Cancer Inst.*, 92: 1740–1752, 2000.

19. McCullough, M.L., Robertson, A.S., Chao, A., Jacobs, E.J., Stampfer, M.J., Jacobs, D.R., Diver, W.R., Calle, E.E., and Thun, M.J. A prospective study of whole grains, fruits, vegetables and colon cancer risk. *Cancer Causes Control*, 14: 959–970, 2003.

20. Key, T.J., Allen, N., Appleby, P.N., Overvad, K., Tjønneland, A., Miller, A., Boeing, H., Karalis, D., Psaltopoulou, T., Berrino, F., Palli, D., Panico, S., Tumino, R., Vineis, P., Bueno-de-Mesquita, H.B., Kieminey, K., Peeters, P., Martinex, D., Dorronsoro, M., Gonzalez, C.A., Chrlaque, M.D., Quiros, J.R., Ardanaz, E., Berglund, G., Egevad, L., Hallmans, G., Stattin, P., Bingham, S., Day, N.E., Gann, P., Kaaks, R., Ferrari,

P., and Riboli, E. Fruits and vegetables and prostate cancer: no association among 1,104 cases in a prospective study of 130,544 men in the European Prospective Investigation into Cancer and Nutrition (EPIC). *Int. J. Cancer*, 109: 119–124, 2004.

21. Smith-Warner, S.A., Spiegelman, D., Yaun, S.S., Albanes, D., Beeson, W.L., van den Brandt, P.A., Folsom, A.R., Fraser, G.E., Freudenheim, J.L., and Giovannucci, E. Fruits, vegetables and lung cancer: a pooled analysis of cohort studies. *Int. J. Cancer*, 107: 1001–1011, 2003.

22. Smith-Warner, S.A., Spiegelman, D., Yaun, S.S., Adami, H.O., Beeson, W.L., van den Brandt, P.A., Folsom, A.R., Fraser, G.E., Freudenheim, J.L., Goldbohm, R.A., Graham, S., Miller, A.B., Potter, J.D., Rohan, T.E., Speizer, F.E., Toniolo, P., Willett, W.C., Wolk, A., Zeleniuch-Jacquotte, A., and Hunter, D.J. Intake of fruits and vegetables and risk of breast cancer: a pooled analysis of cohort studies. *J. Am. Med. Assoc.*, 285: 769–776, 2001.

23. Fahey, J.W., Zalcmann, A.T., and Talalay, P. The chemical diversity and distribution of glucosinolates and isothiocyanates among plants. *Phytochemistry*, 56: 5–51, 2001.

24. Fenwick, G.R., Heaney, R.K., and Mullin, W.J. Glucosinolates and their breakdown products in food and food plants. *CRC Crit. Rev. Food Sci. Nutr.*, 123–200. 1983.

25. Lampe, J.W. and Peterson, S. *Brassica*, biotransformation and cancer risk: genetic polymorphisms alter the preventive effects of cruciferous vegetables. *J. Nutr.*, 132: 2991–2994, 2002.

26. Carlson, D.G., Daxenbichler, M.E., Van Etten, C.H., Tookey, H.L., and Williams, P.H. Glucosinolates in crucifer vegetables: turnips and rutabagas. *J. Agric. Food Chem.*, 29: 1235–1239, 1981.

27. Fahey, J.W., Zhang, Y., and Talalay, P. Broccoli spouts: An exceptionally rich source of inducers of enzymes that protect against chemical carcinogenesis. *Proc. Natl. Acad. Sci., USA*, 94: 10367–10372, 1997.

28. Hecht, S.S., Carmella, S.G., Kenney, P.M.J., Low, S.H., Arakawa, K., and Yu, M.C. Effects of cruciferous vegetable consumption on urinary metabolites of the tobacco-specific lung carcinogen 4-(Methylnitrosamino)-1-(3-Pyridyl)-1-Butanone in Singapore Chinese. *Cancer Epidemiol. Biomarkers Prev.*, 13: 997–1004, 2004.

29. Rosa, E.A.S., Heany, R.K., Fenwick, G.R., and Portas, C.A.M. Glucosinolates in crop plants. *Hort. Rev.*, 19: 99–215, 1997.

30. Vallejo, F., Garcia-Viguera, C., and Tomás-Barberán, F. Changes in broccoli (*Brassica oleracea* L. Var. *italica*) health-promoting compounds with inflorescence development. *J. Agric. Food Chem.*, 51: 3776–3782, 2003.

31. Shapiro, T.A., Fahey, J.W., Wade, K.L., Stephenson, K.K., and Talalay, P. Human metabolism and excretion of cancer chemoprotective glucosinolates and isothiocyanates of *Cruciferous* vegetables. *Cancer Epidemiol. Biomarkers Prev.*, 7: 1091–1100, 1998.

32. Getahun, S.M. and Chung, F.-L. Conversion of glucosinolates to isothiocyanates in humans after ingestion of cooked watercress. *Cancer Epidemiol. Biomarkers Prev.*, 8: 447–451, 1999.

33. Nugon-Baudon, L., Rabot, S., Flinois, J.-P., Lory, S., and Beaune, P.H. Effects of the bacterial status of rats on the changes in some liver cytochrome P450 (EC1.14.14.1) apoproteins consequent to a glucosinolate-rich diet. *Br. J. Nutr.*, 80: 231–234, 1998.

34. Nho, C.W. and Jeffery, E. Crambene, a bioactive nitrile derived from glucosinolate hydrolysis, acts via the antioxidant response element to upregulate quinone reductase alone or synergistically with indole-3-carbinol. *Toxicol. Appl. Pharmacol.*, 198: 40–48, 2004.

35. McDanell, R. and McLean, A.E.M. Chemical and biological properties of indole glucosinolates (glucobrassicans): a review. *Food Chem. Toxicol.*, 26: 59–70, 1988.

36. Riby, J.E., Feng, C., Chang, Y.-C., Schaldach, C.M., Firestone, G.L., and Bjeldanes, L.F. The major cyclic trimeric product of indole-3-carbinol is a strong agonist of the estrogen receptor signaling pathway. *Biochemistry (Mosc).*, 39: 910–918, 2000.

37. Bradfield, C.A. and Bjeldanes, L.F. Modification of carcinogen metabolism by indolylic autolysis products of *Brassica oleraceae. Adv. Exp. Med. Biol.,* 289: 153–163, 1991.

38. Brandi, G., Paiardini, M., Cervasi, B., Fiorucci, C., Filippone, P., De Marco, C., Zaffaroni, N., and Magnani, M. A new indole-3-carbinol tetrameric derivative inhibits cyclin-dependent kinase 6 expression, and induces g1 cell cycle arrest in both estrogen-dependent and estrogen-independent breast cancer cell lines. *Cancer Res.,* 63: 4028–4036, 2003.

39. Conney, A.H. Induction of drug-metabolizing enzymes: a path to the discovery of multiple cytochromes P450. *Annu. Rev. Pharmacol. Toxicol.,* 43: 1–30, 2003.

40. Wattenberg, L.W. Inhibition of polycyclic aromatic hydrocarbon-induced neoplasia by naturally occurring indoles. *Cancer Res.,* 38: 1410–1413, 1978.

41. Pantuck, E.J., Pantuck, C.B., Garland, W.A., Min, B.H., Wattenberg, L.W., Anderson, K.E., Kappas, A., and Conney, A.H. Stimulatory effect of Brussels sprouts and cabbage on human drug metabolism. *Clin. Pharmacol. Ther.,* 25: 88–95, 1979.

42. Pantuck, E.J., Pantuck, C.B., Anderson, K.E., Wattenberg, L.W., Conney, A.H., and Kappas, A. Effects of Brussels sprouts and cabbage on drug conjugation. *Clin. Pharmacol. Ther.,* 35: 161–169, 1984.

43. McDanell, R., McLean, A.E.M., Hanley, A.B., Heaney, R.K., and Fenwick, G.R. Differential induction of mixed-function oxidase activity in rat liver and intestine by diets containing processed cabbage: correlation with cabbage levels of glucosinolates and glucosinolate hydrolysis products. *Food Chem. Toxicol.,* 25: 363–368, 1987.

44. Vang, O., Jensen, M. B., and Autrup, H. Induction of cytochrome P450IA1 in rat colon and liver by indole-3-carbinol and 5,6-benzoflavone. *Carcinogenesis,* 11: 1259–1263, 1990.

45. Vang, O., Jensen, H., and Autrup, H. Induction of cytochrome P-450IA1, IA2, IIB1, and IIE1 by broccoli in rat liver and colon. *Chem. Biol. Interact.,* 78: 85–96, 1991.

46. Vang, O., Frandsen, H., Hansen, K.T., Nielsen, J.B., and Andersen, O. Modulation of drug-metabolising enzyme expression by condensation products of indole-3-ylcarbinol, and inducer in cruciferous vegetables. *Pharmacol. Toxicol.,* 84: 59–65, 1999.

47. Vistisen, K., Loft, S., and Poulsen, H.E. Cytochrome P450 1A2 activity in man measured by caffeine metabolism: effect of smoking, broccoli and exercise. *Adv. Exp. Med. Biol.,* 283: 407–411, 1991.

48. Kall, M.A., Vang, O., and Clausen, J. Effects of dietary broccoli on human *in vivo* drug metabolizing enzymes: evaluation of caffeine, estrone, and chlorzoxazone. *Carcinogenesis,* 17: 793–799, 1996.

49. Lampe, J.W., King, I.B., Li, S., Grate, M.T., Barale, K.V., Chen, C., Feng, Z., and Potter, J.D. *Brassica* vegetables increase and apiaceous vegetables decrease cytochrome P450 1A2 activity in humans: changes in caffeine metabolite ratios in response to controlled vegetable diets. *Carcinogenesis,* 21: 1157–1162, 2000.

50. Bradlow, H.L., Michnovicz, J.J., Halper, M., Miller, D.G., Wong, G.Y.C., and Osborne, M. Long-term responses of women to indole-3-carbinol or a high fiber diet. *Cancer Epidemiol. Biomarkers Prev.,* 3: 591–595, 1994.

51. Fowke, J.H., Longcope, C., and Hebert, J.R. *Brassica* vegetable consumption shifts estrogen metabolism in healthy postmenopausal women. *Cancer Epidemiol. Biomarkers Prev.,* 9: 773–779, 2000.

52. Bjeldanes, L.F., Kim, J.-Y., Grose, K.R., Bartholomew, J.C., and Bradfield, C.A. Aromatic hydrocarbon responsiveness-receptor agonists generated from indole-3-carbinol *in vitro* and in vivo: comparisons with 2,3,7,8-tetrachlorodibenzo-*p*-dioxin. *Proc. Natl. Acad. Sci. USA*, 88: 9543–9547, 1991.

53. Chen, I., McDougal, A., Wang, F., and Safe, S. Aryl hydrocarbon receptor-mediated antiestrogenic and antitumorigenic activity of diindolymethane. *Carcinogenesis*, 19: 1631–1639, 1998.

54. Chen, I., Safe, S., and Bjeldanes, L. Indole-3-carbinol and diindolymethane as aryl hydrocarbon (Ah) receptor agonists and antagonists in T47D human breast cancer cells. *Biochem. Pharmacol.*, 51: 1069–1076, 1996.

55. Murray, G.I., Taylor, M.C., McFadyen, M.C.E., McKay, J.A., Greenlee, W.F., Burke, M.D., and Melvin, W.T. Tumor-specific expression of cytochrome P450 CYP1B1. *Cancer Res.*, 57: 3026–3031, 1997.

56. Wang, H., Griffiths, S., and Williamson, G. Effect of glucosinolate breakdown products on beta-naphthoflavone-induced expression of human cytochrome P450 1A1 via the Ah receptor for Hep G2 cells. *Cancer Lett.*, 114: 121–125, 1997.

57. Conaway, C.C., Yang, Y.M., and Chung, F.L. Isothiocyanates as cancer chemopreventive agents: their biological activities and metabolism in rodents and humans. *Curr. Drug Metab.*, 3: 233–255, 2002.

58. Hecht, S.S. Chemoprevention by isothiocyanates. *J. Cell. Biochem.*, 22: 195–209, 1995.

59. Bacon, J.R., Williamson, G., Garner, R.C., Lappin, G., Langouet, S., and Bao, Y. Sulforaphane and quercetin modulate PhIP-DNA adduct formation in human HepG2 cells and hepatocytes. *Carcinogenesis*, 24: 1903–1911, 2003.

60. Langouët, S., Furge, L.L., Kerriguy, N., Nakamura, K., Guillouzo, A., and Guengerich, F.P. Inhibition of human cytochrome P450 enzymes by 1,2-dithiole-3-thione, oltipraz and its derivatives, and sulforaphane. *Chem. Res. Toxicol.*, 13: 245–252, 2000.

61. Murata, M., Yamashita, N., Inoue, S., and Kawanishi, S. Mechanism of oxidative DNA damage induced by carcinogenic allyl isothiocyanate. *Free Radic. Biol. Med.*, 28: 797–805, 2000.

62. Canistro, D., Croce, C.D., Iori, R., Barillari, J., Bronzetti, G., Poi, G., Cini, M., Caltavuturo, L., Perocco, P., and Paolini, M. Genetic and metabolic effects of gluc
nasturtiin, a glucosinolate derived from cruciferae. *Mutat. Res. Fundam. Mol. Mech. Mutagenesis*, 545: 23–35, 2004.

63. Paolini, M., Perocco, P., Canistro, D., Valgimigli, L., Pedulli, G.F., Iori, R., Croce, C.D., Cantelli-Forti, G., Legator, M.S., and Abdel-Rahman, S.Z. Induction of cytochrome P450, generation of oxidative stress and in vitro cell-transforming and DNA-damaging activities by glucoraphanin, the bioprecursor of the chemopreventive agent sulforaphane found in broccoli. *Carcinogenesis*, 25: 61–67, 2004.

64. Lampe, J.W., Chen, C., Li, S., Prunty, J., Grate, M.T., Meehan, D.E., Barale, K.V., Dightman, D.A., Feng, Z., and Potter, J.D. Modulation of human glutathione S-transferase by botanically defined vegetable diets. *Cancer Epidemiol. Biomarkers Prev.*, 9: 787–793, 2000.

65. Talalay, P. and Zhang, Y. Chemoprotection against cancer by isothiocyanates and glucosinolates. *Proc. Biochem. Soc.*, 24: 806–810, 1996.

66. Talalay, P., Fahey, J.W., Holtzclaw, W.D., Prestera, T., and Zhang, Y. Chemoprotection against cancer by Phase 2 enzyme induction. *Toxicol. Lett.*, 82/83: 173–179, 1995.

67. Verhagen, H., Poulsen, H.E., Loft, S., van Poppel, G.A., Willems, M., and vanBladeren, P.J. Reduction of oxidative DNA-damage in humans by Brussels sprouts. *Carcinogenesis*, 16: 969–970, 1995.

68. Verhagen, H., de Bries, A., Nijhoff, W. A., Schouten, A., van Poppel, G. A., Peters, W. H., and van den Berg, H. Effect of Brussels sprouts on oxidative DNA-damage in man. *Cancer Lett.*, 114: 127–130, 1997.

69. Fowke, J.H., Morrow, J., Motley, S., Bostick, R., and Ness, R. *Brassica* vegetable consumption reduces urinary F2-isoprostane levels, a biomarker of systemic oxidative stress. *Cancer Epidemiol. Biomarkers Prev.*, 14: 546–549, 2005.

70. Ketterer, B. Dietary isothiocyanates as confounding factors in the molecular epidemiology of colon cancer. *Cancer Epidemiol. Biomarkers Prev.*, 7: 645–646, 1998.

71. Kolm, R.H., Danielson, U.H., Zhang, Y., Talalay, P., and Mannervik, B. Isothiocyanates as substrates for human glutathione transferases: structure-activity studies. *Biochem. J.*, 311: 453–459, 1995.

72. Bogaards, J.J., Verhagen, H., Willems, M., van Poppel, G.A., and van Bladeren, P.J. Consumption of Brussels sprouts results in elevated alpha-class glutathione S-transferase levels in human blood plasma. *Carcinogenesis*, 15: 1073–1075, 1994.

73. Nijhoff, W.A., Grubben, M., Nagengast, F.M., Jansen, J., Verhagen, H., van Poppel, G.A., and Peters, W.H. Effects of consumption of Brussels sprouts on intestinal and lymphocytic glutathione S-transferases in humans. *Carcinogenesis*, 16: 2125–2128, 1995.

74. Nijhoff, W.A., Mulder, T.P., Verhagen, H., van Poppel, G.A., and Peters, W.H. Effects of consumption of Brussels sprouts on plasma and urinary glutathione S-transferase class -alpha and -pi in humans. *Carcinogenesis*, 16: 955–957, 1995.

75. Wolf, C.R. Chemoprevention: increased potential to bear fruit. *Proc. Natl. Acad. Sci. USA*, 98: 2941–2943, 2001.

76. Prochaska, H.J., Santamaria, A.B., and Talalay, P. Rapid detection of inducers of enzymes that protect against carcinogens. *Proc. Natl. Acad. Sci. USA*, 89: 2394–2398, 1992.

77. Schmidt, J.V. and Bradfield, C.A. AH receptor signaling pathways. *Annu. Rev. Cell Dev. Biol.*, 12: 55–89, 1996.

78. Bradfield, C.A. and Bjeldanes, L.F. Effect of dietary indole-3-carbinol on intestinal and hepatic monooxygenase, glutathione S-transferase and epoxide hydrolase activities in the rat. *Food Chem. Toxicol.*, 22: 977–982, 1984.

79. Bonnesen, C., Eggleston, I.M., and Hayes, J.D. Dietary indoles and isothiocyanates that are generated from Cruciferous vegetables can both stimulate apoptosis and confer protection against DNA damage in human colon cell lines. *Cancer Res.*, 61: 6120–6130, 2001.

80. Wilkinson, J. and Clapper, M.L. Detoxication enzymes and chemoprevention. *Proc. Soc. Exp. Biol. Med.*, 216: 192–200, 1997.

81. Wark, P.A., Grubben, M., Peters, W.H.M., Nagengast, F.M., Kampman, E., Kok, F.J., and van't Veer, P. Habitual consumption of fruits and vegetables: associations with human rectal glutathione S-transferase. *Carcinogenesis*, 25: 2135–2142, 2004.

82. Zimniak, P., Nanduri, B., Pikula, S., Bandorowicz-Pikula, J., Singhal, S.S., Srivastava, S.K., Awasthi, S., and Awasthi, Y.C. Naturally occurring human glutathione S-transferase GSTP1-1 isoforms with isoleucine and valine in position 104 differ in enzymic properties. *Eur. J. Biochem.*, 224: 893–899, 1994.

83. Lin, H.J., Johansson, A.S., Stenberg, G., Materi, A.M., Park, J.M., Dai, A., Zhou, H., Gim, J.S. Y., Kau, I.H., and Hardy, S.I. Naturally occurring Phe151Leu substitution near a conserved folding module lowers stability of glutathione transferase P1-1. *Biochim. Biophys. Acta — Proteins Proteomics*, 1649: 16–23, 2003.

84. Wu, L., Noyan-Ashraf, M.H., Facci, M., Wang, R., Paterson, P.G., Ferrie, A., and Juurlink, B.H.J. Dietary approach to attenuate oxidative stress, hypertension, and inflammation in the cardiovascular system. *Proc. Natl. Acad. Sci. USA,* 101: 7094–7099, 2004.

85. Zhang, Y.S., Kolm, R.H., Mannervik, B., and Talalay, P. Reversible conjugation of isothiocyanates with glutathione catalyzed by human glutathione transferases. *Biochem. Biophys. Res. Commun.,* 206: 748–755, 1995.

86. Zhang, Y., Wade, K.L., Prestera, T., and Talalay, P. Quantitative determination of isothiocyanates, dithiocarbamates, carbon disulfide, and related thiocarbonyl compounds by cyclocondensation of 1,2-benzenedithiol. *Anal. Biochem.,* 239: 160–167, 1996.

87. Seow, A., Shi, C.-Y., Chung, F.-L., Jiao, D., Hankin, J.H., Lee, H.-P., Coetzee, G.A., and Yu, M.C. Urinary total isothiocyanate (ITC) in a population-based sample of middle-aged and older Chinese in Singapore: relationship with dietary total ITC and glutathione *S*-transferase M1/T1/P1 genotypes. *Cancer Epidemiol. Biomarkers Prev.,* 7: 775–781, 1998.

88. Fowke, J.H., Shu, X.-O., Qi, D., Shintani, A., Chung, F.-L., Conaway, C., Gao, Y.T., and Zheng, W. Urinary isothiocyanate excretion, *Brassica* consumption, and gene polymorphisms among women living in Shanghai, China. *Cancer Epidemiol. Biomarkers Prev.,* 12: 1536–1539, 2003.

89. Walters, D.G., Young, P.J., Agus, C., Knize, M.G., Boobis, A.R., Gooderham, N.J., and Lake, B.G. Cruciferous vegetable consumption alters the metabolism of the dietary carcinogen 2-amino-1-methyl-6-phenylimidazo[4,5-b]pyridine (PhIP) in humans. *Carcinogenesis,* 25: 1659–1669, 2004.

90. Cross, A.J. and Sinha, R. Meat-related mutagens/carcinogens in the etiology of colorectal cancer. *Environ. Mol. Mutagen,* 44: 44–55, 2004.

91. Sinha, R., Kulldorff, M., Swanson, C.A., Curtin, J., Brownson, R.C., and Alavanja, M.C.R. Dietary heterocyclic amines and the risk of lung cancer among Missouri women. *Cancer Res.,* 60: 3753–3756, 2000.

92. Hecht, S.S. Chemoprevention of cancer by isothiocyanates, modifiers of carcinogen metabolism. *J. Nutr.,* 129: 768S–774S, 1999.

93. Hecht, S.S., Chung, F.L., Richie, J.P., Jr., Akerkar, S.A., Borukhova, A., Skowronski, L., and Carmella, S.G. Effects of watercress consumption on metabolism of a tobacco-specific lung carcinogen in smokers. *Cancer Epidemiol. Biomarkers Prev.,* 4: 877–884, 1995.

94. Morse, M.A., LaGreca, S.D., Amin, S.G., and Chung, F.-L. Effects of Indole-3-carbinol on lung tumorigenesis and DNA methylation induced by 4-(Methylnitros-amino)-1-(3-pyridyl)-1-butone (NNK) and on the metabolism and disposition of NNK in A/J mice. *Cancer Res.,* 50: 2613–2617, 1990.

95. Taioli, E., Garbers, S., Bradlow, H.L., Carmella, S.G., Akerkar, S., and Hecht, S.S. Effects of indole-3-carbinol on the metabolism of 4-(methylnitrosamino)-1-(3-pyridyl)-1-butanone in smokers. *Cancer Epidemiol. Biomarkers Prev.,* 6: 517–522, 1997.

96. Lin, H.J., Probst-Hensch, N.M., Louie, A.D., Kau, I.H., Witte, J.S., Ingles, S.A., Frankl, H.D., Lee, E.R., and Haile, R.W. Glutathione transferase null genotype, broccoli, and lower prevalence of colorectal adenomas. *Cancer Epidemiol. Biomarkers Prev.,* 7: 647–652, 1998.

97. Seow, A., Yuan, J.M., Sun, C.L., Van Den Berg, D., Lee, H.P., and Yu, M.C. Dietary isothiocyanates, glutathione S-transferase polymorphisms and colorectal cancer risk in the Singapore Chinese health study. *Carcinogenesis,* 23: 2055–2061, 2002.

98. Solt, D.B., Chang, K.W., Helenowski, I., and Rademaker, A.W. Phenethyl isothiocy-anate inhibits nitrosamine carcinogenesis in a model for study of oral cancer chemo-prevention. *Cancer Lett.*, 202: 147–152, 2003.

99. Chainani-Wu, N. Diet and oral, pharyngeal, and esophageal cancer. *Nutr. Cancer: An International Journal*, 44: 104–126, 2002.

100. Gaudet, M.M., Olshan, A.F., Poole, C., Weissler, M.C., Watson, M., and Bell, D.A. Diet, GSTM1, and GSTT1 and head and neck cancer. *Carcinogenesis*, 25: 735–740, 2004.

101. Spitz, M.R., Duphorne, C.M., Detry, M.A., Pillow, P.C., Amos, C.I., Lei, L., de Andrade, M., Gu, X., Hong, W.K., and Wu, X. Dietary intake of isothiocyanates; evidence of a joint effect with glutathione S-transferasen polymorphisms in lung cancer risk. *Cancer Epidemiol. Biomarkers Prev.*, 9: 1017–1020, 2000.

102. Zhao, B., Seow, A., Lee, E.J.D., Poh, W.-T., Teh, M., Eng, P., Wang, T.-T., Tan, W., Yu, M.C., and Lee, H.-P. Dietary isothiocyanates, glutathione S-transferase -M1, -T1 polymorphisms and lung cancer risk among Chinese women in Singapore. *Cancer Epidemiol. Biomarkers Prev.*, 10: 1063–1067, 2001.

103. Jiao, D., Yu, M., Hankin, J.H., Low, S.-H., and Chung, F.-L. Total isothiocyanate contents in cooked vegetables frequently consumed in Singapore. *J. Agric. Food Chem.*, 46: 1055–1058, 1998.

104. Subar, A.F., Kipnis, V., Troiano, R.P., Midthune, D., Schoeller, D.A., Bingham, S., Sharbaugh, C.O., Trabulsi, J., Runswick, S., Ballard-Barbash, R., Sunshine, J., and Schatzkin, A. Using intake biomarkers to evaluate the extent of dietary misreporting in a large sample of adults: the open study. *Am. J. Epidemiol.*, 158: 1, 2003.

105. Vallejo, F., Tomás-Barberán, F., and García-Viguera, C. Health-promoting compounds in broccoli as influenced by refrigerated transport and retail sale period. *J. Agric. Food Chem.*, 51: 3029–3034, 2003.

106. McNaughton, S.A. and Marks, G.C. Development of a food composition database for the estimation of dietary intakes of glucosinolates, the biologically active constit-uents of cruciferous vegetables. *Br. J. Nutr.*, 90: 687–697, 2003.

107. Mullin, W.J. and Sahasrabudhe, M.R. Glucosinolate content of cruciferous vegetable crops. *Canadian J. Plant Sci.*, 57: 1227–1230, 1977.

108. Mullin, W.J. and Sahasrabudhe, M.R. An estimate of the average daily intake of glucosinolates via cruciferous vegetables. *Nutr. Rep. Int.*, 18: 273–279, 1978.

109. London, S.J., Yuan, J.-M., Chung, F.-L., Gao, Y.-T., Coetzee, G.A., Ross, R.K., and Yu, M.C. Isothiocyanates, glutathioneS-transferase M1 and T1 polymorphisms, and lung-cancer risk: a prospective study of men in Shanghai, China. *Lancet*, 356: 724–729, 2000.

110. Chung, F.-L., Jiao, D., Getahun, S.M., and Yu, M.C. A urinary biomarker for uptake of dietary isothiocyanates in humans. *Cancer Epidemiol. Biomarkers Prev.*, 7: 103–108, 1998.

111. Smith-Warner, S., Willett, W., Spiegelman, D., and Hunter, D. Reply: *Brassica* veg-etables and breast cancer. *J. Am. Med. Assoc.*, 285: 2977, 2001.

112. Terry, P. and Wolk, A. *Brassica* vegetables and breast cancer risk. *J. Am. Med. Assoc.*, 285: 2975–2977, 2001.

113. Zhang, S., Hunter, D., Forman, M.R., Rosner, B.A., Speizer, F.E., Colditz, G.A., Manson, J.E., Hankinson, S.E., and Willett, W.C. Dietary carotenoids and vitamin A, C, and E and risk of breast cancer. *J. Natl. Cancer Inst.*, 91: 547–556, 1999.

114. Fowke, J.H., Chung, F.-L., Jin, F., Qi, D., Cai, Q., Conaway, C., Cheng, J.R., Shu, X.O., Gao, Y.T., and Zheng, W. Urinary isothiocyanate levels, *Brassica*, and human breast cancer. *Cancer Res.*, 63: 3980–3986, 2003.

115 Chiao, J.W., Chung, F.-L., Kancherla, R., Ahmed, T., Mittleman, A., and Conaway, C.C. Sulforaphane and its metabolite mediate growth arrest and apoptosis in human prostate cancer cells. *Int. J. Oncol.*, 20: 631–636, 2002.

116. Chiao, J.W., Wu, H., Ramaswamy, G., Conaway, C.C., Chung, F.-L., Wang, L., and Liu, D. Ingestion of an isothiocyanate metabolite from cruciferous vegetables inhibits growth of human prostate cancer cell xenografts by apoptosis and cell cycle arrest. *Carcinogenesis*, 25: 1403–1408, 2004.

117. Chinni, S.R., Li, Y., Upadhyay, S., Koppolu, P.K., and Sarkar, F.H. Indole-3-carbinol (I3C) induced cell growth inhibition, Gq cell cycle arrest and apoptosis in prostate cancer cells. *Oncogene*, 20: 2927–2936, 2001.

118. Fimognari, C., Nusse, M., Cesari, R., Iori, R., Cantelli-Forti, G., and Hrelia, P. Growth inhibition, cell-cycle arrest and apoptosis in human T-cell leukemia by the isothiocyanate sulforaphane. *Carcinogenesis*, 23: 581–586, 2002.

119. Fimognari, C., Nusse, M., Berti, F., Iori, R., Cantelli-Forti, G., and Hrelia, P. Sulforaphane modulates cell cycle and apoptosis in transformed and non-transformed human T lymphocytes. *Ann. N. Y. Acad. Sci.*, 1010: 393–398, 2003.

120. Gamet-Payrastre, L., Li, P., Lumeau, S., Cassar, G., Dupont, M.-A., Chevolleau, S., Gasc, N., Tulliez, J., and Tercé, F. Sulforaphane, a naturally occurring isothiocyanate, induces cell cycle arrest and apoptosis in HT29 human colon cancer cells. *Cancer Res.*, 60: 1426–1433, 2000.

121. Ge, X., Fares, F.A., and Yannai, S. Induction of apoptosis in MCF-7 cells by indole-3-carbinol is independent of p53 and bax. *Anticancer Res.*, 19: 199–203, 1999.

122. Ge, X., Yannai, S., Rennert, G., Gruener, N., and Fares, F.A. 3,3-diindolylmethane induces apoptosis in human cancer cells. *Biochem. Biophys. Res. Commun.*, 228: 153–158, 1996.

123. Hu, R., Kim, B.R., Chen, C., Hebbar, V., and Kong, A.N.T. The roles of JNK and apoptotic signaling pathways in PEITC-mediated responses in human HT-29 colon adenocarcinoma cells. *Carcinogenesis*, 24: 1361–1367, 2003.

124. Huang, C., Ma, W., Li, J., Hecht, S.S., and Dong, Z. Essential role of p53 in phenethyl isothiocyanate-induced apoptosis. *Cancer Res.*, 58: 4102–4108, 1998.

125. Xiao, D., Srivastava, S. K., Lew, K. L., Zeng, Y., Hershberger, P., Johnson, C. S., Trump, D. L., and Singh, S. V. Allyl isothiocyanate, a constituent of cruciferous vegetables, inhibits proliferation of human prostate cancer cells by causing G2/M arrest and inducing apoptosis. *Carcinogenesis*, 24: 891, 2003.

126. Sarkar, F.H. and Li, Y. Indole-3-carbinol and prostate cancer. *J. Nutr.*, 134: 3493S–3498S, 2004.

127. Rahman, K.M., Li, Y., and Sarkar, F.H. Inactivation of akt and NF-kappaB play important roles during indole-3-carbinol-induced apoptosis in breast cancer cells. *Nutr. Cancer*, 48: 84–94, 2004.

128. Zhu, B.T. and Conney, A.H. Functional role of estrogen metabolism in target cells: review and perspectives. *Carcinogenesis*, 19: 1–27, 1998.

129. Kim, D.J., Han, B.S., Ahn, B., Hasegawa, R., Shirai, T., Ito, N., and Tsuda, K. Enhancement by indole-3-carbinol of liver and thyroid gland neoplastic development in rat medium-term multiorgan carcinogenesis model. *Carcinogenesis*, 18: 377–381, 1997.

130. Bailey, G.S., Hendricks, J.D., Shelton, D.W., Nixon, J.E., and Pawlowski, N. Enhancement of carcinogenesis by natural anticarcinogen indole-3-carbinol. *J. Natl. Cancer Inst.*, 78: 931–934, 1987.

131. Hirose, M., Yamaguchi, T., Kimoto, N., Ogawa, K., Sano, M., Futakuchi, M., and Shirai, T. Strong promoting activity of phenylethyl isothiocyanate and benzyl isothiocyanate on urinary bladder carcinogenesis in F344 male rats. *Int. J. Cancer*, 77: 773–777, 1998.

132. Lubert, R.A., Steele, V.E., Eto, I., Juliana, M.M., Kelloff, G.J., and Grubbs, C.J. Chemopreventive efficacy of anethole trithione, N-acetyl-L-cysteine, miconazole and phenethylisothiocyanate in the DMBA induced rat mammary cancer model. *Int. J. Cancer*, 72: 95–101, 1997.

133. Rao, C.V., Rivenson, A., Simi, B., Zang, E., Hamid, R., Kelloff, G.J., Steele, V., and Reddy, B.S. Enhancement of experimental colon carcinogenesis by dietary 6-phenylhexyl isothiocyanate. *Cancer Res.*, 55: 4311–4318, 1995.

134. Bell, M.C., Crowley-Norwick, P., Bradlow, H.L., Sepkovic, D.W., Schmidt-Grimminger, D., Howell, P., Mayeaux, E.J., Tucker, A., Turbat-Herra, E.A., and Mathis, J.M. Placebo-controlled trial of indole-3-carbinol in the treatment of CIN. *Gynecol. Oncol.*, 78: 123–129, 2000.

135. Rosen, C.A., Woodson, G.E., Thompson, J.W., Hengesteg, A.P., and Bradlow, H.L. Preliminary results of the use of indole-3-carbinol for recurrent respiratory papillomatosis. *Otolaryngol. Head Neck Surg.*, 118: 810–815, 1998.

136. Tang, L. and Zhang, Y. Isothiocyanates in the chemoprevention of bladder cancer. *Curr. Drug Metab.*, 5: 193–201, 2004.

137. Nugon-Baudon, L. and Rabot, S. Glucosinolates and glucosinolate derivatives: implications for protection against chemical carcinogenesis. *Nutr. Res. Rev.*, 7: 205–231, 1994.

138. Beecher, C.W. Cancer preventive properties of varieties of *Brassica oleracea*: a review. *Am. J. Clin. Nutr.*, 59: 1166S–1170S, 1994.

139. Kristal, A.R. and Lampe, J.W. *Brassica* vegetables and prostate cancer risk: a review of the epidemiological evidence. *Nutr. Cancer*, 42: 1–9, 2002.

13 Conclusions and Future Perspectives

Simonetta Friso, Roberto Corrocher, and Sang-Woon Choi

The genetic variability among human beings determines the ability of each individual to meet the challenges of the environment, including those which can induce neoplastic diseases. Different cancer rates within the same population reveal the importance of the individual response to a certain environmental exposure in triggering the carcinogenetic processes. In this regard, the theory of interaction of nutrients and genes in the pathogenesis of disease is among the most fascinating gene–environment interactions known to affect carcinogenesis [1–4]. This remarkable interrelationship between nutrients and genes is especially relevant for public health issues, because the understanding of this relationship will enable us to reduce the risk of cancer more efficiently by adopting targeted dietary recommendations in specific at-risk population subgroups on a genetic basis [5]. Such an approach requires a deep understanding of the biochemical mechanisms underlying the relationship between nutrients and cancer disease as well as a clear knowledge for target genes or genetic pathways in which a certain nutrient is implied for the carcinogenetic process [6]. Moreover, although the dietary approach is conventionally, although not always, considered safe and not toxic, such an assumption should constantly be proven, especially in terms of defining amount requirements, timing, and potential confounding effects through pathways that are not the direct target of the nutritional intervention. All the aforementioned conditions ought to be considered in order to provide safe and effective chemoprevention. In this regard, paradigmatic examples derive from studies evaluating the effects of β-carotene and folate. Supplementation with β-carotene at high dosage may have a procarcinogenic effect vs. a protective effect at low doses [7–11]. As for the folic acid-related carcinogenesis, correct amount and timing are considered essential to exert either protective effects prior the onset of cancer or an effect in promoting tumor development when cancer is established [12].

Even after a decade of studies, however, we still experience certain limited information regarding the mechanisms underlying the relationship between nutrition and cancer as well as insufficient capability to define and measure biomarkers adequately. There are other aspects to be considered such as the heterogeneity in haplotypes and polymorphic genes and the large diversity in tissue, gender, and age specificity for molecular aberrancies, which arise from nutrient and gene interactions.

Indeed, a target for the researchers is to design, through an integrated model, adequate systems for an individually-tailored prevention and treatment approach. Future work, therefore, should pursue the intent of comprehending more precisely how a certain interaction acts to modulate the risk of cancer in each individual when exposed to a particular dietary environment. Only the acquisition of such knowledge will enable us to determine how dietary modulation should be designed on a genetic basis for the cancer prevention or adjuvant treatment.

The relationship among nutrition, genetics, and cancer is very complex. In order to study their interrelationship it seems clear that many different approaches are required. Different sets of study design, including epidemiological studies and mechanistic studies using cultured cells, animal models, and human studies, are indeed warranted.

As described in the introduction to this book, epidemiological studies have contributed much to our knowledge and helped a great deal to lead the directions of further studies. Some of the observational studies on gene–nutrient as well as gene–gene and gene–gene–nutrient interactions, however, are limited also by insufficient sample size. This is a critical issue as it may greatly affect the outcomes of the studies, thus leading to an over- or underestimation of the disease risk estimates if an adequate statistical power is not ensured. Nevertheless, each study design such as ecologic, case–control, and cohort study can surely offer important insights, and randomized controlled interventions can be very effective when a clear association between the status of a certain nutrient and the incidence of a certain cancer is established. As described in each chapter, many different settings of cultured cell, animal, and human studies have investigated the mechanisms by which genes and nutrients interact and thereby enhance or reduce the risk of cancer. Although many biochemical and molecular alterations, as well as many genetic and epigenetic modifications, together with posttranslational mechanisms have been proposed, it emerges undoubtedly that for the better understanding of interaction of nutrients and genes, studies need to be conducted in an integrated fashion, both from the epidemiological and the mechanistic point of view.

Among the main mechanisms involved in the nutrition and cancer relationships addressed in the present book, a fundamental role emerged for foods and nutrients with antioxidant properties. Oxidative damage to DNA plays a major role in carcinogenesis, and all cells adopt defense mechanisms by way of antioxidant compounds to contrast this phenomenon because it alters the nucleic acid structure and perturbs the biological processes, eventually inducing mutations and ultimately setting off carcinogenesis. To know the precise role of the interaction between antioxidants and related genes on cancer development, integration is needed among epidemiological studies on antioxidants and the risk of cancer, studies of molecular epidemiology on the putative pathways involved in carcinogenesis through oxidative DNA damage, and genetically engineered animal or cultured cell studies. However, limitations in such studies are often derived from measurement errors that may obfuscate associations between the procarcinogenic or protective factors and the outcomes [13].

One of the most extensively studied gene–nutrient relationship affecting cancer risk is that of *MTHFR* and folic acid in one-carbon metabolism [14–16]. The

MTHFR–folate interaction model should help us open new areas of interest for gene–nutrient, as well as gene–gene interactions, and may also serve as a paradigm to investigate potential novel intragene or haplotype–nutrient interactions and nutrient–nutrient interactions. The function of *MTHFR* gene is essential within one-carbon metabolism for its central role in this pathway, which is strictly related to the mechanisms involved in carcinogenesis, namely the epigenetic control of gene expression via methylation of DNA and the regulation of nucleotide synthesis. Epidemiological studies have suggested that each of the *MTHFR* genotypes conveys a different risk as it refers to several types of cancer and, even more interestingly, that this risk could be modified by folate status. Mechanistic studies have also supported these observations by showing an altered DNA methylation status, a well described epigenetic mechanism in carcinogenesis, in subjects carrying the variant allele in homozygosity compared to those with the wild-type genotype but only under inadequate folate conditions. This finding strongly suggests that the major factor in determining an altered DNA methylation is not due to folate status or to the presence of the polymorphic gene *per se* but to the interaction between the two components: folate and *MTHFR* genotype [17]. The hypotheses that have been formulated so far need further verification in appropriate *in vitro* and animal models and in large, well-designed intervention studies and longitudinal investigations.

On the aspect of chemoprevention, several data strongly suggest that a different strategy should be adopted according to each genotype of *MTHFR* and, in the future, we might prevent or treat cancers differently according to each person's genotype of critical genes, therefore avoiding unanimous modifications of the folate amount in the diet by food fortification. This strategy may exert, in fact, a potentially harmful effect by enhancing cancer risk or by inducing other side effects in certain subgroups of population not originally targeted by the program and unintentionally exposed to a higher amount of folate [12]. It should be also taken into account that nutrients consumed either by food fortification or supplementation may have different metabolic effects from those supplied by the diet, i.e., together with other nutritional factors. This could give a reason, also, for the apparent contradictory observation of the beneficial effect of diets rich in fruits and vegetables against cancer development and, on the other hand, the higher risk observed after supplementation with certain selected nutrient components [8]. Furthermore, considering the role of one-carbon metabolism as an important mechanism related to carcinogenesis, more studies are needed to identify other possible gene–nutrient as well as gene–gene or nutrient–nutrient interactions within one-carbon metabolism.

In general, we could state that the study of genetic variability within essential pathways related to carcinogenesis will strengthen data offered by nutrition and will provide an important complement for dietary studies. The understanding of genetic susceptibility will help researchers highlight stronger associations suggested by epidemiological studies and identify new links between nutrition, genetics, and dietary patterns within genetically defined specific subgroups. Considering that the magnitude of an association is essential to define a causal relationship, the studies integrating data on both nutrition and genetics are likely to generate more conclusive findings that will affect public health policies. Such studies may be very helpful to also provide potential hypotheses for the mechanisms and pathways underlying such relationships and, thus, provide a guide in more powerful mechanistic studies. In this regard, although much has been done, still a large number of areas within gene–nutrient interactions affecting carcinogenesis are to be explored.

REFERENCES

1. Giovannucci, E. Nutritional factors in human cancers. *Adv Exp Med Biol.* 472: 29–42, 1999.
2. Mathers, J.C. Nutrition and cancer prevention: diet–gene interactions. *Proc Nutr Soc.* 62(3): 605–610, 2003.
3. McCullough, M.L. and Giovannucci, E.L. Diet and cancer prevention. *Oncogene.* 23(38): 6349–6420, 2004.
4. Vineis, P. Individual susceptibility to carcinogens. *Oncogene.* 23(38): 6477–6483, 2004.
5. Vineis, P. Diet, genetic susceptibility and carcinogenesis. *Public Health Nutr.* 4(2B): 485–491, 2001.
6. Mathers, J.C. The biological revolution — towards a mechanistic understanding of the impact of diet on cancer risk. *Mutat Res.* 551(1-2): 43–49, 2004.
7. Department of Health, Nutritional Aspects of the Development of Cancer, Report on Health and Social Subjects 48, The Stationery Office, London, 1998.
8. Beta Carotene Cancer Prevention Study Group. The Alpha-Tocopherol. The effect of vitamin E and beta-carotene on lung cancer incidence and other cancers in male smokers. *N Engl J Med.* 330: 1029, 1994.
9. Palozza, P., Serini, S., Maggiano, N., Angelini, M., Boninsegna, A., Di Nicuolo, F., Ranelletti, F.O., Calviello, G. Induction of cell cycle arrest and apoptosis in human colon adenocarcinoma cells by β-carotene through down regulation of cyclin A and Bcl-2 family proteins. *Carcinogenesis.* 23, 11, 2002.
10. Russell, R.M. The enigma of beta-carotene in carcinogenesis: what can be learned from animal studies. *J Nutr.* 134(1): 262S–268S, 2004.
11. Wang, X.D. and Russell, R.M. Procarcinogenic and anticarcinogenic effects of beta-carotene. *Nutr Rev.* 57(9 Pt. 1): 263–72, 1999.
12. Kim, Y.I. Will mandatory folic acid fortification prevent or promote cancer? *Am J Clin Nutr.* 80(5): 1123–1128, 2004.
13. Bingham, S. and Riboli, E. Diet and cancer — the European prospective investigation into cancer and nutrition. *Nat Rev.* 4: 206–215, 2004.
14. Choi, S.W. and Mason, J.B. Folate and carcinogenesis: an integrated scheme. *J Nutr.* 130(2): 129–132, 2000.
15. Friso, S. and Choi, S.W. Gene–nutrient interactions and DNA methylation. *J Nutr.* 132(8 Suppl.): 2382S–2387S, 2002.
16. Robien, K. and Ulrich, C.M. 5,10-Methylenetetrahydrofolate reductase polymorphisms and leukemia risk: a HuGE minireview. *Am J Epidemiol.* 157(7): 571–582, 2003.
17. Friso, S., Choi, S.W., Girelli, D., Mason, J.B., Dolnikowski, G.G., Bagley, P.J., Olivieri, O., Jacques, P.F., Rosenberg, I.H., Corrocher, R., Selhub, J. A common mutation in the 5,10-methylenetetrahydrofolate reductase gene affects genomic DNA methylation through an interaction with folate status. *Proc Natl Acad Sci U.S.A.* 99(8): 5606–5611, 2002.

Index